CRITICAL THINKING *and*
CLINICAL JUDGMENT

ELSEVIER

evolve

⋮• *To access your Student Resources, visit:*

http://evolve.elsevier.com/Alfaro-LeFevre/CT

Evolve Student Learning Resources for *Alfaro-LeFevre: Critical Thinking and Clinical Judgment: A Practical Approach to Outcome-Focused Thinking, fourth edition,* offers the following features:

Resources

- **Chapter Worksheets**
  Each worksheet provides chapter descriptions, expected learning outcomes, major content headings, and links to references and recommended resources available online.

- **Printable Clinical and Study Tools from the Book**
  Print several tools from the book for quick and easy reference and portability!

- **Resources from www.AlfaroTeachSmart.com**
  Direct links to the complete Evidence-Based Critical Thinking Indicators document, PowerPoint slides, and other handouts.

CRITICAL THINKING *and* CLINICAL JUDGMENT

A Practical Approach to Outcome-Focused Thinking

Fourth Edition

Rosalinda Alfaro-LeFevre, RN, MSN
President
Teaching Smart/Learning Easy
Stuart, Florida
www.AlfaroTeachSmart.com

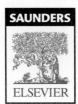

SAUNDERS

ELSEVIER

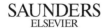

SAUNDERS
ELSEVIER

11830 Westline Industrial Drive
St. Louis, Missouri 63146

CRITICAL THINKING AND CLINICAL JUDGMENT: ISBN-13: 978-1-4160-3948-8
A PRACTICAL APPROACH TO OUTCOME-   ISBN-10: 1-4160-3948-1
FOCUSED THINKING, FOURTH EDITION

Notice

Neither the Publisher nor the Authors assume any responsibility for any loss or injury and/or damage to persons or property arising out of or related to any use of the material contained in this book. It is the responsibility of the treating practitioner, relying on independent expertise and knowledge of the patient, to determine the best treatment and method of application for the patient.

The Publisher

Previous editions copyrighted 2004, 1999, and 1995

Library of Congress Control Number: 2007943473

Acquisitions Editors: Robin Carter, Kristin Geen
Developmental Editors: Deanna Davis, Jamie Horn
Editorial Assistants: Mary Parker, Jennifer Stoces
Publishing Services Manager: Jeff Patterson
Project Manager: Clay S. Broeker
Design Direction: Kim Denando

Printed in Canada

Last digit is the print number: 9 8 7 6 5 4 3 2 1

Working together to grow
libraries in developing countries

www.elsevier.com | www.bookaid.org | www.sabre.org

ELSEVIER   BOOK AID International   Sabre Foundation

DEDICATION

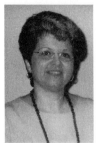

Jo-Ann Rossitto, DNSc
March 8, 1951 to January 25, 2006

"When you were born, you cried and the world rejoiced.
Live your life so that when you die, the world cries and you rejoice."

Dr. Jo-Ann Rossitto lived her life as a tribute to all who loved her. As Director of Nursing and Associate Dean at San Diego City College from 1988 to 2006, she was beloved by faculty, students, and colleagues for her dedication to improving and expanding nursing education and opportunities. Born in New York City, she earned her Vocational Nurse Certification at Mesa College in 1970 and then graduated in the first ADN class of nursing students at City College in 1972. She earned her BSN from the University of San Diego in 1976, her MA in Education with an emphasis in Nursing from New York University in 1981, and her Doctorate of Nursing Science at the University of San Diego in 1997. Although she enjoyed practicing as a nurse, she found her real passion in teaching. She was highly regarded for her leadership and administrative skills. While a practicing nurse, she noted a "gap" in nursing education and dedicated her career to educating students "how" to be a good nurse. Her proven methods allowed most of her nursing students to secure jobs before they even graduated. Dr. Rossitto also worked to ensure that nurses had a voice in the decision-making process. She readily offered her time, expertise, and membership to professional groups, including the American Nurses' Association, Association of California Community College Administrators, National League for Nursing, California Association of Associate Degree Nursing Program Directors, New York Alumni Association, American Association of University Women, American Educator's Research Organization, NCLEX-RN Task Force of the California Board of Registered Nursing, Sigma Theta Tau, Zeta Mu Chapter-At-Large, and National League for Nursing Accrediting Commission.

CONTRIBUTORS, ADVISORS, AND REVIEWERS

A note of thanks: Without the timely and insightful reviews and advice of the experts listed on these pages, this book would not have been possible. The author wishes to also acknowledge the translators of previous editions: Aiko Emoto (Japanese), Maria Teresa Luis (Spanish), and Maria Augusta Soares, Miriam de Abreu Almeida, and Valéria Giordami Araújo (Portuguese).

Contributor to the Third Edition
Donna D. Ignatavicius, RN, MS, AFEN
Author and Consultant
President, DI Associates
Placitas, New Mexico

Advisors and Reviewers
United States

Carolyn Adams, EdD, RN, CNAA, BC
Robert H. Hoy III Distinguished Professor
School of Nursing
University of Texas at El Paso
El Paso, Texas

Dee Allen, MEd
Educational Consultant
New Orleans, Louisiana

Coral Andino-Natal, RN, MSN
Inter-American University of Puerto Rico
Metropolitan Campus
Carmen Torres de Tiburcio School of
    Nursing
San Juan, Puerto Rico

Ann Strong Anthony, PhD(c), RN
Associate Dean, Nursing Department
Tulsa Community College
Tulsa, Oklahoma

Ledjie Ballard, CRNA, ARNP, MSN
Independent Practitioner
Out Patient and Office Anesthesia
Affiliate Clinical Faculty
University of Washington
Seattle, Washington

Suzanne C. Beyea, RN, PhD, FAAN
Director of Nursing Research
Dartmouth-Hitchcock Medical Center
Lebonan, New Hampshire

Deanne A. Blach, MSN, RN
Nurse Educator
DB Productions
Green Forest, Arkansas

Susan A. Boyer, MEd, RN
Director
Vermont Nurse Internship Project
Windsor, Vermont

Hilda H. Brito, RN, BC, MSN
Director of Education
Kendall Medical Center
Miami, Florida

Eleanor T. Campbell, EdD, RN
Assistant Professor, Nursing
Herbert Lehman College, CUNY
Bronx, New York

Susan Carper, RN, BS.
Case Manager
Community Aging & Retirement Services
Port Richey, Florida

Ellen Ceppetelli, MS, RN
Director of Nursing Education
Dartmouth-Hitckcock Medical Center
Lebanon, New Hampshire

Phyllis Class, RN
Editorial Director
Nursing Spectrum (FL Division)
Pembroke Pines, Florida

Darnell H. Cockram, EdD, RN
Educational Consultant
Martinsville, Virginia

Barbara Janson Cohen, MEd
Author and Educator
Broomall, Pennsylvania

Bette Case Di Leonardi, PhD, RN, BC
Independent Consultant
Chicago, Illinois

Pamela Di Vito-Thomas, PhD, RN
Site Coordinator
Langston University-Tulsa
School of Nursing and Health Professions
Tulsa, Oklahoma

Beverly L. Edmonds, MSN, RN, CHCR
Nurse Recruiter
University of Pennsylvania Health System
Philadelphia, Pennsylvania

Karen Elechko, RN, MSN
Golden Memory Clinic Coordinator
Veteran Affairs Medical Center, Coatesville
Coatesville, Pennsylvania

Bonnie Eyler, MSN, RN, JD
Boca Raton, Florida

Ann B. Fives, RN, MS
Professor Emeritus
Raritan Valley Community College
North Branch, New Jersey

Rebecca S. Frugé, RN, PhD
Director, Graduate Nursing Program
Universidad Metropolitana
San Juan, Puerto Rico

Karen L. Gorton, MSN, APRN, BC, MS
Director, Nursing Program
Carroll College
Waukesha, Wisconsin

Cecelia G. Grindel, PhD, RN, CMSRN, FAAN
Associate Director, Undergraduate
  Programs
Byrdine F. Lewis School of Nursing
Georgia State University
Atlanta, Georgia

Elizabeth E. Hand, MS, RN
Adjunct Faculty
Collaborative BSN Program
Tulsa Community College
Tulsa, Oklahoma

Dan Hankison
CONSULTING Dragons
Stuart, Florida

Ruth I. Hansten, RN, MBA, PhD, FACHE
Principal
Hansten Healthcare PLLC
Port Ludlow, Washington

Cheryl Herndon, ARNP, CNM, MSN
Director Aesthetic Services
Women's Health Specialists
Jensen Beach, Florida

Deborah J. Hess, PhD, RN
Assistant Professor
Department of Teacher Education
Wright State University
Dayton, Ohio

Robert Hess, RN, PhD
Senior Vice President
Continuing Education
Nursing Spectrum
Bala Cynwyd, Pennsylvania

Carol Hutton, EdD, ARNP
Associate Professor
Department of Management
Miami Gardens, Florida

Marilynn Jackson, PhD, RN
Intuitive Options
Kasilof, Alaska

Frances J. Jessup, RN, BSN
Wound Care Specialist
Valdosta, Georgia

Sharon Johnson, MSN, RNC, CNA
Director of Home Health
The Home Care Network
Jefferson Health System
Wayne, Pennsylvania

Suzanne Hall Johnson, MN, RN, CNS
Director
Hall Johnson Consulting
Lakewood, Colorado

Elaine Bishop Kennedy, EdD, RN
Professor, Nursing
Wor-Wic Community College
Salisbury, Maryland

Kathie J. Kulikowski, MSN, RN-BC
Faculty Associate
Arizona State University
Academy of Continuing Education
Phoenix, Arizona
Clinical Faculty
Gonzaga University
Spokane, Washington

Corrine R. Kurzen, RN, MEd, MSN
Author and Consultant
Lafayette Hill, Pennsylvania

Heidi Pape Laird
Systems Designer
Partners HealthCare
Boston, Massachusetts

Kathleen C. Langille, BSN, RN
Emergency Department
Staff RN & DHMC Student Affairs
    Manager
Dartmouth-Hitchcock Medical Center
Lebonan, New Hampshire

**Jody M. Masterson, RN, MSN, CRRN,
    FIALCP**
Adjunct Professor, College of Nursing
Villanova University
Villanova, Pennsylvania
Rehabilitation Nurse Consultant
Nursing Consultation Services, LTD
Plymouth Meeting, Pennsylvania

Angélica Y. Matos-Ríos, RN, DNS
Professor and Director
Graduate Department of Nursing
Medical Sciences Campus
University of Puerto Rico
San Juan, Puerto Rico

Barbara Maxwell, MSN, MS, CNS, RN
Associate Professor of Nursing and
    Program Coordinator
SUNY Ulster
Stone Ridge, New York

Patricia McCarthy, RN, MS
Associate Chief Nursing Service for
    Education
VA Health Care System
Palo Alto, California

Marycarol McGovern, PhD, RN
Assistant Professor
College of Nursing
Villanova University
Villanova, Pennsylvania

Melanie McGuire, RN, BSN
Staff Nurse
Emergency Department
Paoli Hospital
Paoli, Pennsylvania

Judith C. Miller, RN, MS
Nursing Tutorial & Consulting Services
Henniker, New Hampshire

**Kathleen B. Murphy, RN, MSN, CRRN,
    FIALCP**
Rehabilitation Nurse Consultant
Nursing Consultation Services, LTD
Plymouth Meeting, Pennsylvania

Barbara A. Musinski, RN, C, BS
Nursing Consultant
West Palm Beach, Florida

Jan Nash, RN, MS, PhD
Vice President Patient Services
Paoli Hospital
Paoli, Pennsylvania

Charles L. Nola
Aerospace Engineer
Madison, Alabama

Marilyn H. Oermann, PhD, RN, FAAN
Professor, College of Nursing
Wayne State University
Detroit, Michigan

Lourdes Maldonado Ojeda, EdD, RN
Dean, School of Health Sciences
Universidad Metropolitana
San Juan, Puerto Rico

Kathleen D. Pagana, PhD, RN
Professor Emeritus, Lycoming College
Pagana Seminars & Presentations
Williamsport, Pennsylvania

Terri Sue Patterson, RN, MSN, CRRN, FIALCP
President
Nursing Consultation Services
Plymouth Meeting, Pennsylvania

William F. Perry, MA, RN
Informatics Consultant
Creekspace Informatics
Beavercreek, Ohio

James Riley
Richmond, Virginia

Mathew Riley, BA
Therapeutic Staff Support
Chester County Regional Educational
    Services Inc.
Downingtown, Pennsylvania

Michael Riley, LMSW, LPC, EMT-Paramedic
Safety Analyst
Praesidium Inc.
Arlington, Texas

Mary Anne Rizzolo, EdD, RN, FAAN
Senior Director of Professional
    Development
National League for Nursing
New York, New York

Gina Rybolt, RN, BSN
Author of www.codeblog.com
Milpitas, California

Jacqui Scipio-Bannerman, RNC, BSN, CCE
Women and Childrens Health Services
Philadelphia, Pennsylvania

Roz Seymour, EdD, RN
Editor-in-Charge of Informatics Education
Online Journal of Nursing Informatics
Professor Emeritus
East Tennessee State University
Johnson City, Tennessee

Rose Sherman, EdD, RN, CNAA
Nursing Leadership Institute Director
Florida Atlantic University
Boca Raton, Florida

Darlene N. Silver, MSN, RN, IBCLC
Nursing Department
Bowie State University
Bowie, Maryland

Bill Skehan
Media Specialist
Comstock Elementary School
Miami, Florida

Jean Smith, RN, BSN, CCRN
Level 3 Staff Nurse
Intensive Care Units
Paoli Hospital
Paoli, Pennsylvania

Melva J. Solon, BSN, MSN, RN
Danville, Illinois

Maria Sophoclies, MD
Princeton, New Jersey

Kathleen R. Stevens, RN, EdD, FAAN
Professor and Director
Academic Center for Evidence-Based
    Practice (ACE)
The University of Texas Health Science
    Center at San Antonio
San Antonio, Texas

Jenifer K. Storms, CMT
Lebanon, Pennsylvania

Sandy Swearingen, RN, PhD
Nursing Leadership Development
Florida Hospital
Orlando, Florida

Carol Taylor, RN, PhD
Director, Center for Clinical Bioethics
Assistant Professor, Nursing
Georgetown University
Washington, District of Columbia

Brent W. Thompson, DNSc, RN
Associate Professor
Department of Nursing
West Chester University
West Chester, Pennsylvania

Elizabeth M. Tsarnas, APRN, BC
Clinical Director
Volunteers in Medicine Clinic
Stuart, Florida

Theresa M. Valiga, EdD, RN, FAAN
Director of Professional Development
National League for Nursing
New York, New York

Linda S. Weinberg RN, MSN
Nursing Faculty
West Chester University
Community and Diabetes Educator
Chester County Hospital
West Chester, Pennsylvania

Sheila Quilter Wheeler, RN, MS
President, TeleTriage Systems
San Anselmo, California

Toni C. Wortham, RN, BSN, MSN
Professor
Madisonville Community College
Health Campus
Madisonville, Kentucky

International

Miriam de Abreu Almeida, RN, PhD
Professor, School of Nursing
Federal University of Rio Grande do Sul
Porto Alegre, Brazil

Emilia Campos de Carvalho, RN, PhD
Professor, Colllege of Nursing
University of Sao Paulo at Ribeirao Preto
Ribeirao Preto, Brazil

Dame June Clark, PhD, RN, FRCN
Professor Emeritus
School of Health Science
University of Wales Swansea
Wales, United Kingdom

Judy Boychuk Duchscher, RN, PhD
Executive Director, Nursing The Future
Faculty, Nursing Education
Saskatchewan Institute of Applied Science
    & Technology (SIAST)
Saskatoon, Saskatchewan, Canada

Aiko Emoto
Professor Emeritus
Saniku Gakuin College
Chiba, Japan

Bernie Garrett, PhD, BA (Hons), RN
Assistant Professor
University of British Columbia
School of Nursing,
Vancouver, British Columbia, Canada

Ana M. Giménez, RN
Professor of Medical-Surgical Nursing
Puerta de Hierro School of Nursing
Universidad Autónoma de Madrid
Madrid, Spain

Maria Teresa Luis, RN
Professor of Medical-Surgical Nursing
Univeristy of Barcelona
Barcelona, Spain

Isabel Amélia Costa Mendes
Director
WHO Collaborating Center for Nursing
    Reseach Development
Professor, College of Nursing
University of São Paulo at Ribeirão Preto
Ribeirão Preto, Brazil

Jeanne Michel, RN, MSN
Assistant Professor,
Department of Nursing
University of São Paulo
São Paulo, Brazil

Nico Oud, RN, MNSc, Dipl N Adm
Consultant and Trainer of Aggression
    Management
"CONNECTING"
Amsterdam, The Netherlands

Ann Paterson, RN, MA, MRCNA,
Senior Lecturer in Nursing & Midwifery
RMIT University
Bundoora West Campus
Melbourne, Australia

Joanne Profetto-McGrath, PhD, RN
Interim Dean and Associate Professor
Nursing Department
University of Alberta
Edmonton, Alberta, Canada

Laura Sherburn, BA, MsC
Head of Urgent Care
Leeds Primary Care Trust
Leeds, West Yorkshire, United Kingdom

Yvonne Stillwell, RN, BA, PG Dip, MBS
Nurse Manager
Nursing Practice Development
MidCentral District Health Board
Palmerston North, New Zealand

**Catherine Jean Thorpe, RN, RM, DipIC,
Health Nursing, BAdmin**
Deputy Director, Nursing
Groote Schuur Hospital Observatory
Capetown, South Africa

PREFACE

What's Practical about This Approach?

Critical thinking—your capacity to focus your thinking to get the results you need—determines whether you succeed or fail. It makes the difference between keeping patients safe and putting them in harms way. For this reason, accreditation bodies such as *The Joint Commission* and *National League for Nursing Accrediting Commission* increasingly stress the need to use evidence-based approaches to improve critical thinking. Many nurses, however, use the term *critical thinking* as a buzzword. You can't improve thinking based on gut feelings or by using vague terms. You must be *specific* and know the evidence that supports your approaches. Compare the following examples and note how using specific, evidence-based terms brings the clarity that can help everyone be "on the same page" about what you have to do to think critically.

- **Example of buzzwords:** You've got to learn to think critically.
- **Example of specific evidence-based terms**: According to the literature and most experts, one of the first things you must learn is that critical thinking is *systematic* and that it *changes with circumstances*—one size doesn't fit all. You need to learn how to *assess systematically in the context of each situation*, paying attention to unique patient circumstances.

Using an engaging style and giving you the latest evidence on improving thinking, this book gives you the language and tools you need to move from buzzwords to *specifics*. It gives you a frame of reference to put your thinking into words and dialogue about reasoning with students, nurses, educators, and leaders. Ultimately, you learn how to develop specific critical thinking skills needed to keep patients safe, achieve desired outcomes, and improve patient and nurse satisfaction.

Who Should Read This Book?

You should read this book if:

- You're a student or beginning nurse and want to be more confident and competent in making patient care decisions.
- You're a preceptor or a mentor and need strategies and tools to work together to promote critical thinking.
- You're an educator or a leader who wants to prepare for accreditation visits or Magnet status.
- You want to make the shift from simply "fixing problems" to "fixing problems in ways that give you the best outcomes."
- You need to prepare for standard tests like the National Council Licensure Examinations (NCLEX®).

Whether you're a student, a new graduate, or an expert nurse, the following content organization is designed to help you connect with what you already know, and move quickly to developing the complex thinking skills needed to succeed today.

- **Chapters 1 and 2** examine critical thinking in daily life, with some reference to nursing situations. Whether you want to improve your ability to handle personal or professional matters, this section helps you focus your thinking to get results using your own particular talents.
- **Chapters 3 and 4** are designed to help you meet the challenges of acquiring the thinking skills required to succeed in six common nursing situations: reasoning in the clinical setting (clinical judgment), moral and ethical reasoning, evidence-based practice, teaching others, teaching ourselves, and taking tests. If you are a beginner, you may want to read the sections on *teaching ourselves* and *taking tests* before reading other sections. This is a good example of making learning meaningful by reading what you're most interested in first.
- **Chapter 5** gives opportunities to practice skills needed for clinical reasoning, nursing process, and clinical judgment, using case scenarios based on real experiences.
- **Chapter 6** helps you gain skills needed to work in any position that demands collaboration. When you have skills like *managing conflict* and *working as a team*, you can use your brainpower to resolve unique, rather than common "human nature," problems. This section helps you learn how to build empowered partnerships with patients, families, peers, and colleagues. You also learn how to work smarter, not harder—how to set priorities and manage your time.

Because of the depth and breadth of content, you can use this book to guide a specific course on critical thinking or as an adjunct to numerous courses. You get the best results if you begin to use it in beginning courses and continue to refer to as you progress through various stages of learning. You may even consider making parts of the book required reading *before* starting nursing school, when motivation to begin to learn about nursing is high. For example, students can benefit greatly from reading Chapter 1 and the sections on teaching, learning, and test taking in Chapter 4.

What's New to This Edition

Here's what's new:

- **A NEW TITLE!** Now includes *Outcome-Focused* in the title to reflect more emphasis on identifying desired outcomes *early*, together with patients and families.
- **A NEW DESIGN!** Inspired by the beautiful continent of Africa, giraffe icons 🦒 were chosen because of the giraffe's ability to look ahead and see the big picture. Elephant icons 🐘 were chosen because of the elephant's celebrated memory and social and emotional connections.
- Applies brain-based learning principles (uses strategies that get your brain plugged in to learning).
- Addresses the roles of preceptors in helping novices learn.

- Helps you prioritize your thinking to make sound clinical decisions in a timely way
- Applies evidence-based critical thinking indicators (CTIs) and a 4-circle model to promote CT.
- Gives maps, memory-jogs, decision-making tools, and strategies for how to map to promote CT.
- Focuses on today's health care realities, including giving more on:
  - Institute of Medicine's (IOM) competencies and delegation strategies based on the ANA's *Principles for Delegation.*
  - Using the nursing process as a critical thinking tool, according to *ANA Standards.*
  - The role of logic, intuition, and creativity in critical thinking and clinical judgment.
  - How multidisciplinary practice, use of computers, and critical paths affect thinking.
  - How personality, upbringing, and culture affect thinking and teamwork.
  - The importance of paying attention to context (circumstances).
  - Making sure your documentation reflects critical thinking.
  - How to use the ACE Star Model to transform knowledge to evidence-based practice.
  - Developing a culture of safety and healthy work environments.
  - How to promote and evaluate critical thinking in diverse nurses and situations.
- Has new information on how to make educated guesses and pass standard tests on the first try (includes NCLEX practice questions).

The following content was completely updated:

- The importance of moving to a predictive model—*Predict, Prevent, Manage, Promote*—rather than using a more reactive *Diagnose and Treat* approach.
- How the nursing process continues to evolve to a more proactive and dynamic model.
- Detailed information on key workplace skills such as how to:
  - Set priorities and manage your time.
  - Access and use information.
  - Prevent and deal with mistakes.
  - Manage conflict constructively.

Additional Benefits

With this edition you also get access to Evolve resources, which include the following:

Student Resources:

1. The following tools from the book, printable as handouts or worksheets:
- Clinical Decision Making map (page 90)
- Body Systems Assessment (page 104)
- Systematic Problem Analysis Worksheet (page 178)

- Neurologic Focus Assessment Guide (page 157)
- Writing Outcomes for Problems diagram (page 186)
- Writing Outcomes for Interventions diagram (page 186)
- Individualizing Interventions diagram (page 189)

2. Chapter Worksheets (in Word Format) to help you study or make presentations.

- Each worksheet includes chapter title, chapter purpose, learning outcomes, major headings, and direct links for all online references and resources cited in this book.
- You also get direct links for Internet resources for studying, test-taking, and preparing for NCLEX and other standard tests.

3. Direct links to the complete *Evidence-Based Critical Thinking Indicators* document and other handouts and PowerPoint slides available at *www.AlfaroTeachSmart.com*.

Faculty Resources:

1. Analyzing Assignments to Include Elements that Promote Critical Thinking
2. Creating a Climate to Promote Critical Thinking
3. Clinical Cards Guide (Guide to Promoting Reflective Thinking)
4. Pre-Course Assessment Tool
5. Test Bank

We'll continue to add resources as they are developed. Check us out at *http://evolve.elsevier.com/Alfaro-LeFevre/CT*.

What's the Same

The following features are retained from previous editions:

- Great pains were taken to include design elements that motivate you to learn in meaningful ways (see *The Best Way to Read This Book* on the next page)
- You get practical information and strategies in a concise format (gives theory, strategies, and exercises to apply content).
- To ensure up-to-date, cutting edge information, content was reviewed by experts from various disciplines, specialties, and nationalities.
- HMO (Help Me Out) cartoons return to this edition, with new art. HMO addresses the funny things that happen to care givers and receivers. If you have a story—one that involves the care of a patient, friend, family member, or pet—to share, please contact me at the address given at the end of this preface.

THE BEST WAY TO READ THIS BOOK

The Best Way to Read This Book Is However You Choose to Read It

1. If you like the traditional approach, read it from beginning to end. You'll enjoy the narrative, logical approach, and numerous scenarios and examples designed to help you understand and remember content.

2. If you like to use your own unique approach—for example, the back to front approach (read summaries before text), the "skip around to the stuff that looks interesting" approach, or the "read the stuff that will be on the test first approach"—here are some of the features that help you focus on what's most important.

Preceding Each Chapter

- **This Chapter at a Glance:** Allows you to scan major headings.
- **Prechapter Self-Tests:** Help you focus on learning outcomes and decide where you stand in relation to what needs to be learned.

Following Each Chapter

- **Critical Thinking Exercises:** Direct you to use content, helping you clarify understanding and move information into long-term memory.
- **Key Points:** Give a detailed summary of the most important content.

Other Features You Need to Know about

- **Glossary:** Provides definitions of key terms. If you don't understand words, look them up or you may miss major points.
- **Critical Moments:** Give simple strategies that can make a BIG difference in results, in accordance with our African theme.
- **Other Perspectives:** Offer interesting (and sometimes amusing) points of view.
- **Response Key:** When appropriate, you get example responses for Critical Thinking/Practice Exercises to help you evaluate your responses (all exercises that have an example response are marked with an asterisk). This is called a *response key*, rather than an *answer key*, to avoid implying that there's only one right answer to each question. In many cases, a variety of responses are acceptable. (Great minds don't always think alike!) The main point of the exercises isn't necessarily to come up with one *right* response; rather, the point is to get in touch with the thinking that led you to your response and to be able to evaluate and correct your thinking as needed.

Reading Efficiently

However you choose to read, keep in mind the following steps, which provide an organized and efficient way to master content.

- **Survey:** Scan the abstract, major headings, tables, and illustrations.
- **Question:** Turn major headings into questions.
- **Read:** Read, taking notes and answering your questions.
- **Review, Recite, and Reread:** Review the chapter (or your notes), reciting key content out loud, and then ask yourself, "What's still not clear here?" Read the sections you don't understand again, and raise questions to ask in class or discuss with your peers.

A Word about Patients, Clients, Stakeholders, and "He/She"

To keep in mind that patients and clients are *individuals* with unique needs, values, perceptions, and motivations, whenever possible, a fictitious name, or "someone," "person," "consumer," or "individual" is used (instead of "patient" or "client"). The term *stakeholder* is now used when talking about *all the individuals and groups* who have a vested interest in how care is given. (Examples of *stakeholders* include patients, significant others, caregivers, and insurance companies.) *He* and *she* are used interchangeably to avoid the awkwardness of using "he/she."

Please Tell Us What You Think

We want to hear your struggles and concerns. Whether you're a student, a staff nurse, leader, or educator, if you have a problem with something, it's likely that others do too. Your problems are our opportunities to learn, improve, and help others with the same concerns. Please let us know what you think. Address comments to myself or to Robin Carter, Nursing Editorial, Elsevier, 11830 Westline Industrial Drive, St. Louis, MO 63146.

Rosalinda Alfaro-LeFevre, RN, MSN
www.AlfaroTeachSmart.com

ASSUMPTIONS AND PROMISES

Before I began to write this book, I made some assumptions:
- You want to learn.
- Your time is valuable, and you don't want to waste it.
- You like to learn the most important things first.
- You learn better when you're motivated, know why information is relevant, and choose your own way of learning.
- You know yourself best, so it's inappropriate for *me* to tell *you* how to think.
- You feel a sense of accomplishment when you gain the knowledge and skills that help you be more independent.

Because of these assumptions, I promise to:
- Let you know what's most important.
- Use lots of examples and present information in a usable way.
- Give the "reasons behind the rules."
- Encourage you to choose what works for you.
- Help you develop the skills required to be a better thinker, independent learner, and more effective nurse.

ACKNOWLEDGMENTS

I want to thank my husband, Jim, for his love, support, and sense of humor and fun. I also want to thank the rest of my family and the following people for their ongoing support and contribution to my personal and professional growth: Louise Rochester, Heidi Laird, Terri Patterson, Ledjie Ballard, Grace and Frank Nola, Charlie Nola, Chuck and Pat Morgan, Loraine Locasale, Dan Hankison, Karen Smith, Virginia McFalls, Bill Perry, Carol Taylor, Terry Valiga, Mary Ann Rizzolo, Annette Sophocles, Melani McGuire, Maria Sophocles, Barbara Cohen, Patti Cleary, Michael Ledbetter, the Villanova College of Nursing Faculty, and the past and present staff nurses of Paoli Hospital, Paoli, Pennsylvania. I can't thank those of you who have been willing to advise and give so freely of your time and expertise enough.

My special thanks go to the following people at Elsevier: Robin Carter, Acquisitions Editor; Kristin Geen, Acquisitions Editor; Deanna Davis, Developmental Editor; Jamie Horn, Developmental Editor; Mary Parker, Editorial Assistant, Jennifer Stoces, Editorial Assistant; Clay Broeker, Project Manager; and the sales and marketing staff for their vital roles in making this book successful.

Rosalinda Alfaro-LeFevre RN, MSN
www.AlfaroTeachSmart.com

CONTENTS

CHAPTER 1   What Is Critical Thinking and Why Do We Care?

Why Focus on Critical Thinking?, 2
How This Book Helps You Improve Thinking, 3
   Brain-Based Learning, 3
   Organized for Novices and Experts, 5
What's the Difference between Thinking and Critical Thinking?, 5
Critical Thinking: Some Different Descriptions, 6
   A Synonym: Reasoning, 6
   Frequently Quoted Critical Thinking Descriptions, 6
   Applied Definition, 6
Problem-Focused Versus Outcome-Focused Thinking, 7
What about Common Sense?, 7
What Do Critical Thinkers Look Like?, 8
Critical Thinking Indicators (CTIs), 9
What's Familiar and What's New?, 9
   What's Familiar, 12
   What's New, 13
Critical Thinking, Nursing Process, and Clinical Judgment, 15
4-Circle CT Model: Get the Picture?, 15
Thinking Ahead, Thinking-in-Action, and Thinking Back (Reflecting), 16
Key Points/Summary, 22

CHAPTER 2   How to Think Critically

Gaining Insight and Self-Awareness, 26
   Connecting with Your Learning Style, 26
   How Your Personality Affects Thinking, 28
   Effects of Birth Order, Upbringing, and Culture, 29
   Male Versus Female Thinking, 31
Developing Trust in Relationships, 32
Mentoring and Building Empowered Partnerships, 33
Factors Influencing Critical Thinking Ability, 34
   Personal Factors Influencing Thinking, 34
   Situational Factors Influencing Thinking, 37
   Habits Creating Barriers to Critical Thinking, 38
   Habits Promoting Critical Thinking, 40
Outcome-Focused (Results-Oriented) Thinking, 42
   Goal (Intent) Versus Outcome (Result), 42
   Clarifying Outcomes, 42
Critical Thinking Strategies, 43
   10 Key Questions, 43
   Using Logic, Intuition, and Trial and Error, 45

Focusing on Details and Big Picture, 46
Drawing Maps, Diagrams, and Decision Trees, 46
Simulated Learning Experiences, 47
Other Useful Strategies, 47
CTIs for Knowledge and Intellectual Skills, 48
Developing Character and Acquiring Knowledge and Skills, 51
Assessing and Evaluating Thinking, 52
Basic Principles of Evaluating Thinking, 52
Self-Assessment, 53
Peer Review, 53
Using Tests and Instruments, 53
Key Points/Summary, 59

CHAPTER 3   Critical Thinking and Clinical Judgment in Nursing

Critical Thinking and Clinical Judgment, 64
Applied Definition, 64
What Other Nurses Say, 64
Mapping Critical Thinking, 65
Improving Practice and Performance, 67
Critical Thinking Indicators and 4-Circle Model, 68
Goals and Outcomes of Nursing, 68
Major Goals of Nursing, 68
Major Outcomes of Nursing, 69
What Are the Implications?, 69
Novice Versus Expert Thinking, 69
Paying Attention to Context, 70
Changes in Health Care Impacting on Thinking, 71
Institute of Medicine (IOM) Competencies, 71
Empowering Patients and Families: Nurses as Stewards for Safe Passage, 73
Diagnose and Treat Versus *Predict, Prevent, Manage, and Promote*, 74
Disease Management, 76
Outcome-Focused, Evidence-Based Care, 77
Clinical, Functional, and Other Outcomes, 79
Dynamic Relationship of Problems and Outcomes, 80
A Changing Nursing Process, 82
Proactive, Dynamic, and Outcome-Focused, 84
Interplay of Intuition and Logic, 85
Ready, Fire, Aim, 86
What about Creativity?, 86
Using Standard Tools to Improve Thinking, 87
Collecting Versus Analyzing Data, 88
Computerized Decision-Support Tools, 88
Is the Care Plan Dead?, 89
Expanding Roles Related to Diagnosis and Management, 89
Growing Responsibilities, 89
Legal Implications of Diagnosis, 92

Defining Nursing Diagnosis, 82
Accountability for Diagnosis, 93
Frequently Encountered Diagnoses and Complications, 95
Using Standard or Recognized Terms, 97
Developing Clinical Reasoning Skills, 99
Activating the Chain of Command, 99
Scope of Practice Decisions, 100
Decision Making and Nursing Standards and Guidelines, 100
Applying Delegation Principles, 101
How to Develop Effective Clinical Judgment, 101
10 Strategies for Developing Clinical Judgment, 101
Charting That Shows Critical Thinking, 105
Key Points/Summary, 110

CHAPTER 4   Critical Thinking in Nursing: Beyond Clinical Judgment

Moral and Ethical Reasoning, 118
Clarifying Values, 118
Moral Versus Ethical Reasoning, 119
How Do You Decide?, 119
Seven Ethical Principles, 120
Standards, Ethics Codes, and Patients' Rights, 120
Steps for Moral and Ethical Reasoning, 122
Evidence-Based Practice (EBP), 123
Relationship of Research to EBP, 123
Transforming Knowledge to EBP, 124
Clinical Summaries, 124
ACE Star Model of Knowledge Transformation, 124
Nursing Research, EBP, and Critical Thinking, 125
Scanning before Reading Research Articles, 129
Questioning Care Practices: Promoting Inquiry and Creativity, 129
Surveillance and Quality Improvement, 130
Teaching Others: Promoting Independence, 134
10 Steps for Teaching Others, 134
Teaching Yourself: Grab the Spoon, 135
Memorizing Effectively, 136
Learning and Memorization Strategies, 136
Test Taking: Improving Grades and Passing the First Time, 137
Strategies for Successful Test Taking, 138
Strategies for NCLEX and Other Standard Tests, 141
Key Points/Summary, 144

CHAPTER 5   Practicing Clinical Judgment Skills: Up Close and Clinical

Chapter Overview, 150
Clinical Judgment (Clinical Reasoning) Skills: Dynamic and Interrelated, 150

Why Practice These Skills Separately?, 150
How to Get the Most out of This Section, 151
  1. Identifying Assumptions, 152
    Definition, 152
    Why This Skill Promotes Clinical Judgment, 152
    Guidelines: How to Identify Assumptions, 152
    Practice Exercises: Identifying Assumptions, 153
  2. Assessing Systematically and Comprehensively, 155
    Definition, 155
    Why This Skill Promotes Clinical Judgment, 155
    Guidelines: How to Assess Systematically and Comprehensively, 155
    Practice Exercises: Assessing Systematically and Comprehensively, 158
  3. Checking Accuracy and Reliability (Validating Data), 159
    Definition, 159
    Why This Skill Promotes Clinical Judgment, 159
    Guidelines: How to Check Accuracy and Reliability, 159
    Practice Exercises: Checking Accuracy and Reliability (Validating Data), 160
  4. Distinguishing Normal from Abnormal and Identifying Signs and Symptoms, 160
    Definition, 160
    Why This Skill Promotes Clinical Judgment, 161
    Guidelines: How to Distinguish Normal from Abnormal and Identify Signs and Symptoms, 161
    Practice Exercises: Distinguishing Normal from Abnormal and Identifying Signs and Symptoms, 161
  5. Making Inferences (Drawing Valid Conclusions), 162
    Definition, 162
    Why This Skill Promotes Clinical Judgment, 162
    Guidelines: How to Make Inferences (Draw Valid Conclusions), 162
    Practice Exercises: Making Inferences (Drawing Valid Conclusions), 163
  6. Clustering Related Cues (Data), 162
    Definition, 163
    Why This Skill Promotes Clinical Judgment, 164
    Guidelines: How to cluster Related Cues (Data), 164
    Practice Exercises: Clustering Related Cues (Data), 164
  7. Distinguishing Relevant from Irrelevant, 165
    Definition, 165
    Why This Skill Promotes Clinical Judgment, 165
    Guidelines: How to Distinguish Relevant from Irrelevant, 165
    Practice Exercises: Distinguishing Relevant from Irrelevant, 166
  8. Recognizing Inconsistencies, 167
    Definition, 167
    Why This Skill Promotes Clinical Judgment, 167
    Guidelines: How to Recognize Inconsistencies, 167
    Practice Exercises: Recognizing Inconsistencies, 168

9. **Identifying Patterns, 169**
  Definition, 169
  Why This Skill Promotes Clinical Judgment, 169
  Guidelines: How to Identify Patterns, 169
  Practice Exercises: Identifying Patterns, 170
10. **Identifying Missing Information, 170**
  Definition, 170
  Why This Skill Promotes Clinical Judgment, 170
  Guidelines: How to Identify Missing Information, 170
  Practice Exercises: Identifying Missing Information, 171
11. **Promoting Health by Identifying and Managing Risk Factors, 171**
  Definition, 171
  Why This Skill Promotes Clinical Judgment, 171
  Guidelines: How to Identify and Manage Risk Factors, 171
  Practice Exercises: Promoting Health by Identifying and Managing Risk Factors,
    173
12. **Diagnosing Actual and Potential Problems, 173**
  Definition, 173
  Why This Skill Promotes Clinical Judgment, 173
  Guidelines: How to Diagnose Actual and Potential Problems, 175
  Identifying Actual Problems, 175
  Predicting Potential (Risk) Problems, 177
  Practice Exercises: Diagnosing Actual and Potential Problems, 179
13. **Setting Priorities, 180**
  Definition, 180
  Guidelines: How to Set Priorities, 180
  Practice Exercises: Setting Priorities, 183
14. **Determining Client-Centered (Patient-Centered) Outcomes, 184**
  Definition, 184
  Why This Skill Promotes Clinical Judgment, 185
  Guidelines: How to Determine Client-Centered (Patient-Centered) Outcomes, 185
  Practice Exercises: Determining Client-Centered (Patient-Centered) Outcomes, 187
15. **Determining Individualized Interventions, 188**
  Definition, 188
  Why This Skill Promotes Clinical Judgment, 188
  Guidelines: How to Determine Specific Interventions, 188
  Practice Exercises: Determining Individualized Interventions, 191
16. **Evaluating and Correcting Thinking (Self-Regulating), 192**
  Definition, 192
  Why This Skill Promotes Clinical Judgment, 192
  Guidelines: How to Evaluate and Correct Thinking (Self-Regulate), 192
17. **Determining a Comprehensive Plan and Evaluating and Updating the Plan, 194**
  Definition, 194
  Why this Skill Promotes Clinical Judgment, 194
  Guidelines: How to Develop a Comprehensive Plan/Update the Plan, 194
  Practice Exercises: Determining a Comprehensive Plan and Updating the Plan, 196

CHAPTER 6 Mastering Common Workplace Skills

How to Use This Chapter, 199
  1. Navigating and Facilitating Change, 199
    Definition, 199
    Learning Outcomes, 199
    Thinking Critically about Change, 200
    How to Navigate and Facilitate Change, 200
  2. Communicating Bad News, 203
    Definition, 203
    Learning Outcomes, 203
    Thinking Critically about Giving Bad News, 203
  3. Dealing with Complaints Constructively, 206
    Definition, 206
    Learning Outcomes, 206
    Thinking Critically about Complaints, 207
    How to Deal with Complaints Constructively, 207
  4. Developing Empowered Partnerships, 209
    Definition, 209
    Learning Outcomes, 209
    Thinking Critically about Empowered Partnerships, 209
    How to Develop Empowered Partnerships, 210
  5. Giving and Taking Constructive Criticism, 212
    Definition, 212
    Learning Outcomes, 212
    Thinking Critically about Giving and Taking Constructive Criticism, 212
  6. Managing Conflict Constructively, 216
    Definition, 216
    Learning Outcomes, 216
    Thinking Critically about Conflict, 216
    How to Manage Conflict Constructively, 216
  7. Managing Your Time, 221
    Definition, 221
    Learning Outcomes, 221
    Thinking Critically about Managing Your Time, 221
    How to Manage Your Time, 221
  8. Preventing and Dealing with Mistakes Constructively, 226
    Definition, 226
    Learning Outcomes, 226
    Thinking Critically about Preventing and Dealing with Mistakes, 226
    How to Prevent and Deal with Mistakes Constructively, 229
    What to Do When Mistakes Happen, 231
  9. Transforming a Group into a Team, 233
    Definition, 233
    Learning Outcomes, 234
    Thinking Critically about Teamwork, 234
    How to Transform a Group into a Team, 234

10. **Accessing and Using Information Effectively, 238**
Definition, 238
Learning Outcomes, 238
Thinking Critically about Accessing and Using Information, 238
How to Access and Use Information Effectively, 238
11. **Outcome-Focused Writing (Writing to Get Results), 243**
Definition, 243
Learning Outcomes, 243
Thinking Critically about Writing, 243
How to Write to Get Results, 243

RESPONSE KEY FOR EXERCISES IN CHAPTERS 1 TO 5, 249

APPENDIX A   Mind Mapping (Concept Mapping): Getting in the "Right" State of Mind, 263
APPENDIX B   Patients' Rights, 266
APPENDIX C   DEAD ON!! A Game to Promote Critical Thinking, 267
APPENDIX D   Example Critical Pathway, 268
APPENDIX E   Admission Tool, 272
APPENDIX F   Nursing Interventions Classification (NIC) and Nursing Outcomes Classification (NOC) Examples, 276
APPENDIX G   American Nurses Association (ANA) Standards of Practice and Professional Performance Related to Registered Nurses, 277
APPENDIX H   NCLEX® Practice Questions, 279

GLOSSARY, 287

INDEX, 293

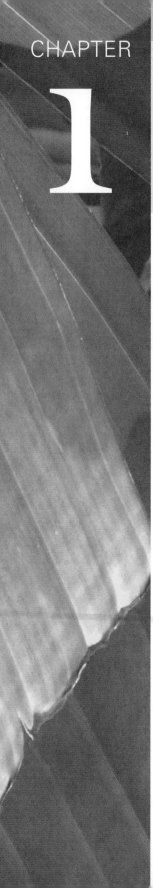

CHAPTER

1

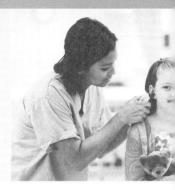

What Is Critical Thinking and Why Do We Care?

This chapter at a glance...

- Why Focus on Critical Thinking?
- How This Book Helps You Improve Thinking
    Brain-Based Learning
    Organized for Novices and Experts
- What's the Difference between Thinking and Critical Thinking?
- Critical Thinking: Some Different Descriptions
    A Synonym: Reasoning
    Frequently Quoted Critical Thinking Descriptions
    Applied Definition
- Problem-Focused Versus Outcome-Focused Thinking
- What about Common Sense?
- What Do Critical Thinkers Look Like?
- Critical Thinking Indicators (CTIs)
- What's Familiar and What's New?
    What's Familiar
    What's New
- Critical Thinking, Nursing Process, and Clinical Judgment
- 4-Circle CT Model: Get the Picture?
- Thinking Ahead, Thinking-in-Action, and Thinking Back (Reflecting)
- Critical Thinking Exercises
- Key Points / Summary

Decide where you stand in relation to each of the following learning outcomes:

Learning Outcomes

After completing this chapter, you should be able to:

1. Describe critical thinking in your own words, based on the descriptions in this chapter.
2. Give at least three reasons why critical thinking is essential for nurses.
3. Address how critical thinking is similar to and different from problem solving.
4. Identify four principles of the scientific method that are evident in critical thinking.
5. Compare and contrast the terms *problem-focused thinking* and *outcome-focused thinking.*
6. Clarify the term *critical thinking indicator* (CTI).
7. Use CTIs, together with the 4-circle CT model, to identify five critical thinking characteristics you'd like to improve.
8. Explain the relationship between the nursing process and critical thinking in the context of American Nurses Association (ANA) standards.
9. Address how creating healthy workplaces, healthy learning environments, and a culture of safety promote critical thinking.
10. Compare and contrast the terms *thinking ahead, thinking-in-action,* and *thinking back (reflective thinking).*

Why Focus on Critical Thinking?

Have you noticed how complicated life is today? Doesn't it seem like you constantly juggle priorities, face new challenges, and struggle with information overload? Critical thinking—your ability to focus your thinking to get the results you need—can make the difference between whether you succeed or fail. Whether you're trying to resolve a conflict, gain new skills, or streamline a plan of care, critical thinking—deliberate, informed thought—is the key.

Learning what critical thinking is—what it "looks like" and how you "do it" in various circumstances—helps you:

- **Gain confidence**, a trait that's crucial for critical thinking; lack of confidence is a "brain drain" that impedes your performance
- **Be autonomous**, as it helps you decide when to take initiative and act independently, and when to get help
- **Improve patient outcomes and job satisfaction**, because nothing's more rewarding than seeing patients and families thrive because you made a difference

Yet thinking isn't "like it always was." Workplace expectations are changing. Consider how the following points relate to the importance of gaining broad-based critical thinking skills:

- In communities, in schools, and at work, we're expected to accept more responsibilities, collaborate with diverse individuals, and make more independent decisions (Box 1-1).
- Critical thinking is the key to preventing and resolving problems. If you can't think critically, you become a part of the problems.
- Nurses are involved in complex situations that require in-depth consideration. We must view ourselves as knowledge workers, who are thought-oriented rather than task-oriented. For the public to value the need for nurses, we must change our image from being simply "a caring, helpful hand" to one that shows that we have specific knowledge that's vital to keeping patients safe, and helping them get and stay well. We must "wear not only our hearts, but also our brains on our sleeves."[1]
- Critical thinking is crucial to passing tests that demonstrate that you are qualified to practice nursing—for example, certification tests, the National Council Licensure Examination (NCLEX) and the Canadian Nurse Registered Examination (CNRE).
- Critical thinking skills are key to establishing the foundation for lifelong learning, a healthy workplace, and an organizational culture that's more concerned with reporting errors and promoting safety than "pointing fingers" and "blaming" (Box 1-2 on page 4).
- Patients and families must be active participants in making decisions—as the saying goes, "Nothing about me, without me." Knowing how to advocate, and how to teach and empower patients and families to manage their own care, requires highly developed critical thinking and interpersonal skills.

BOX 1-1	WORKPLACE SKILLS REQUIRED TODAY

To succeed in the workplace and as learners, you must know how to do the following:
- Be a self-starter: Take initiative, ownership, and responsibility.
- Engage in independent and group planning and problem solving.
- Teach yourself and others; advocate for yourself and others.
- Use resources: allocate time, money, materials, space, and human resources.
- Establish positive interpersonal relationships: work on teams, lead, negotiate, and work well with diverse individuals.
- Find, evaluate, and use information: organize and maintain files, interpret and communicate information, use computers to process data, and apply relevant principles to the "real" world.
- Assess social, organizational, and technologic systems.
- Apply professional and ethical standards to guide decision making.
- Monitor and correct performance; design and improve systems.
- Use technology: select equipment and tools; apply technology to tasks; maintain and trouble-shoot equipment.

Accomplishing the above requires you to have the following:
- Basic skills: reading, writing, speaking, listening, mathematics
- Thinking skills: knowing how to learn, reason, and think creatively, generate and evaluate ideas, see things in the mind's eye, make decisions, and solve problems
- Personal qualities: responsibility, self-esteem, self-confidence, self-management, sociability, and integrity

How This Book Helps You Improve Thinking

To keep your interest and help you understand and remember what you read, this book is designed based on principles of brain-based learning.[2,3,4]. The following section explains brain-based learning and how this book helps both novices and experts improve thinking.

Brain-Based Learning

Brain-based learning centers on using strategies that help your brain get "plugged in to learning mode." For example:

1. You learn best when there's logical progression of content, and you're engaged by a conversational style that gives lots of examples, strategies, and exercises to help you connect with how the content applies to you and the "real world."
2. Gaining deep understanding requires intensive analysis, which means thinking about the same topics in various ways.
3. Understanding and retaining what you read requires that you make learning meaningful by using your own unique way of processing how content relates to you personally.
4. Humor reduces stress, keeps your interest, and helps you learn.

5.　Thinking is like any skill (e.g., music, art, athletics)—we each have our own styles and innate or learned capabilities. We can all improve by gaining insight, acquiring instruction and feedback, and constantly practicing to improve.

BOX 1-2	LEARNING ENVIRONMENTS, HEALTHY WORKPLACES, AND SAFETY

What Makes a Good Learning Environment?

Students identify that the following makes a good learning environment: (1) Staff and teachers are approachable and promote self esteem and confidence, relating to learners with kindness and showing genuine interest in them as people. (2) A good team spirit is present where everyone works together towards common goals in an atmosphere of trust and respect, making students feel they belong to a team. (3) High standards are maintained through the use of efficient and flexible approaches that are tailored to individuals, not tasks. (4) Teaching and learning are key features and an integral part of daily activities of the organization. (5) Staff and teachers are keen to learn, and ongoing development is actively promoted. Information is shared, and learning opportunities are created and used well.[13]

Standards for Establishing and Sustaining a Healthy Workplace Environment

Standards form the foundation for a climate that fosters critical thinking by providing an atmosphere that's respectful, healing, and humane. These standards stress the need for the following: (1) effective communication, (2) true collaboration, (3) effective decision making, (4) appropriate staffing, (5) meaningful recognition, and 6) authentic leadership. A safe and respectful environment requires each standard to be maintained, because studies show that you don't get effective outcomes when any one standard is considered optional.[14]

Establishing a Culture of Safety

When an organization has a culture of safety, everyone feels responsible for safety and pursues it on a regular basis. Everyone—for example, nurses, physicians, and technicians—looks out for one another and feels comfortable pointing out unsafe behaviors (e.g., when hand sanitation has been missed or when safety glasses should be worn). Safety takes precedence over egos or pressures to complete tasks with little help or time. The organization values and rewards such actions.

Recommended Resources

- Centers for Disease Control and Prevention website links for healthy workplace, violence and injury, prevention, and other topics: www.cdc.gov
- Workplace Violence Prevention Position Statement. Retrieved May 8, 2006, from https://www. aacn.org/AACN/pubpolcy.nsf/Files/Workplace%20Violence %20Position%20Statement/$file/W orkplace%20Violence%204.12.04.pdf
- AACN Testimony to the IOM Committee on Work Environment for Nurses and Patient Safety. Retrieved May 8, 2006, from www.aacn.org/aacn/pubpolcy.nsf/92712bceed60b1878825688e00776 c1f/1138e880af4cafe788256cc60001ff73?OpenDocument

---

Organized for Novices and Experts

Whether you're a novice or an expert, the following organization helps you connect with what you already know, and readily move on to developing the complex skills you need to succeed today.

- **This chapter and Chapter 2** examine critical thinking in daily life with some reference to nursing situations. Whether you want to improve your ability to handle personal or professional matters, this section helps you focus your thinking to get results using your own particular talents.
- **Chapters 3 and 4** are designed to help you gain the knowledge and skills required to succeed in six common nursing situations: reasoning in the clinical setting (clinical judgment), moral and ethical reasoning, evidence-based practice, teaching others, teaching ourselves, and taking tests. Beginning students sometimes like to jump to Chapter 4, where *teaching others, teaching ourselves,* and *taking tests* are discussed, before reading other chapters. This is a good example of making learning meaningful. Read what you are most interested in first.
- **Chapter 5** gives opportunities to practice skills needed for clinical reasoning, nursing process, and clinical judgment, using case scenarios based on real experiences.
- **Chapter 6** helps you gain skills needed to work in any position that demands collaboration. When you have skills like *managing conflict* and *working as a team,* life is easier because you're less stressed and more productive. This section helps you learn how to build empowered partnerships with patients, families, peers, and colleagues. You also learn how to work smarter, not harder—how to set priorities and manage your time.

You'll find many useful Internet resources and references throughout this book. For direct links to the URLs, go to http://evolve.elsevier.com/Alfaro-LeFevre/CT or www.AlfaroTeachSmart.com (click on "Links & Resources").

What's the Difference between Thinking and Critical Thinking?

The main difference between thinking and critical thinking is *purpose and control.* Thinking refers to any mental activity—it can be "mindless," like when you're daydreaming or doing routine tasks like brushing your teeth. On the other hand, critical thinking is controlled and purposeful, using well-reasoned strategies to get the results you need.

Critical Thinking: Some Different Descriptions

Because critical thinking is a complex process that can be described in more than one way, there's no one *right* definition. Many authors (including me) develop their own descriptions to complement and clarify someone else's (which is, by the way, a good example of thinking critically: critical thinking requires you to "personalize" information—to analyze it and decide what it means to you rather than simply memorizing someone else's words). Think about the following synonym and commonly seen descriptions.

A Synonym: Reasoning

A good synonym for critical thinking is *reasoning*. Today, schools stress "four Rs" instead of three: reading, 'riting, 'rithmetic, and *reasoning*. From as early as the first grade, students learn the "how to's" of effective reasoning.

Now you know a synonym. But, since reasoning is a highly individualized, complex activity that involves distinct ideas, emotions, and perceptions, let's move on to a deeper discussion.

Frequently Quoted Critical Thinking Descriptions

Here are some commonly quoted descriptions of critical thinking:

- "Knowing how to learn, reason, think creatively, generate and evaluate ideas, see things in the mind's eye, make decisions, and solve problems"[5]
- "Reasonable, reflective thinking that focuses on what to believe or do"[6]
- "The ability to solve problems by making sense of information using creative, intuitive, logical, and analytical mental processes … and the process is continual"[7]
- "Thinking about your thinking, while you're thinking, to make it better, more clear, accurate, and defensible"[8]
- "The process of purposeful, self-regulatory judgment … the cognitive engine that drives problem solving and decision making"[9]
- "Knowing how to focus your thinking to get the results you need (includes intuitive, logical, and creative thinking)"[10]

All of the previous descriptions are helpful. There isn't *one* right description; rather, each one sheds light on the other. Think about the one that makes most sense to you.

Applied Definition

To understand what's involved in thinking critically in the clinical setting—a setting that's challenging, complex, and regulated by laws and standards—study the definition in the following box. Remember that *critical thinking* is a process and that *clinical judgment* is the *result* of the process (forming an opinion or making a decision).

APPLIED DEFINITION

Critical thinking and clinical judgment in nursing is purposeful, informed, outcome-focused (results-oriented) thinking that:[15,16]

- ❑ Is guided by professional standards, ethics codes, and laws (individual state practice acts)
- ❑ Carefully identifies the key problems, issues, and risks involved, including patients, families, and caregivers *early* in the process.
- ❑ Is based on principles of nursing process, problem solving, and the scientific method (requires forming opinions and making decisions based on evidence).
- ❑ Applies logic, intuition, and creativity and is grounded in specific knowledge, skills, and experience.
- ❑ Is driven by patient, family, and community needs, as well as nurses' needs to give competent, efficient care (e.g., streamlining paperwork to free nurses for patient care).
- ❑ Calls for strategies that make the most of human potential and compensates for problems created by human nature (e.g., applying technology, finding ways to prevent errors, and overcoming the powerful influence of personal views).
- ❑ Requires constantly reevaluating, self-correcting, and striving to improve.

Problem-Focused Versus Outcome-Focused Thinking

Many nurses don't understand the difference between problem-focused thinking and outcome-focused thinking. Think about the following points.

- **Problem-focused thinking is an important part of outcome-focused thinking:** You have to prevent, control, and resolve *problems* in order to achieve *outcomes.*
- **There are many ways to solve a problem.** There are quick fixes, "one-size-fits-all" solutions, temporary and long-term solutions, and solutions that are satisfactory but could be better. Outcome-focused thinking aims to fix problems in ways that get you *the best results.*
- **Sometimes there are so many problems that you decide to focus on** *outcomes* **rather than** *problems.* For example, if you work on a team with many interpersonal problems, your manager might say, "We have a long history of problems and it will take forever to fix them. I want to see us all working as a team. I'm asking you to put the problems aside and get agreement on roles, responsibilities, and behavior, so that our patients get good care and we enjoy coming to work."

What about Common Sense?

Some people believe that critical thinking is simply *common sense*, something that can't be taught. However, this belief is grounded on superficial understanding of what critical thinking is and how you get common sense. Although some people are born with common sense, a lot of it is *learned from experience.* You can put someone with great common sense in a new or stressful situation and you're likely to see behaviors that don't seem at all sensible. Think about the following scenario.

Scenario **CRITICAL THINKING: SIMPLY COMMON SENSE?**	As an evening supervisor, I stopped to check on a new graduate who was in charge for the first time. She appeared to be "in over her head," nervous and running around. Calmly, I asked how things were going. She replied, "Fine, except for the man in Room 203. His temperature was 104° an hour ago. We drew blood cultures, gave aspirin, and started him on antibiotics." I asked, "What's the temperature now?" She replied, "He's not due until 8 pm" (3 hours later). It seemed common sense to me that you would check the temperature more frequently when it was that high. Wanting to set a collaborative tone, I stressed the need to check it more frequently, and asked her to keep me informed. I also made sure I came back frequently to see how things were going. At the time I believed this nurse had no common sense, but she went on to be an excellent clinician with a track record of success. She was simply inexperienced, nervous, and overwhelmed in a new situation. She may even have been subconsciously defending an oversight. Although some people are blessed with an innate ability to focus on what's practical, a lot of common sense comes from knowledge, experience, and an ability to stay focused and pay attention. What may be common sense to you, based on your upbringing, schooling, or experience, may not be so to someone else. If you encounter someone who seems to have no common sense, don't jump to conclusions. Dig a little deeper to determine the real problems: Is there a knowledge, confidence, communication, or organizational skills problem? Is the person simply inexperienced or stressed by a new environment? Has the person become complacent? Could a learning disability be contributing to the problem? Like critical thinking, common sense often can be taught if you determine the underlying problems and do something about them.

What Do Critical Thinkers Look Like?

Research shows that most critical thinkers have high foreheads and furrowed brows, probably because of all the thinking they do. If you're not questioning this statement, then you're not thinking critically about what you're reading. When we ask, "What do critical thinkers look like?" we mean, "What characteristics do we see in someone who thinks critically?" Consider the following description:

> *"The ideal critical thinker is habitually inquisitive, self-informed, trustful of reason, open-minded, flexible, fair-minded in evaluation, honest in facing personal biases, prudent in making judgments, willing to reconsider, clear about issues, orderly in complex matters, diligent in seeking relevant information, reasonable in selection of criteria, focused in inquiry, and persistent in seeking results that are as precise as the subject and the circumstances of inquiry permit."*[11]

Now that you have a somewhat lengthy description of the ideal critical thinker, let's look at another way of describing critical thinkers. The next section describes behaviors that critical thinkers display.

Critical Thinking Indicators (CTIs)

Studying *behavior*—what good thinkers *do and say*—helps us to learn what critical thinkers "look like." The next page shows behaviors that evidence suggests promote critical thinking. These behaviors are called *critical thinking indicators* (CTIs) because they *indicate* characteristics or attitudes of critical thinkers. Keep in mind that no one is perfect—there's no ideal critical thinker who demonstrates *all* of the characteristics. Realize that even the best thinkers' characteristics vary, depending on circumstances such as confidence level and familiarity with the people and situations at hand. What matters are *patterns of behavior* over time (is the behavior usually evident?). Also remember that CTIs focus on critical thinking from a *nursing* perspective, which explains why things like "managing stress through healthy behaviors" are on the list. If you're unhealthy or stressed out, you're likely to have trouble thinking critically.

In Chapter 2, we'll address other CTIs—indicators of knowledge and intellectual skills. For now, decide where you stand in relation to the list of CTIs in the box on the next page. Rate how well you demonstrate each behavior, using a 0-10 scale as follows:

0 = This indicator is very difficult for me

10 = This indicator is pretty much a habit for me

As you evaluate yourself, remember that some of you, due to your nature, will be harder on yourselves than others (and vice versa). If you have some trusted friends, peers, or family members, it's a good idea to get their input on how they see your behavior. You may be surprised—or reaffirmed! Also remember that ability to demonstrate the CTIs varies with your familiarity and comfort level with the situation at hand. If you're in an unfamiliar, uncomfortable situation, the CTIs are more difficult to accomplish.

Box 1-3 (page 11) shows how other authors describe critical thinking traits. These traits were incorporated into the CTIs using simpler terms. Table 1-1 (page 12) gives examples of what critical thinking *is* and what it's *not*.

What's Familiar and What's New?

We understand something best by comparing it with something we already know: How is it the same and how is it different? This section first addresses critical thinking concepts you're likely to find familiar; then it addresses concepts that are likely to be new. Turn to page 12 and read on.

CRITICAL THINKING INDICATORS (CTIs): Behaviors Demonstrating CT Characteristics / Attitudes

Note: Indicators listed are in the context of clinical practice.

- **Self-aware:** Clarifies biases, inclinations, strengths, and limitations; acknowledges when thinking may be influenced by emotions or self-interest
- **Genuine:** Shows authentic self; demonstrates behaviors that indicate stated values
- **Self-disciplined:** Stays on task as needed; manages time to focus on priorities
- **Healthy:** Promotes a healthy lifestyle; uses healthy behaviors to manage stress
- **Autonomous and responsible:** Shows independent thinking and actions; begins and completes tasks without prodding; expresses ownership of accountability
- **Careful and prudent:** Seeks help when needed; suspends or revises judgment as indicated by new or incomplete data
- **Confident and resilient:** Expresses faith in ability to reason and learn; overcomes disappointments
- **Honest and upright:** Seeks the truth, even if it sheds unwanted light; upholds standards; admits flaws in thinking
- **Curious and inquisitive:** Looks for reasons, explanations, and meaning; seeks new information to broaden understanding
- **Alert to context:** Looks for changes in circumstances that warrant a need to modify thinking or approaches
- **Analytical and insightful:** Identifies relationships; expresses deep understanding
- **Logical and intuitive:** Draws reasonable conclusions ("If this is so, then it follows that..., because...."); uses intuition as a guide to search for evidence; acts on intuition only with knowledge of risks involved
- **Open and fair-minded:** Shows tolerance for different viewpoints; questions how own viewpoints are influencing thinking
- **Sensitive to diversity:** Expresses appreciation of human differences related to values, culture, personality, or learning style preferences; adapts to preferences when feasible
- **Creative:** Offers alternative solutions and approaches; comes up with useful ideas
- **Realistic and practical:** Admits when things aren't feasible; looks for user-friendly solutions
- **Reflective and self-corrective:** Carefully considers meaning of data and interpersonal interactions, asks for feedback, corrects own thinking, alert to potential errors by self and others, finds ways to avoid future mistakes
- **Proactive:** Anticipates consequences, plans ahead, acts on opportunities
- **Courageous:** Stands up for beliefs, advocates for others, doesn't hide from challenges
- **Patient and persistent:** Waits for right moment; perseveres to achieve best results
- **Flexible:** Changes approaches as needed to get the best results
- **Empathetic:** Listens well; shows ability to imagine others' feelings and difficulties
- **Improvement-oriented (self, patients, systems): (1) self**—Identifies learning needs, finds ways to overcome limitations, seeks out new knowledge; **(2) patients**—Promotes health, maximizes function, comfort, and convenience; **(3) systems**—Identifies risks and problems with health care systems; promotes safety, quality, satisfaction, and cost containment

BOX 1-3	HOW OTHER AUTHORS DESCRIBE CRITICAL THINKING TRAITS

Scheffer and Rubenfeld's Habits of the Mind*

- **CONFIDENCE:** Assurance of one's reasoning abilities
- **CONTEXTUAL PERSPECTIVE:** Consideration of the whole situation, including relationships, background, and environment relevant to some happening
- **CREATIVITY:** Intellectual inventiveness used to generate, discover, or restructure ideas. Imagining alternatives
- **FLEXIBILITY:** Capacity to adapt, accommodate, modify, or change thoughts, ideas, and behaviors
- **INQUISITIVENESS:** An eagerness to know, demonstrated by seeking knowledge and understanding through observation, and thoughtful questioning to explore possibilities and alternatives
- **INTELLECTUAL INTEGRITY:** Seeking the truth through sincere, honest processes, even if the results are contrary to one's assumptions and beliefs
- **INTUITION:** Insightful sense of knowing without conscious use of reason
- **OPEN-MINDEDNESS:** A viewpoint characterized by being receptive to divergent views and sensitive to one's biases
- **PERSEVERANCE:** Pursuit of a course with determination to overcome obstacles
- **REFLECTION:** Contemplation upon a subject, especially on one's assumptions and thinking for the purposes of deeper understanding and self-evaluation

Facione and Facione's Critical Thinking Dispositions†

- **TRUTHSEEKING:** A courageous desire for the best knowledge, even if such knowledge fails to support or undermines one's preconceptions, beliefs, or self-interest
- **OPEN-MINDEDNESS:** Tolerance of divergent views, self-monitoring for possible bias
- **ANALYTICITY:** Demanding the application of reason and evidence, alert to problematic situations, inclined to anticipate consequences
- **SYSTEMATICITY:** Valuing organization, focusing, and being diligent about problems of all levels of complexity
- **CRITICAL THINKING SELF-CONFIDENCE:** Trusting of one's own reasoning skills and seeing oneself as a good thinker
- **INQUISITIVENESS:** Curious and eager to acquire knowledge and learn explanations even when the applications of the knowledge are not immediately apparent
- **MATURITY:** Prudence in making, suspending, or revising judgment; awareness that multiple solutions can be acceptable; appreciation of the need to reach closure even in the absence of complete knowledge

Paul and Elder's Intellectual Traits*

- **INTELLECTUAL HUMILITY:** Consciousness of limits of your knowledge; willingness to admit what you don't know
- **INTELLECTUAL COURAGE:** Awareness of the need to face and fairly address ideas, beliefs, or viewpoints to which you haven't given serious hearing
- **INTELLECTUAL EMPATHY:** Consciousness of the need to imaginatively put yourself in the place of others to genuinely understand them
- **INTELLECTUAL AUTONOMY:** Having control over your beliefs, values, and inferences; being an independent thinker
- **INTELLECTUAL INTEGRITY:** Being true to your own thinking; applying intellectual standards to thinking; holding yourself to the same standards you hold others; willingness to admit when your thinking may be flawed
- **CONFIDENCE IN REASON:** Confidence that, in the long run, using your own thinking and encouraging others to do the same gets the best results
- **FAIRMINDEDNESS:** Awareness of the need to treat all viewpoints alike, with awareness of vested interest

*Descriptions quoted from Scheffer, B., & Rubenfeld, M. (2000). A consensus statement on critical thinking in nursing. *Journal of Nursing Education, 39*(8), 353.
†Descriptions quoted from Facione, P. Critical thinking: A statement of expert consensus for purposes of educational assessment and instruction. Retrieved January 17, 2007 from www.insightassessment.com.

TABLE 1-1   CRITICAL THINKING: WHAT IT *IS* AND WHAT IT'S *NOT*

Critical Thinking	Not Critical Thinking	Example of Critical Thinking
Organized and explained well by using words, examples, pictures, or graphics	Disorganized and vague	Persisting until you find a way to make your ideas easy to understand; using examples and illustrations to facilitate understanding
Critical for the sake of improvement, new ideas, and doing things in the best interest of the key players involved	Critical for the sake of attacking without being able to suggest new ideas and alternatives; critical for the sake of having it your way	Determining key players affected, then looking for flaws in the way something is done and figuring out ways to achieve the same outcomes more easily or better
Inquisitive about intent, facts, and reasons behind an idea or action; thought- and knowledge-oriented	Unconcerned about motives, facts, and reasons behind an idea or action; task-oriented, rather than thought-oriented	Raising questions to deeply understand what happened, why it happened, and what was being attempted when it happened
Sensitive to the powerful influence of emotions, but focused on making decisions based on what's morally and ethically the right thing to do	Emotion-driven	Finding out how someone feels about something, then moving on to discuss what's morally and ethically right
Communicative and collaborative with others when dealing with complex issues	Isolated, competitive, or unable to communicate with others when dealing with complex issues	Seeking multidisciplinary approaches to planning care as indicated by client needs

What's Familiar

Problem Solving. Knowing specific problem-solving strategies is a key part of critical thinking. For example, if you're caring for someone after heart surgery, you must know strategies to prevent and treat complications. Be aware, however, that using *problem solving* interchangeably with *critical thinking* can be a "sore subject." *Problem solving* is missing the important concepts of prevention, creativity, improvement, and aiming for the best results. Even if there are no problems, you should be thinking creatively, asking, "What could we be doing better?" and "How can we prevent problems before they happen?"

Analyzing. Although being analytical is important, critical thinking requires more than analyzing. It requires coming up with new ideas (right-brain thinking) and judging the worth of those ideas (left-brain thinking). Some overly analytical people suffer from "analysis paralysis," over-thinking problems when they should be taking action.

    Decision Making. *Decision making* and *critical thinking* are sometimes used interchangeably. This is because making decisions is an important part of critical thinking.

    The Scientific Method. This is an excellent tool for critical thinking, as it has been well studied and applies the following principles of scientific investigation:

- **Observing:** Continuously observing and examining to collect data, check for changes, and gain understanding
- **Classifying data:** Grouping related information so that patterns and relationships emerge
- **Drawing conclusions** that follow logically: "If this is so, then...."
- **Conducting experiments:** Performing studies to examine hypotheses (hunches or suspicions) and identify ways to improve
- **Testing hypotheses (hunches):** Determining whether we have factual evidence to support our hunches, assumptions, or suspicions

    Nursing Process. Experienced nurses often use the terms nursing process and critical thinking interchangeably. This is discussed in depth beginning on page 15.

What's New

    Strategies to Maximize Human Potential. We're only just beginning to learn how to maximize the human potential to think critically. For example, as children, we did a lot of memorizing. Yet, few of us know how to memorize in ways that promote comprehension and retention. Memorizing a list of facts can be a dead end for our minds. It doesn't help us understand information, and it doesn't help us retain it in the long term. We also didn't know much about learning style preferences or the need to use different learning strategies depending on your preferences. (If you aren't familiar with various learning styles and useful strategies, see page 58.) Now we realize the importance of learning in ways that get your brain "plugged in" to make connections that help you understand and remember in deep ways. For example, concept mapping (mind mapping) is an excellent tool to promote deep, personal understanding. *Mind-Mapping (Concept Mapping): Getting in the "Right" State of Mind* on page 263 summarizes how to draw concept maps.

    New Thinking on Error Prevention. We acknowledge that error prevention is a complex issue. We have changed thinking from "we can't make mistakes" to "because we're human we *will* make mistakes." Instead of looking only at *who's involved* in the mistakes, we study *who's involved and all contributing factors* (for example, fatigue, look-alike drugs, understaffing), so that we can develop *comprehensive approaches* to error prevention.

    More Importance Given to Developing What-if Strategies. We pay more attention to developing detailed approaches, policies, and procedures to cover what-if scenarios. For example with threats of bioterrorism and new diseases, we now continually work to fine-tune policies and procedures to prevent problems and to respond in a rapid, effective way.

Evidence-Based Thinking Emphasized. Clinicians are expected to provide evidence that supports opinions, solutions, and courses of action. We must be confident when we're asked questions like *What evidence do you have that this will work?* or *What data are you using to support that this is the problem or that this is a good solution?*

More Emphasis on Being Very Specific about How to Measure Outcomes (Results). Critical thinking makes it necessary to develop very specific ways to measure progress and results. For example, in the case of pain management, you don't ask a general question, like *Are you more comfortable?* You ask, "Can you rate your pain on a scale of 0 to 10, with 0 meaning pain-free, and 10 meaning the worst possible pain?"

Interpersonal Skills and Promoting Collaborative Thinking. We continue to work on developing interpersonal skills and identifying approaches that bring diverse thinkers together. Only then can we facilitate "meetings of the minds" to get the collaborative approaches that are so important to giving quality care.

Box 1-4 summarizes additional advances in promoting critical thinking.

BOX 1-4   RECENT ADVANCES ON IMPROVING THINKING

- Research suggests that intelligence quotient (IQ) tests may not really measure IQ: that there is more to intelligence that what's on IQ tests. For example, having a high EQ (emotional intelligence) is crucial to critical thinking. (See Chapter 2.)
- The idea that thinking can and must be taught—that practicing thinking skills is key to improving thinking
- Studies suggest that the brain is like a muscle: The more you use it, the more capable it becomes
- The belief that personal interests, passions, and commitments, as well as a sense of aesthetics (beauty), mystery, and wonder, play a crucial role in developing attitudes necessary for thinking
- Increased concern about the reasoning process: It's as important to know *how* a conclusion or decision was made as it is to know *what* the conclusion or decision is
- More emphasis on understanding other perspectives and using several different perspectives (collaboration) to come to better conclusions. Great minds don't always think alike: Different viewpoints enhance our thinking
- More acceptance of "There's more than one way" and "Sometimes there are no right answers" (each answer is correct in its own way)
- Acknowledgment that there are useful mistakes (occasional failure is the price of improvement) and that sharing mistakes is a responsible action that helps others avoid the same errors
- The identification of strategies that help us take advantage of how our brains work, including how to do the following:
  1. Get information into long-term memory
  2. Use both right (creative) and left (logical) sides of our brains
  3. Form good habits of inquiry
  4. Enhance creativity

Critical Thinking, Nursing Process, and Clinical Judgment

The terms *critical thinking, nursing process,* and *clinical judgment* are often used interchangeably. To understand these terms better, think about the following rule and also see Figure 1-1.

RULE

The nursing process is a tool that helps nurses to think critically. American Nurses Association (ANA) standards stress two points:
1. The nursing process—*assessment, diagnosis, outcome identification, planning, implementation,* and *evaluation*—serves as a critical thinking model that promotes a competent level of care.
2. Principles of the nursing process provide the basis for decision making and underpin virtually all care models.[12]

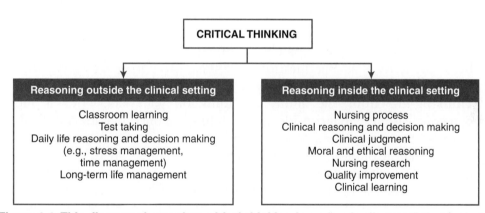

Figure 1-1 **This diagram shows that critical thinking is an "umbrella term"** that includes many aspects of reasoning both *inside and outside* of the clinical setting. Your ability to reason outside of the clinical setting—your ability to learn in class, manage stress, and maintain a healthy lifestyle—affects your ability to think critically in the clinical setting. (Copyright 2006-2008 by R. Alfaro-LeFevre. Workshop handouts. www.Alfaro TeachSmart.com.)

4-Circle CT Model: Get the Picture?

Whereas CTIs give verbal explanations of behaviors needed to promote critical thinking, the 4-circle CT model on the inside front cover *creates a picture* of what critical thinking involves. Study the four circles. Note that critical thinking (CT) requires a blend of CT characteristics, theoretical and experiential knowledge, inter-personal skills, and technical skills. Realize that the top circle—CT characteristics—corresponds with the CTIs listed on page 10. Take a highlighter or pencil and shade in that top circle. Then, put into the circle some of the CTIs from page 10 that you'd like to develop. In the next chapters, we'll address the other circles in more depth. For now, remember that if you develop the CT characteristics and attitudes in the *top* circle (e.g., confidence, resilience, and being proactive) developing the skills in the other *three* circles of the model will be easier.

Thinking Ahead, Thinking-in-Action, and Thinking Back (Reflecting)

Critical thinking is contextual, which means it changes depending on circumstances. Let's finish this chapter by addressing the importance of looking at critical thinking from three perspectives: thinking ahead, thinking in action, and thinking back (reflective thinking). Consider the following descriptions and think about the differences in each circumstance.

- **Thinking Ahead:** The ability to be proactive—to anticipate what might happen and to identify what you can do to be prepared. For novices, being proactive is difficult and sometimes restricted to reading procedure manuals and textbooks to anticipate what might happen. An important part of being proactive is asking questions like *What can I bring with me to help jog my memory and stay focused and organized?*

- **Thinking-in-Action:** The ability to "think on your feet." This is rapid, dynamic reasoning that considers several things at once, making it difficult to describe. For example, suppose you find your stove on fire. Your mind races, thinking all at once about what's fueling the flames, where the fire extinguisher is, whether you can put it out, whether you need to evacuate, and how to get help. Thinking-in-action *is highly influenced by previous knowledge and hands-on experience.* To improve outcomes and keep safety first, in all important situations, you need experts nearby who have extensive experiential knowledge stored in their brains. In the example above, wouldn't you like to have a fireman standing at your side? *Thinking-in-action* is prone to "knee-jerk" responses and decisions. To use the fire example again, an untrained person may throw water on a grease fire, which can make it worse.

- **Thinking Back (Reflective Thinking):** The ability to reflect on your reasoning to look for flaws, gain better understanding, and correct and improve thinking. Experienced nurses double-check their thinking in a dynamic way during thinking-in-action. However, this doesn't replace reflective thinking that happens *after the fact.* Deliberate, methodical reflective thinking that happens after the fact, using specific strategies and tools (e.g., journaling, chart reviews, honest dialogue with others), brings new insights, more depth, and greater accuracy—you can more objectively identify "lessons learned" from experience.

Before going on to review the end of chapter key points, study the diagram below, showing the key parts of your brain involved in thinking, and page 18, which gives a visual summary of questions that can help you evaluate your potential to think critically.

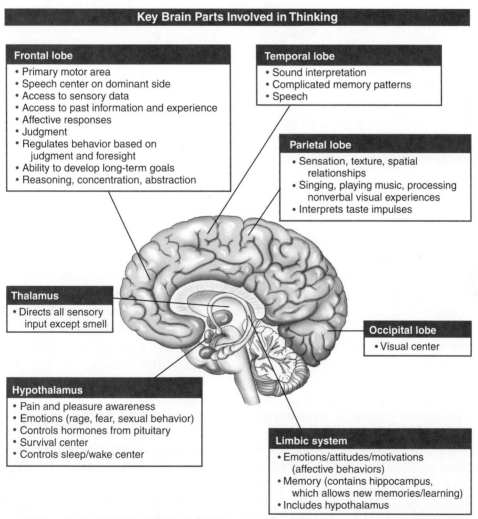

Key Brain Parts Involved in Thinking

Frontal lobe
- Primary motor area
- Speech center on dominant side
- Access to sensory data
- Access to past information and experience
- Affective responses
- Judgment
- Regulates behavior based on judgment and foresight
- Ability to develop long-term goals
- Reasoning, concentration, abstraction

Temporal lobe
- Sound interpretation
- Complicated memory patterns
- Speech

Parietal lobe
- Sensation, texture, spatial relationships
- Singing, playing music, processing nonverbal visual experiences
- Interprets taste impulses

Thalamus
- Directs all sensory input except smell

Occipital lobe
- Visual center

Hypothalamus
- Pain and pleasure awareness
- Emotions (rage, fear, sexual behavior)
- Controls hormones from pituitary
- Survival center
- Controls sleep/wake center

Limbic system
- Emotions/attitudes/motivations (affective behaviors)
- Memory (contains hippocampus, which allows new memories/learning)
- Includes hypothalamus

References: Cohen, B. (2005). *Memmler's the human body in health and disease* (10th ed.). Philadelphia: Lippincott Williams & Wilkins; Ignatavicius, D., & Workman, L. (Eds.). (2005). *Medical-surgical nursing: Critical thinking for collaborative care* (5th ed.). Philadelphia: Saunders.

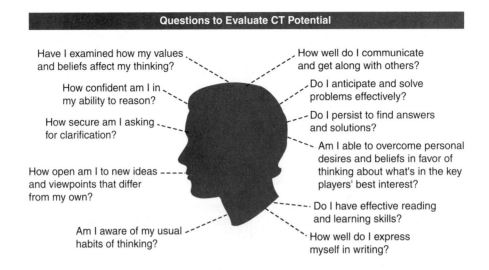

Questions to Evaluate CT Potential

Have I examined how my values and beliefs affect my thinking?

How confident am I in my ability to reason?

How secure am I asking for clarification?

How open am I to new ideas and viewpoints that differ from my own?

Am I aware of my usual habits of thinking?

How well do I communicate and get along with others?

Do I anticipate and solve problems effectively?

Do I persist to find answers and solutions?

Am I able to overcome personal desires and beliefs in favor of thinking about what's in the key players' best interest?

Do I have effective reading and learning skills?

How well do I express myself in writing?

Instructions for Completing Critical Thinking Exercises

Prioritize your learning and improve your understanding of each chapter by "personalizing information" and " making it yours." Together with your instructor or classmates:

- Discuss what information you *personally* found to be *most* helpful, and what information you found to *least* helpful.
- Use strategies like drawing pictures, diagrams, and maps to make connections between concepts. See *Mind Mapping (Concept Mapping): Getting in the "Right" State of Mind* on page 263.
- Apply strategies that use your own learning style preferences (see page 58 for style-specific strategies). For example, if you have trouble writing and do better verbally, tape your response; then play it and write it down. This will save you time in the long run. Or, use a voice-activated software program, such as *Naturally Speaking*.
- When writing responses, at first be more concerned with substance than grammar (as you would if you were writing a diary or sending e-mail). However, as you progress, work to make your responses clear to others. Making your responses clear to others helps you clarify your thoughts.
- Don't be afraid to paraphrase. Paraphrasing helps you gain understanding because you explain what you read using familiar language (your own). To avoid concerns of plagiarism, cite the page numbers you're paraphrasing.
- Exercises followed by an asterisk (*) have example response(s) listed in the *Response Key* beginning on page 249. Compare your responses with the responses of others and those in the *Response Key*. Remember that these are *examples of* responses, not the *only* responses. You may have a creative response that's different, but equally good as, the example response. The main point is that you *learn* by *evaluating your thinking* in relation to the exercise and the content in each chapter. If you have questions about whether your responses are appropriate, check with your instructor.

- Think about how the exercises can be improved: Give suggestions to your instructor, and send them to us, by clicking on "Contact Us" at www.AlfaroTeachSmart.com. If your suggestion is unique, we will post it on the Web and cite you as the contributor of the exercise.

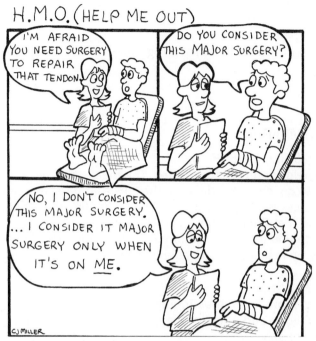

Showing your human side and using humor can help you make human connections with patients.

CRITICAL THINKING EXERCISES

Note: Exercises followed by asterisks (*) have example responses listed in the Response Key *beginning on page 249.*

1. What is the relationship between *achieving outcomes* and *identifying problems, issues, and risks involved?*
2. Complete the following sentences and then compare your responses with those of others:
    - If I were to explain to someone else what critical thinking is, I would say that…
    - I do my best thinking when…
    - I do my worst thinking when...
3. Study Box 1-1 (page 3), addressing workplace skills. Identify three skills you'd like to improve, and then think of some ways you can develop them.
4. Compare and contrast the traits of confidence, critical thinking self-confidence, and confidence in reason, listed in Box 1-3 on page 11.*

5. When you form an opinion, you draw a conclusion from *facts* (evidence).
   a. What's the difference between facts and opinions?*
   b. How can you determine if an opinion is valid?*
6. Study the brain diagram on page 17 and decide how thinking ability would be influenced if you had brain damage in frontal lobe or hippocampus.*
7. Discuss the effect "mind games" (worrying too much or focusing on the negatives) can have on thinking and performance.
8. Decide where you stand in relation to being able to achieve the *Learning Outcomes* listed on page 1.

CRITICAL MOMENTS

APPLYING 80/20 RULE HELPS YOU PRIORITIZE

The 80/20 rule helps you to set priorities. The idea is that when you're faced with 100% of things to do, narrow it down to the 20% that *must* be done. You can apply this rule in many ways. For example: (1) You wear 20% of your clothes 80% of the time (think about that the next time you clean out your closet or want to buy new clothes. (2) When you look after patients, be sure you identify the 20% that must be done to stay on task and keep patients safe.

QUESTIONS, PLEASE

Socrates learned more from questioning others than he did from reading books. Seek others' opinions and question deeply to gain understanding. Develop your ability to ask questions.

LOOK FOR AHA'S!

We say "aha!" when we suddenly realize something or have our suspicions confirmed. We say, "aha!" when we connect with something that was in the back of our minds but never put into words. As you read this book, do some "hemming and hawing" about what you read. Look for "ahas." These moments of "light bulbs going off in your head" are energizing. They bring new ideas and stimulate you to learn more.

BOOT CAMPS FOR BRAINS?

Today we have brain imaging techniques, such as Positron Emission Tomography (PET) scans that let us actually see the brain "in action": We can see exactly what parts of the brain are being used in various thinking and tasks. People have survived brain injuries that used to be fatal, and we continue to learn from their rehabilitation. For example, some people who have had strokes cannot speak, but they can sing words. We now know how to use brain techniques not only to learn, but also to promote healing, stress reduction, and wellness. Get in touch with your brain and how it works. Keep your mind open to trying new strategies. Try brain exercises that promote "brain fitness." (See *Take Your Brain to Boot Camp*, available at www.aarp. org/about_aarp/nrta/livelearn/staying_sharp_boot_camp.html, and *Eight Essentials for Keeping Your Mind Sharp*, available at www.drgarysmall.com/eight_essentials.)

OTHER PERSPECTIVES

HOW TO THINK LIKE EINSTEIN

"It's not that I'm smart, it's just that I stick with problems longer."

—*Albert Einstein*

CRITICAL THINKING MAY BE TRIGGERED BY POSITIVE EVENTS, NOT JUST PROBLEMS

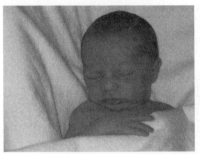

When a baby is born in some hospitals, everyone shares in the celebration. With each birth the public address system plays Brahms' Lullaby. Patients love it—even oncology patients, who say it lifts their spirits and allows them to share someone else's joy. Parents who have just lost their baby are given the option of playing the lullaby or not. Many of them choose to have it played for their baby.

"Playing the music is a simple thing that can be done for patients and families that costs virtually nothing and brings a great deal of pleasure."—*Jean Young, ICU patient care manager*

YOU ARE YOUR OWN COACH

"If you don't talk to yourself and give yourself pep talks, start now. Time was, only crazies talked to themselves; now, you miss the boat if you don't. Our minds are tricky things. We know now that attitude is the base on which knowledge and ability stand."—*Jean T. Penny, PhD, ARNP*

SIGN HANGING IN CAFÉ

 Unattended children get double espressos and a free puppy.

KEY POINTS / SUMMARY

- This book is designed using brain-based learning—principles that help you get your brain "plugged in" to learn.
- Because critical thinking is a complex activity that can be described in more than one way, there's no one right definition—there are several that complement and clarify one another.
- Critical thinking is an "umbrella term" that includes reasoning inside and outside of the clinical setting.
- There's a lot about critical thinking that's similar to principles of science and the scientific method.
- Critical thinking requires right-brain thinking (generating new ideas) and left-brain thinking (analyzing and judging the worth of those ideas).
- *Critical thinking* refers to purposeful, informed, results-oriented thinking in any situation, and is often used interchangeably with *clinical reasoning, clinical judgment, nursing process, problem solving,* and *decision making.*
- ANA standards stress that the nursing process—*assessment, diagnosis, outcome identification, planning, implementation,* and *evaluation*—underpins all care models, providing the basis for critical thinking. To pass licensing and competency tests and be a safe, effective clinician, you need to be very familiar with how to use the nursing process as a tool to promote critical thinking (addressed in detail in Chapters 3 through 5).

- Page 10 shows critical thinking indicators (CTIs)—behaviors that demonstrate characteristics that promote critical thinking. Although ability to demonstrate these behaviors varies, depending on circumstances such as familiarity with the people and situations at hand, these are the behaviors that you should work to develop.
- The 4-circle CT model on the inside front cover gives you "a picture" of what it takes to think critically. If you demonstrate CT characteristics (top circle), you will easily develop skills related to the other circles.
- Critical thinking is like any skill (e.g., music, art, athletics). We each have our own styles and innate or learned capabilities. Further, we can all improve by gaining awareness, acquiring instruction, and consciously practicing to improve.
- It's important to look at critical thinking from three different perspectives: thinking ahead, thinking-in-action, and thinking back (reflective thinking).

REFERENCES

1. Gordon, S. (2006). What do nurses really do? *Topics in Advanced Nursing eJournal, 6*(1). Retrieved July 24, 2006, from www.medscape.com/viewarticle/520714?src=mp.

2. Caine, R., & Caine, G. (2002). *Making connections: Teaching and the human brain.* Reading, MA: Addison-Wesley.

3. Hart, L. (2002). *Human brain, human learning* (3rd ed.). Covington, WA: Books for Educators.

4. On Purpose Associates. Brain-based learning. Retrieved May 8, 2006, from www.funderstanding.com/brain_based_learning.cfm.

5. The Secretary's Commission on Achieving Necessary Skills [SCANS], The U.S. Department of Labor. (1992). *Learning a living: A blueprint for high performance, a SCANS report for America 2000.* Washington, DC: Author.

6. Ennis, R., & Milman, J. (1985). *Cornell tests of critical thinking: Theory and practice.* Pacific Grove, CA: Midwest Publications.

7. Snyder, M. (1993). Critical thinking: A foundation for consumer-focused care. *The Journal of Continuing Education in Nursing, 24*(5), 206-210.

8. Paul, R. (1995). *Critical thinking: How to prepare students for a rapidly changing world.* Santa Rosa, CA: Foundation for Critical Thinking.

9. Facione, P. Critical thinking: A statement of expert consensus for purposes of educational assessment and instruction. Retrieved January 17, 2007, from www.insight-assesment.com.

10. Alfaro-LeFevre, R. (2007). Evidenced-based critical thinking indicators. Retrieved January 24, 2007 from www.alfaroteachsmart.com/cti.htm.

11. The Delphi Report. (1990). Retrieved May 14, 2006, from www.insightassessment.com/pdf_files/DEXadobe.PDF.

12. American Nurses Association. (2004). *Nursing scope and standards of performance and standards of clinical practice.* Washington, DC: American Nurses Publishing.

13. Hand, H. (2006). Promoting effective teaching and learning in the clinical setting. Nursing Standard, *20*(39), 55-63. Retrieved June 18, 2006 from www.nursing-standard.co.uk/archives/ns/vol20-39/pdfs/v20n39p5563.pdf.

14. American Association of Critical Care Nurses. Healthy work environment backgrounder. Retrieved May 8, 2006, from https://www.aacn.org/AACN/pubpolcy.nsf/Files/HWEPosStat/$file/HWE%20BG%20Color%206.21.04.pdf.

15. Alfaro-LeFevre, R. (2006). *Applying nursing process: A tool for critical thinking* (6th ed.). Philadelphia, PA: Lippincott Williams & Wilkins.

16. Alfaro-LeFevre, R. (2008). Evidence-based critical thinking indicators. Retrieved January 17, 2007, from www.alfaroteachsmart.com/cti.htm.

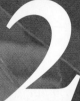

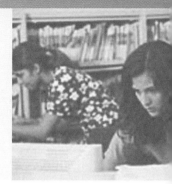

CHAPTER 2

How to Think Critically

This chapter at a glance...

- Gaining Insight and Self-Awareness
  - Connecting with Your Learning Style
  - How Your Personality Affects Thinking
  - Effects of Birth Order, Upbringing, and Culture
  - Male Versus Female Thinking
- Developing Trust in Relationships
- Mentoring and Building Empowered Partnerships
- Factors Influencing Critical Thinking Ability
  - Personal Factors Influencing Thinking
  - Situational Factors Influencing Thinking
- Habits Creating Barriers to Critical Thinking
- Habits That Promote Critical Thinking
- Critical Thinking Exercises
- Outcome-Focused (Results-Oriented) Thinking
  - Goal (Intent) Versus Outcome (Result)
  - Clarifying Outcomes
- Critical Thinking Strategies
  - 10 Key Questions
  - Using Logic, Intuition, and Trial and Error
  - Focusing on Details and Big Picture
  - Drawing Maps, Diagrams, and Decision Trees
  - Simulated Learning Experiences
  - Other Useful Strategies
- CTIs for Knowledge and Intellectual Skills
- Developing Character and Acquiring Knowledge and Skills
- Assessing and Evaluating Thinking
  - Basic Principles of Evaluating Thinking
  - Self-Assessment
  - Peer Review
  - Using Tests and Instruments
- Critical Thinking Exercises
- Key Points / Summary

Decide where you stand in relation to each of the following learning outcomes:

Learning Outcomes

After completing this chapter, you should be able to:

1. Explain the three main steps to improving thinking.
2. Describe how personality, learning style, upbringing, and culture affect critical thinking.
3. Explain why building trust and following a code of conduct promote critical thinking.
4. Discuss how human habits influence critical thinking.
5. Address how answering the questions listed on the inside back cover promotes critical thinking.
6. Identify the roles of logic, intuition, and trial and error in critical thinking.
7. Decide where you stand in relation to being able to demonstrate critical thinking indicators (CTIs) for knowledge and intellectual skills.
8. Decide where you stand in relation to what's required for critical thinking as described by the 4-circle CT model on the inside front cover.
9. Explain the relationship between evaluating thinking, improving performance, and ensuring patient safety.
10. Discuss how analyzing a nurse's outcomes and behavior helps you evaluate critical thinking.

Gaining Insight and Self-Awareness

A first-grade teacher I know tells the following great story: One of my kids came bouncing into class looking very pleased. He pointed to the middle of his forehead and announced, "I just realized that I can read my own mind!" Another teacher I know likes to talk to herself. If someone asks, "Why are you talking to yourself?" she replies, "Because I'm the only one who makes any sense around here." Many people have little understanding of their own thinking, and even *less* understanding of *others'* thinking. Although I can't promise that reading this chapter will stop you from talking to yourself, it *will* help you gain insight into how and why you think the way you do…and how and why *others* think the way *they* do. Whether you want to improve your ability to handle personal or professional matters, this chapter helps you learn how to focus your approach to get the results you need in your own way.

As you read this chapter, keep the following points in mind:

- Thinking is a skill like any other (e.g., music, art, athletics).
- As with any skill, we each have our own styles—innate and learned capabilities.
- Improving thinking requires three main steps: (1) Gain insight and self-awareness. (2) Get agreement on a code of conduct (see the next page) and what critical thinking entails. (3) Make the choice to practice and develop the attitudes, knowledge, and skills that promote critical thinking.

Let's start the discussion on gaining insight and self-awareness by looking at how and why you think and learn the way you do.

Connecting with Your Learning Style

Your ability to connect with your preferred learning style makes the difference between learning efficiently (feeling energized and capable and wanting more) and wasting time (feeling tired, useless, and frustrated). Many people believe they are poor learners. However, the reality is that they're simply unaware of their own learning preferences. For example, my sister once said: "What I like best about computers is that I never was a good learner…but with computers, it doesn't matter because you just have to figure things out for yourself…and I'm good at that." Learning is *figuring things out for yourself*. When you figure things out for yourself, it's *learning at its best* because you "own the material and make it yours." You understand deeply, and your brain retains more.

CODE OF CONDUCT

As a member of this team or group, I agree to work to make the following a part of my daily routine.

1. To promote empowered partnerships by:
- Valuing your time and the contribution you make to the team or group
- Accepting the diversity in our styles—recognizing that you know yourself best and should be allowed to choose your own approaches
- Promising to be honest, and treating you with respect and courtesy
- Promoting independence and mutual growth by applying the "Platinum Rule" (Treat others as they want to be treated, not assuming they have the same desires you do)*
- Listening openly to new ideas and other perspectives
- Attempting to walk a mile in your shoes
- Committing to resolving conflict without resorting to the use of power
- Taking responsibility for my own emotional well-being (if I feel bad about something, it's my responsibility to do something about it)
- Ensuring that we both:
  - Stay focused on our joint purpose and responsibilities for achieving it
  - Make decisions together as much as possible
  - Realize that we're accountable for the outcomes (consequences) of our actions
  - Have the right to say no, so long as it doesn't mean neglecting my responsibilities

2. To foster open communication and a positive work environment by:
- Addressing specific issues and behaviors
- Acknowledging and/or apologizing if I've caused inconvenience or made a mistake
- Doing my "homework" before drawing conclusions
- Maintaining confidentiality when I'm used as a sounding board
- Using only ONE person as my sounding board before I decide to either give feedback or drop the issue
- Determining the validity of any rumors I hear
- Redirecting co-workers who are talking about someone to speak directly to the person
- Addressing unsafe or unethical behavior directly and according to policies
- Offering feedback as indicated:
  - Within 72 hours
  - Using "I" statements ("I feel..." rather than "You make me feel...")
  - Describing behaviors and giving specific examples
  - Limiting discussion to the event at hand and not discussing past history and telling you honestly and openly the impact of the behavior

3. To be approachable and open to feedback by:
- Taking responsibility for my actions and words
- Taking time to reflect on what was said, rather than blaming, defending, or rejecting
- Asking for clarification of the perceived behaviors
- Remembering that there's always a little bit of truth in every criticism
- Staying focused on what I can learn from the situation

*Retrieved Jan. 22, 2007, from www.alessandra.com/abouttony/aboutpr.asp.

> ### RULE
>
> **There are no right or wrong ways to learn.** There are only *differences.* You're responsible for connecting with your preferred style and the learning strategies that can help you learn efficiently *in your own way.* When you figure things out in your own way, you're thinking critically. Improving your ability to think and learn requires you to do two things:
> 1.   Believe in your ability to be a good thinker and learner.
> 2.   Learn strategies that can help you think and learn more efficiently in your own way.

If you don't know how you learn best—whether you're a doer, observer, or whatever—study page 58, which gives an overview of various learning styles and corresponding strategies to promote learning. You can also find resources like the following by entering "learning style preferences" into Google:

- Learning Styles Questionnaire: www.engr.ncsu.edu/learningstyles/ilsweb. html
- Learning Styles Inventories: www.stylesoflearning.com/trial_inventory.html
- www.learning-styles-online.com

How Your Personality Affects Thinking

Personality plays a major role in how you think and learn. Your personality determines what information you notice and recall, the way you make decisions, and how much structure and control you like. Connecting with your own particular personality's needs helps you understand how and why you think the way you do. It helps you get in touch with your talents and blind spots and find ways to improve. Understanding personality types different from your own helps you realize how and why *others* think the way they do. Armed with this information, you can facilitate "meetings of the minds."

To better understand your personality and thinking style, study *What's Your Thinking Style?* on page 29 (Box 2-1) and *Do You Know What to Do When Someone Turns Blue?* on page 30. Think about where you and others who are close to you "fit into" the various styles described on those pages. Keep in mind that no one style is better than another. They are all good styles, with specific strengths and limitations. What's important is that you know that there are distinct style differences and that you (1) connect with your own style, celebrating your strengths and working to overcome limitations, and (2) learn to connect with people with styles that are different from your own, respecting their need to approach things in their *own* way. Box 2-2 shows the benefits of being sensitive to personality differences.

BOX 2-1	WHAT'S YOUR THINKING STYLE? (MYERS-BRIGGS TYPE)*

Extrovert	**Introvert**
Thinks out loud	Thinks inside
Draws energy from being with people	Draws energy from being quiet
Sensate	**Intuitive**
Perceives the world discretely through the five senses	Perceives the world overall
Looks for facts	Looks for meaning
Thinking	**Feeling**
Uses objective data	Uses subjective data
Seeks just decisions	Seeks fair decisions
Judging	**Perceiving**
Orders the environment	Keeps things flexible and open
Likes to plan	Likes to be spontaneous

*Data from www.humanmetrics.com/#Jtype. You can find various style inventories at www.humanmetrics.com.

BOX 2-2	BENEFITS OF SENSITIVITY TO PERSONALITY TYPES

Partnering and Team Building
- Helps diverse personalities come together with understanding and respect, promoting solid relationships
- Keeps the focus on common goals, improving quality and efficiency
- Helps identify strategies to reduce and resolve conflicts
- Facilitates collaboration and makes the most of individual and team talents

Performance and Retention
- Promotes critical thinking (people think better when they understand and trust one another)
- Reduces stress, allowing more brainpower for finding solutions
- Increases self-confidence by providing style-specific strategies
- Promotes an environment that nurtures professional and personal growth

Customer and Patient Satisfaction
- Facilitates communication with "difficult" patients and families
- Improves outcomes by helping you tailor approaches to consider different personalities' wants and needs
- Patients and families feel understood, empowered, and motivated by receiving care that's "in sync" with their own specific styles

Effects of Birth Order, Upbringing, and Culture

Your birth order—whether you were the eldest who was expected to lead or the "baby" who had few responsibilities—impacts on how you think, as does your parents' "parenting style." If you were raised by strict, authoritarian parents who insisted that you "do as you are told, without asking questions," it's likely that you'll find it difficult to approach teachers or leaders to discuss problems, ask for feedback, or offer suggestions. Some of you need to muster courage to overcome deep-seated insecurities that come from lessons learned as a child.

Where you grew up and the culture you embrace also impacts on thinking. For example, in some countries, questioning teachers is considered rude. However, when students ask questions, everyone learns.

DO YOU KNOW WHAT TO DO WHEN SOMEONE TURNS BLUE?

Here's a theory that gives new meaning to turning blue, red, white, or yellow (no, it doesn't mean becoming cyanotic, inflamed, shocky, or jaundiced). Psychologist Taylor Hartman uses colors to represent personality types. (By the way, he says you can't really turn one color or another—you are what you are born.) Hartman believes that each of us, from birth, is blessed with a core motive—a drive to approach life from a certain perspective. Using colors as labels, here's how he describes four distinct personality types:

REDS have a drive for power. They know how to take charge and make things happen. Red strengths are that they are confident, determined, logical, productive, and visionary. However, they can be bossy, impatient, arrogant, argumentative, and self-focused.

BLUES are driven to achieve intimacy. They love getting to know people well, have strong feelings, and like talking about the daily details of life. Blues are creative, caring, reliable, loyal, sincere, and committed to serving others. On the flip side, they can be judgmental, worry-prone, doubtful, and moody, and often have unrealistic expectations.

WHITES strive for peace. They're independent, contented people who ask little of those around them. Whites are insightful, flexible, tolerant, easy-going, patient, and kind. But Whites tend to avoid conflict at all costs, are indecisive, silently stubborn, and may "explode" because they hold things in until there are so many things bothering them that just one more problem pushes them over the edge.

YELLOWS are driven to have fun. They wake up happy, know how to enjoy life in the present moment, and are simply fun to be around. Yellows are outgoing, enthusiastic, optimistic, popular, and trusting. However, they tend to avoid facing facts and can be impulsive, undisciplined, disorganized, and uncommitted.

Applying the *Color Code* principles helps you connect with inner drives that often lie dormant, waiting to be harnessed in positive ways. Armed with this knowledge, you can make better "people decisions," like how to nurture a team, or get along with difficult people. Imagine how you could apply this theory to help a group come together to give a presentation. You might get a productive, visionary Red to coordinate and lead the project; a caring, detail-oriented Blue to do the handouts; a peace-loving, insightful White to be a "human suggestion box" (no one's afraid to approach a White); and a fun-loving Yellow to make sure that the class is more than serious stuff (a little fun, humor, and refreshment make it an enjoyable, memorable, learning experience).

Think about what could happen in the above situation if you switched some of those personalities and tasks around! *The Color Code* facilitates a crucial first step to improving thinking—understanding how and why we think the way we do (and how and why others think they way they do). These are challenging times that require us to think and work in teams. Applying these principles helps us spend less time spinning wheels and more time "in gear," fully engaged in progress. **To take the Color Code test, or order the book,** go to www.theColorCode.com. For a CEU article on this topic, go to www.nurse.com/ce/CE236.

Summarized with permission from Hartman, T. (1998). *The color code.* New York, New York: Scribner.
Source: Adapted from Alfaro-LeFevre, R. Do you know what to do when someone turns blue? Copyright 1998. *Nursing Spectrum Nurse Wire* (www.nurse.com). All rights reserved. Used with permission.

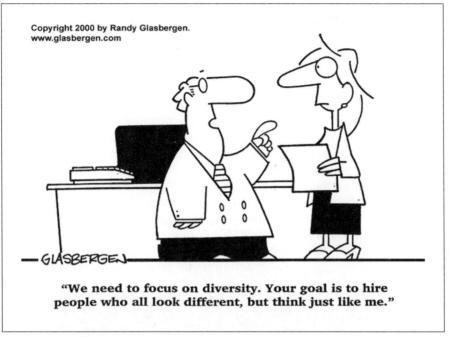

Copyright 2000 by Randy Glasbergen.
www.glasbergen.com

GLASBERGEN

"We need to focus on diversity. Your goal is to hire
people who all look different, but think just like me."

Reprinted with special permission from www.glasbergen.com.

Male Versus Female Thinking

Understanding differences between male and female thinking is especially important for nursing. We have more males in nursing, but historically, nursing is a female profession. Think about the following *Other Perspectives*, addressing how culture and male-female differences can affect thinking.

OTHER PERSPECTIVES

IN SOME CULTURES, QUESTIONING SHOWS WEAKNESS
"I have trouble asking questions because in my culture, asking questions is discouraged and is a sign of weakness and embarrassment. What I'm working on and want to know is how to become more confident and capable in asking questions, for I realize it's essential to critical thinking."—*One of my workshop participants*

MEN IN NURSING HAVE DIFFERENT NEEDS
"My doctoral research opened my eyes to the struggles of male nursing students. Men learn differently from women, have different backgrounds on entering nursing school, and have different experiences once *in* school. For instance, guys are less likely to be assigned to female patients in med-surg units. Their peers, and sometimes their instructors, seek them out to assist with moving and positioning patients. Some men feel they must be 'extra' professional to avoid misconceptions by patients. Men approach teamwork differently from what they experience in nursing.

They tend to address issues directly, whereas women often talk around issues and avoid the person with whom they have a conflict. Learning to care is a big deal for guys. Men are socialized to not express emotion. Yet when we teach therapeutic communication, what do we expect? We want them to maintain eye contact and use touch to show connection. We want interactive responses that show engagement— 'really?' 'uh huh,' head nods, and of course, reflective restatements. We talk about maintaining an open posture without crossing our arms, and leaning in to show attention. But, what are guys' normal responses to conversation? They may rest against the wall with arms crossed and respond to patients' concerns with humor. Too often, instructors regard this type of communication as nonattentive, nonconnected, and nontherapeutic (that's not how we females interact). Guys may be just as connected and therapeutic in their approaches. We have to be careful not to judge their performance based on our female expectations for communication." (You can read more on this topic in Anthony, A. [2006]. Retaining men in nursing—Our role as nursing educators. In Oermann, M., & Heinrich, K. [Eds.], *Annual Review of Nursing Education [4th ed.],* 211-234. New York: Springer.[9])

—Ann Anthony RN, MSN, Tulsa Community College

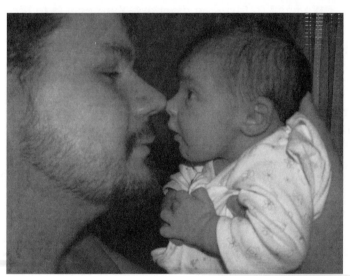

You are born with unique and inherited personality traits. Your birth order, upbringing, and culture also impact on your personality and learning preferences.

Developing Trust In Relationships

From dealing with patients to dealing with peers and professionals, developing trust in relationships is essential to getting the results you need. Without trust, you're likely to have superficial—rather than meaningful—discussion, since people are afraid to speak their minds. Improving thinking requires honest, open dialogue—something that only happens when there's trust between the two people. Remember the following rule:

People think best when they like and trust one another. Adopt a code of conduct, be sensitive to style differences, and follow the *Platinum Rule* ("Treat others as they want to be treated"), rather than the *Golden Rule* ("Do unto others as you would have them do unto you").[1] This changes your thinking from "this is what I want, so I'll give everyone the same thing" to "let me first understand what others want so I can give it to them."

Mentoring and Building Empowered Partnerships

Think about the following quotes:

> "Early in my career, I was powerfully influenced by a nursing instructor who saw potential in me that I did not recognize. Under the watchful, yet caring, tutelage of this person, I began to find my professional self."[2]
> —*Patricia Thompson, RN, EdD, President, Sigma Theta Tau International*

> "Expert nurses are made, not born. Remember your first code, your first day in charge, the sadness with the death of your primary patient, or feeling alone? These experiences are all common to the novice nurse. The perception of the experience, as well as what is brought forward to future career events, can be shaped by an experience with a mentor."[3]
> —*Margaret M. Ecklund, RN, MS, CCRN*

Most nurses can identify people in their lives who have impacted on their thinking. Often, these individuals are parents, teachers, co-workers, or friends. Today, because we know the value of improving thinking and performance through on-the-job partnerships, many organizations assign mentors (also called preceptors) to help students and novice nurses.[4] Mentors are nurses with exemplary skills whose role it is to teach, nurture, and empower new nurses on a one-to-one basis. Learning how to be a mentor (acquiring the skills needed to nurture novices) and how to be a "mentee" (knowing how to learn from a more experienced person) is an important step in critical thinking. When choosing mentor-novice partnerships, it's important to give thought to the pair's "fit". When matched well, mentors experience the reward of making a difference in someone else's life. Under competent, caring guidance from a well-matched mentor, novices "spread their wings." If matched poorly, for example, if the two nurses are very different thinkers or personalities, the end result can be frustration, disappointment, and damaged spirits on both sides. Remember that mentoring isn't a "one size fits all" situation. Build empowered partnerships, pay attention to personal style differences, and address these early (see *Developing Empowered Partnerships* on page 209).

Factors Influencing Critical Thinking Ability

Have you ever found yourself saying, "I just wasn't thinking" or "Boy, that really got me thinking—I came up with some great ideas"? We all feel this way at one time or another. Our ability to think well varies, depending on personal factors and the circumstances that are present at the time. This section addresses personal and situational factors that influence thinking.

Personal Factors Influencing Thinking

In addition to learning styles, personality, birth order, culture, up-bringing, and male versus female differences as described earlier, think about how the following personal factors influence your thinking.

Fair-Mindedness and Moral Development. People who are fair-minded and have a mature level of moral development are more likely to think critically. It makes sense that those who are keenly aware of their own values, have a good sense of right and wrong, and approach situations with an attitude of "I must consider all viewpoints and make decisions in the key players' best interests," already are critical thinkers.

Effective Communication and Interpersonal Skills. You must be able to understand others, be understood by others, and gain others' trust to get the facts required for sound reasoning. Keep in mind that communication is more than talking and listening: Consider the messages sent by your behavior over time. For example, if you say that you're committed to giving good care, but consistently arrive late for work with excuses, the real message you send is quite different from your *words*. The following gives communication strategies to promote critical thinking.

COMMUNICATION STRATEGIES TO PROMOTE CRITICAL THINKING

1. **Work to understand what other people are trying to say before trying to get them to understand *you*.** Apply the *Platinum Rule* ("Treat others the way they want to be treated").[8] For example: Don't assume everyone likes "a caring hand" on their shoulder. If someone is formal and reserved, respect this.
2. **Point out that your intent is not to judge but to understand** (e.g., "I'm not here to judge. I just want to understand what's going on").
3. **Use strategies that help you see other points of view.**
   - Ask for clarification (e.g., "I don't mean to be difficult, but I still don't understand. Can you clarify further?" or "Help me understand what you're trying to do").
   - Use phrases like, "From your way of looking at it" or "From your perspective."
   - Paraphrase in your own words. (e.g., "It seems to me that you're saying... Is that correct?"

COMMUNICATION STRATEGIES TO PROMOTE CRITICAL THINKING—cont'd

4. **Listen empathetically** (with the intent of understanding the other person's way of looking at the situation). This is called imagining what it's like to "walk in someone else's shoes," and can be done by taking the following steps:
   a. Clear your mind of thoughts about how you view the situation or concerns about how you're going to respond.
   b. Focus on listening to the person's feelings and perceptions.
   c. Rephrase the feelings and perceptions as you understand them to be.
   d. Detach and come back to your own frame of reference.
5. **Apply strategies that help you get accurate and comprehensive information**.
   • Use open-ended questions (those requiring more than a one-word answer). For example, "How do you feel about leaving tomorrow?"
   • Avoid closed-ended questions (those requiring only a one-word answer). For example, "Are you ready to leave tomorrow?"
   • Use exploratory statements that lead the person to expand on certain issues. For example, "Tell me more about..."
   • Don't use leading questions (those that lead someone to a desired answer). For example, "You don't smoke, do you?"
   • Put body language into words. For example, "You looked a little sad..."
   • Use silence. Allow the person time to gather his thoughts.
   • Remember the value of using written communication (letters and diaries really help).
   • Record the information you gathered, and then look to see what's missing and check for inconsistencies.
   • Ask the person to keep a log or diary, or keep one yourself.
6. **Use strategies that help you get your point across**.
   • Make sure the time and place are appropriate.
   • Wait until the person is ready to listen.
   • When voicing an opinion, use phrases that convey that you're voicing an opinion, rather than dictating what is so (e.g., "From my way of looking at it... From my perspective...").
   • Ask the person to paraphrase what you've said (e.g., "I need to know you understand. Explain to me what I just said.")
7. **Demonstrate behaviors that send messages** like *I'm responsible, I can be trusted,* and *I want to do a good job.* For example, keep promises, be punctual, accept responsibility, and respect others' time.
8. **Apologize** when you've caused inconvenience, been careless, made a mistake, or offended someone.
9. **Respect others' territory;** ask permission (e.g., "May I listen to your chest?" rather than, "Sit up and let me listen to your chest.").

Age/Maturity. Most authors agree that age correlates with critical thinking ability: The older you get, the better a thinker you become. There are two logical reasons for this: (1) Moral development usually comes with maturity. (2) Most older people have had more opportunities to practice reasoning in various situations. Realize, however, that sometimes older nurses are rigid and set in their ways—in this case, age impedes critical thinking.

Dislikes, Prejudices, and Biases. These can be subtle but powerful factors that hinder critical thinking. If you don't recognize these factors—put them out on the table, so to speak—and overcome them, you're unlikely to think critically in situations where you have to function in spite of your dislikes, prejudices, and biases.

Emotional Intelligence. This is frequently called EQ (emotional quotient), which is as important as IQ (intelligence quotient). EQ is the ability to recognize emotions and make them work in positive ways. A high EQ enhances critical thinking because how you feel about something significantly impacts on how you think. Many of us aren't aware of deep, strong feelings. Clarifying emotions and giving them the attention they deserve helps us adjust our behavior and improve results. You must "name emotions to tame them" (Box 2-3).

Self-Confidence. For the most part, self-confidence aids thinking. If you aren't confident, you use much of your brain power worrying about failure, reducing the energy available for productive thinking. *Occasionally* self-confidence hinders critical thinking; some people become overly confident and believe they can't be wrong or have little to learn from others.

BOX 2-3	USING EMOTIONAL INTELLIGENCE TO PROMOTE CRITICAL THINKING

1. **Connect with emotions.** Put your feelings into words and, through dialogue, help others to do the same ("I feel... because..."). Never assume you know what someone else is feeling or expect others to know what you're feeling.
2. **Accept true feelings** for what they are. No one's to blame for what he feels.
3. **Learn mood management.** Recognize the importance of connecting with how emotions are affecting thinking. Learn to manage feelings like anger, anxiety, fear, and discouragement.
4. **Don't be too concerned with isolated events.** Patterns of behavior are what matter. Don't sweat the small stuff.
5. **Keep in mind that emotions are "catching."** If you're depressed, you may trigger depression in someone else. If you're enthusiastic, you may trigger enthusiasm.
6. **Do something to reduce stress.** Take time out, use humor, play a game, take a walk, learn to use yoga or guided imagery.

Recommended: Visit the Web page of Daniel Goleman, who is recognized internationally as a pioneer in EQ: www.daniel-goleman.info/blog.

Knowledge of Problem Solving, Decision Making, Nursing Process, and Research Principles. Because critical thinking is based on many of these same principles, familiarity with the methods enhances critical thinking.

Early Evaluation and Reflection. When you make it a habit to evaluate early—reflecting on your thinking and checking whether your information is accurate, complete, and up-to-date—you can make corrections early. You avoid making decisions based on outdated, inaccurate, or incomplete information. This is a combination of *thinking-in-action* and *reflective thinking*, as described on page 16.

Past Experience. Most authors view *experience as an enhancing factor*, since you remember best what you learn from experience. If, however, your past experience is a bad one, it may be an *inhibiting* factor. For example, if a mother had a bad experience breast-feeding her firstborn child, it may be difficult for her to think clearly about breast-feeding subsequent children.

Effective Writing Skills. When you learn how to make yourself clear in writing, you learn to apply critical thinking principles like identifying an organized approach, deciding what's relevant, and focusing on others' perspectives.

Effective Reading and Learning Skills. Because critical thinking often requires that you use resources independently, you must know how to read and learn well. Having effective reading skills doesn't mean knowing how to read rapidly. It means knowing how to read efficiently, identifying what's important, and drawing conclusions about what the material implies.

Situational Factors Influencing Thinking

Anxiety, Stress, and Fatigue. Anxiety and stress, often the first to drain your brain power, make concentration difficult. When you're fatigued, you're already operating on a "low battery." A low anxiety level, however, like being a little nervous about a test, can promote critical thinking by motivating you to prepare.

Awareness of Risks. Usually this is an enhancing factor. When you know the risks, you think more carefully (you "think before acting"). Sometimes awareness of the risks can increase anxiety to a level that impedes critical thinking. For example, most of us remember how hard it was to think critically when we gave our first injection.

Knowledge of Related Factors. The more you know about a situation, the better you'll be able to reason. For example, you might know about diabetes, but if you don't know *the person* you're going to teach about diabetes—the person's lifestyle, desires, and motivations—you'll be unlikely to design a plan that the person will follow.

Awareness of Resources. Awareness of resources is the key to thinking critically. You can't know it all, but it's your responsibility to determine where you can get reliable help.

Positive Reinforcement. Positive reinforcement promotes critical thinking by building confidence and focusing on what's being done *right*.

Negative "Talk." Having someone focus too much on what you're doing wrong—or worrying yourself too much about what you might do wrong—can impede thinking, as it drains your confidence and takes your attention away from what you need to do *right*.

Evaluative or Judgmental Styles. An evaluative or judgmental style impedes critical thinking. When you think someone is judging or evaluating you, you spend more brain power worrying about what the *other person* is thinking than what *you* are thinking.

Presence of Motivating Factors. When you have motivating factors (things that make you *want* to think critically), you feel enticed to get your brain "in gear." An example of a common motivating factor for critical thinking is knowing why you're asked to do something. Think how motivated you are to learn when someone says, "You must know this because it will be on the test."

Time Limitations. This can be an enhancing or impeding factor. Time limitations can be motivating factors—deadlines stimulate us to get things done. If there's too little time, however, you may make decisions more quickly than you'd like and come up with less than satisfactory answers. It's interesting to note that the courts give more leeway to decisions that were made in emergency situations than to those made with plenty of time for thinking.

Distractions. These impede critical thinking for obvious reasons—the more distractions, the more difficult it is to stay focused. For example, it's best to do your charting in a quiet place, where there are few interruptions and distractions.

Habits Creating Barriers to Critical Thinking

As humans, many of us have habits that create barriers to critical thinking. Think about the habits in the following box, then read on to learn more about how they impede thinking.

BARRIERS TO CRITICAL THINKING

❑ Self-Focusing	❑ Mine-Is-Better*	❑ Tunnel Vision
❑ Choosing-Only-One	❑ Face-Saving*	❑ Resistance to Change*
❑ Conformity*	❑ Stereotyping*	❑ Self-Deception*

*You can find more on these habits in Ruggerio, V. (2006). *The art of thinking: A guide to critical and creative thought* (8th ed.). New York: Longman.

Keep in mind that these habits are simply a result of human nature. Whether we realize it or not, we're all victims of these behaviors to some extent at one time or another.

Self-Focusing. Focusing on ourselves is a carry-over from primitive survival instincts. In the early days of man, humans had to be keenly centered on their own needs to survive. We still have this instinct. Critical thinking requires you to overcome this natural tendency and work to understand needs, perspectives, and challenges that are *different* from our own.

Mine-Is-Better. We tend to regard our ideas, values, religions, cultures, and points of view as being superior to others. To think critically, recognize when you are biased and have strong personal "pro" or "con" views that may influence your opinions.

Tunnel Vision. Tunnel vision is a universal problem. We see what we *expect* to see, often misinterpreting what's before us. A classic example of tunnel vision is when a psychiatric nurse fails to consider whether someone's confusion is related to a *medical problem,* and vice versa (a medical-surgical nurse fails to consider whether someone's confusion is related to a *psychiatric problem).*

Choosing-Only-One. When faced with more than one choice, we tend to choose only one. We forget to think about things like, Are there other, better choices? Can we do *both*? Do we have to do *either*? Beginners are most vulnerable to the *choosing-only-one* habit. They tend to blindly accept that if they've chosen at least one option, they've made a good decision. They also tend to make the assumption that there must be *one best way* to do something, rather than thinking that there probably are several good ways of getting things done and that each has advantages and disadvantages, depending on circumstances. You can overcome this tendency by remembering to ask, Must I choose only one? or Is this the only way? What approaches can we combine?

Face-Saving. We have a strong instinct to protect our image—we try to save face. Critical thinking requires us to learn and grow. As we learn and grow, we'll make mistakes or realize that our old ways of thinking or doing things can be improved. To be a critical thinker, we must be comfortable saying things like *I'm not sure, I was wrong,* or *I have to think about that.*

Resistance to Change. We all tend to resist change. Too often change is considered "guilty until proven innocent." Overcoming this barrier doesn't mean embracing every new change uncritically. It means being willing to suspend judgment long enough to make an informed decision on whether the change is worthwhile (see *Navigating and Facilitating Change* on page 199).

Conformity. Although some conformity—like following policies and procedures—is *good,* there's also harmful conformity. Harmful conformity is when we conform to group thinking just to avoid being viewed as "different." Conforming without thought stifles the ability to be creative and improve. An example of harmful conformity is following policies blindly, even if there are circumstances that clearly indicate that the policy doesn't apply in *this* particular situation.

Stereotyping. We stereotype when we make fixed and unbending overgeneralizations about others (e.g., *homeless people aren't very bright*). When our minds are fixed and unbending, we're unlikely to see what's really before us. By recognizing our tendency to stereotype, we can make a conscious effort to overcome this habit.

Self-Deception. This is the subconscious forgetting of things about ourselves we don't particularly feel good about. An example of this is experienced nurses who deceive themselves into believing they were never as shy, nervous, or insecure as the students they encounter today.

Habits Promoting Critical Thinking

As discussed in Chapter 1, developing habits that promote critical thinking is a constant "work in progress." For example, making the behaviors listed in the critical thinking indicators (CTIs) on page 10 into habits of performance requires ongoing self-reflection, self-correction, and practice.

Stephen Covey, author of *The 7 Habits of Highly Effective People*, stresses the need to develop the following habits to bring balance to your life and get the best long-term results*:

1. **Be Proactive.**® Choose to be responsible for your own life, anticipate responses, and act before things happen.
2. **Begin With the End in Mind.**® Develop goals and make your expectations explicit.
3. **Put First Things First.**® Decide what's important and stick to priorities moment by moment, day by day.
4. **Think Win-Win.**® Seek mutual benefit in all human interactions.
5. **Seek First to Understand, Then to Be Understood.**® Communicate effectively.
6. **Synergize.**® Recognize that the whole is greater than the sum of its parts: Collaborate, bringing diverse ideas and talents together to create new and better ideas.
7. **Sharpen the Saw;**® Look after yourself physically, emotionally, and spiritually. Covey explains sharpening the saw by telling a story about a man who is sawing a tree trunk for hours: The saw is dull, and the man is exhausted. Someone suggests that he might do better if he sharpens the saw. The man responds, "I don't have time" and continues to work ineffectively.

If you want to know where you stand in relationship to Covey's habits, you can take *The Self-Scoring Seven Habits Profile* at www.FranklinCovey.com.

---

*Habits are summarized from Covey, S. (1989). *The 7 habits of highly effective people*. New York: Simon & Schuster. All trademarks of Franklin Covey are used with permission. All rights reserved. www.FranklinCovey.com.

CRITICAL THINKING EXERCISES

Note: Exercises followed by asterisks (*) have example responses listed in the Response Key *beginning on page 249.*

1. Study *What's Your Thinking Style?* on page 29 and *Do You Know What to Do When Someone Turns Blue?* on page 30. In a group or in a personal journal, discuss the following:
   a. Your thinking style and main motive according to Myers-Briggs and Hartman's *Color Code*
   b. How your style and innate motives affect your ability to think clearly
   c. What personalities and thinking styles are difficult for you to work with…and how you can improve your ability to work with these styles
   d. How other factors such as birth order, culture, and upbringing affect how you think
   e. How you would feel about taking a personality test for your own personal knowledge versus taking one for use by your teachers at school or supervisors at work
2. Compare and contrast the *Golden Rule* and the *Platinum Rule.**
3. Emotive thinking is thinking that's driven by feelings: How does this relate to critical thinking?*
4. Write a paragraph explaining how intelligent use of emotions helps improve thinking.*
5. In a personal journal, write about the influence of feelings on your thinking. Are you ruled more by your heart than your head, or vice versa, and what difference does that make? Identify at least one thing you can do to improve your ability to have more balanced thinking (thinking that considers both "heart" and "head").
6. Respond to the following from the pre-chapter self-test:
   a. Explain the three main steps to improving thinking.*
   b. Describe how personality, learning style, upbringing, and culture affect critical thinking.*
   c. Explain why building trust and following a code of conduct promote critical thinking.*
   d. Discuss how human habits influence critical thinking.*

Outcome-Focused (Results-Oriented) Thinking

As addressed in Chapter 1, critical thinking is outcome-focused (results-oriented) thinking: You must give careful thought to exactly what *benefits* and *ultimate results* you expect to achieve. This section clarifies the relationship between goals and outcomes. It also explains why focusing on outcomes promotes better thinking.

Goal (Intent) Versus Outcome (Result)

The terms *goal*, *objective*, and *outcome* are often used interchangeably because these terms have similar meanings. There is, however, a significant difference among them.

- **Goal or objective:** Indicates **general intent**, what you *aim* to do. Example: My goal (or objective) is to teach Steve about diabetes.
- **Outcome:** Indicates specific, **measurable results**. Example: At discharge, Steve will be able to demonstrate insulin injection and explain how he will keep his blood sugar within normal range through diet, exercise, and medication.

Goals are often vague, and can be idealistic. Outcomes center on *clearly observable benefits and desired ultimate results*, forcing you to be realistic and think things through from the beginning. Use the following memory jog to help you remember these two terms.

$$G = G \qquad \text{(Goals / objectives = General intent)}$$
$$O = O \qquad \text{(Outcomes = Observable results)}$$

Clarifying Outcomes

To some people, outcome-focused thinking is just a buzzword that gets too much attention—it seems obvious that you need to focus on end results to reason well. But, consider the following scenario that shows how clarifying end results isn't always obvious.

Scenario
CLARIFYING OUTCOMES (END RESULTS): NOT ALWAYS EASY

A group gathers to discuss building a bridge in a rural town. Someone says, "Let's first be sure that we all agree on the end result." Several members consider this a dumb statement because the end result, obviously, is that the town will have a bridge. A bridge is a clear and observable outcome, right? How about if I tell you this is very limited thinking? The real end result you need to focus on is that *whoever wants to get across that bridge is able to do so*. To think critically, you have to pay attention to the end users—the people who will use the bridge. You must start by asking questions like, "Who will use this bridge?" "How much room will they need to get their vehicles across?" "When will there be the most traffic, and how much will that traffic weigh?" "Where is the best place for this bridge?" If these questions aren't raised in the beginning, it's likely that you'll end up with a costly, useless, inconvenient, or even dangerous bridge.

Remember the following two rules:

RULE

Determining outcomes requires you to stay centered on the *key people who will demonstrate that the desired end result has been achieved.* In the previous scenario, the key people are those who travel the bridge. In health care, it's patients, families, clients, and consumers.

RULE

Critical thinking requires you to ask two main questions: (1) What exactly are the major results you need? and (2) What are the problems, issues, or risks that must be addressed to get the results? (Sometimes the results you *need* may be in conflict with the results you *want.* For example, you may want things done your way. But if you allow people to do things their way, you may get better results.)

In later chapters, we'll go into detail about how to determine outcomes in nursing situations. For now, just remember that if you haven't given enough thought to exactly what *end results* you need, you aren't thinking critically.

Critical Thinking Strategies

This section first summarizes 10 questions key to critical thinking, and then it addresses the use of logic, intuition, and trial and error. It also points out the importance of using specific strategies such as mind mapping (concept mapping) and simulation.

10 Key Questions

There are 10 key questions you must ask to determine your approach to critical thinking in various situations. These are summarized on the inside back cover and addressed in detail in the following list.

1. **Exactly what major outcomes (observable beneficial results) do you expect to achieve?** Be as specific as possible. For example, compare the vague outcome in the first situation below, with the more specific outcome in the second situation.

Situation 1: Jody will be discharged home in 2 days.

Situation 2: Jody will be discharged home in 2 days in the care of her mother, who will be able to demonstrate sterile dressing change by then.

2. **Exactly what problems, issues, or risks must be managed to achieve the major outcomes?** Clearly identifying the problems, issues, and risks that may impede progress is 60% of the critical thinking challenge. Asking this question

helps you prioritize. You have only so much time—assign top priority to addressing problems, issues, or risks that may *impede progress* toward getting results. Using the previous example, Jody's mother tells you that she knows nothing about changing sterile dressings and also wants to know how she can improve her parenting skills. If time is short, give top priority to teaching her about dressing changes, and handle the issue of how to be a better parent by giving her information on reference materials and support groups.

3. **What are the circumstances (what is the context)?** The approach to critical thinking changes, depending on the circumstances (context). For example, imagine that you're in class and you're asked how to manage a patient in shock. You aren't sure, but you think you know, so it's appropriate for you to answer. If you're in the clinical setting, however, trying to manage shock based on uncertain knowledge may be dangerous.

4. **What knowledge and skills are required?** Having discipline-specific knowledge and skills is crucial to critical thinking. For example, how can you think critically about managing cardiac pain if you don't know the causes and common treatments of cardiac pain? If you don't know what knowledge and skills are required, you probably don't know enough to get involved—get help.

5. **How much room is there for error?** When there's less room for error, we must carefully assess the situation, examine all possible solutions, and make every effort to make prudent decisions. For example, which situation below has less room for error, and how might your approach to decision making change in each situation?
   Situation 1: You need to decide whether to give an over-the-counter antihistamine to someone who is usually in good health.
   Situation 2: You need to decide whether to give an over-the-counter antihistamine to someone with multiple health problems.
   Obviously, the first situation has more room for error because the person is less likely to have preexisting conditions or be taking medications that might be affected by an antihistamine. The second situation requires consultation with a physician. If there's plenty of room for error—if there are few or no risks involved—you can be more creative and spontaneous.

6. **How much time do you have?** If you have plenty of time, you can take time to think independently, using resources such as textbooks. If you don't have much time, you may need to refer the problem to an expert immediately to ensure timely attention. **Patient safety and welfare is #1.**

7. **What human and information resources can help?** Identifying resources (e.g., textbooks, computers, or experts) is essential to getting the information you need to think critically. For example, you don't have to know every side effect of every drug in a drug manual. Rather, know when you need detailed information. Look the drug up in a manual or check with a pharmacist to carefully review *all* side effects.

8. **Whose perspectives must be considered?** Critical thinking requires you to consider the perspectives of all of the key players involved; otherwise you

risk having conflicting purposes. For example, to develop an effective plan for home care, you must consider the perspectives of the patient, other household members, and other key members of the health care team. Imagine what could happen if you sent a grandmother home with many brightly colored medications and everyone forgot to consider the perspective of a toddler in the home!

9. **What's influencing thinking?** Recognizing influencing factors such as personal biases helps us identify vested interests, an important step in making fair-minded choices. For example, a nurse who is strongly against abortion may avoid working in gynecology, where women's decisions might make it difficult to give objective nursing care.

10. **What must be done to monitor, prevent, manage, or eliminate the problems, issues, and risks identified in question 2** (and who's accountable for doing it)? Getting results depends on your ability to identify specific strategies to prevent or manage problems that may be barriers to outcome achievement. For example, if you have a bedridden patient who has surgery, preventing skin breakdown is a problem that *must* be managed to ensure timely discharge. Deciding *who* is accountable for *what* is essential to ensure that nothing "falls through the cracks."

Using Logic, Intuition, and Trial and Error

Let's consider how logic, intuition, and trial and error relate to critical thinking.

Logic—sound reasoning that's based on facts (evidence)—is the foundation for critical thinking. It's the safest, most reliable approach. For all important decisions and opinions, make sure you can explain the logic of your thinking.

Intuition—a valuable part of thinking—is best described as "knowing something without evidence." For experts, intuitive hunches speed up problem solving, since they have a lot of experiential knowledge in their heads. For them, thinking-in-action is rapid, dynamic, and intuitive. Novices must rely more on step-by-step logic. Keep in mind that sometimes things are counterintuitive—the *opposite* of what your intuition tells you. In important situations, bring logic to your thinking and look for evidence to support gut feelings. If you have no evidence to support your intuition, consider the risks of acting on intuition alone. For example, can you remember a time when you did something on your computer based on intuition and ended up with a disaster? This can also happen with patients.

Trial and error—trying several solutions until you find one that works—is risky but sometimes necessary. Use trial and error only when there's plenty of room for mistakes, when the problem can be monitored closely, and when the solutions have been logically thought through. A common example of useful trial and error in nursing is determining the best way for a dressing to be applied to an awkward wound—it may take several tries before the best way is determined.

OTHER PERSPECTIVES

TRIAL AND ERROR: A CONTINUOUS PROCESS

"Trial and error, the process of trying one thing and observing the outcome, and then analyzing the result and making changes, is an important learning experience. It takes a great deal of critical thinking. Call it what you want, but individuals and health care organizations must continue to interact with the world, learn from experience, and then use that experience to improve the next attempt. However, remember that trial and error is a continuous cycle. You must constantly try to improve care quality based on what you learn from experience—it isn't just a one-time thing."

—*Workshop participant, a quality improvement expert*

Focusing on Details and Big Picture

Whether you see yourself a "details" person or a "big picture" person, it's important to realize that critical thinking requires focusing on *both* the big picture *and* the details—the whole and the parts. Think about the following examples.

- **Mr. Martinez has cardiac problems.** He tells you he has chest pain and is afraid he might die. Treating both "the whole" (Mr. Martinez's pain and anxiety) and "the parts" (Mr. Martinez's oxygen-deprived heart) is essential to resolving the chest pain (and, perhaps, to saving his life).

- **You're trying to teach Tonya how to care for her newborn.** You're well-prepared with lots of nice pamphlets. She seems interested, but she keeps yawning and doesn't seem to retain information very long. Finally you say, "Is there a better time we could do this?" She admits that she hasn't slept all night and is too tired. You come back later after Tonya's had a good rest. She learns readily. In this case, paying attention to an important detail (fatigue) helped you be a more effective teacher.

Remember to ask questions like *What's the big picture here? Am I considering both the parts and the whole?* and *Am I paying attention to key details?*

Drawing Maps, Diagrams, and Decision Trees

Drawing maps, diagrams, and decision trees promotes critical thinking by helping your brain grasp complex relationships. When you draw your own map, diagram, or decision tree, it helps you "personalize" information and "make it your own." When you study well-designed maps, diagrams, or decision trees, you learn more quickly, because your brain does better with "pictures" than words. For example, study the map of how the brain works on page 264 of *Mind Mapping (Concept Mapping): Getting in the "Right" State of Mind.* Get in touch with how your brain handles information by deciding whether the list of percentages, the graph, or the circle on the next page is easiest for you to grasp.

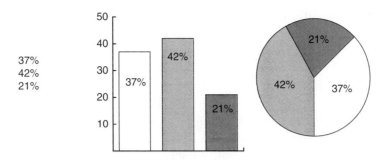

Simulated Learning Experiences

The use of simulated learning experiences provides a safe, powerful, way to learn problem-solving and other critical thinking skills (e.g., setting priorities, juggling technical skills together with other thinking). You retain best what you experience. With highly sophisticated training patient simulators, you can practice on your own or in groups, correcting mistakes in real time. Simulated learning is especially valuable for learning how to "think on your feet." In a safe environment, you can challenge your knowledge and skills to determine if you are ready for a variety of "what-if" scenarios.

Other Useful Strategies

The following summarizes other useful strategies for critical thinking.

Anticipate questions others might ask. These may include: What will my instructor want to know? What do patients need to know? What will the doctor want to know? This helps identify a wider scope of questions that have to be answered to gain relevant information.

Ask what-else questions. For example, change *Have we done everything?* to *What else do we need to do?* Asking what-else questions pushes you to look further and be more complete.

Think out loud or write your thoughts down. When you put your thinking into words, you make your ideas, reasons, and logic explicit, making it easier to assess and correct yourself.

Ask an expert to think out loud. When you ask experts to think out loud, you often learn organized systematic approaches to solving problems and making decisions.

Look for flaws in your thinking. Ask questions like *What's missing?* and *How could this be made better?* If you don't go looking for flaws, you'll be unlikely to find them. Once you've found them, you can make corrections early.

Ask someone else to look for flaws in your thinking. This offers a "fresh eye" for evaluation and may bring new ideas and perspectives.

Ask what-if questions. These may include: *What if the worst happens?* or *What if we try another way?* This helps you be proactive instead of reactive. It enhances your creativity and helps you put things in perspective.

Ask *why?* To fully understand something, you must know what it is and *why* it's so. There's a saying: "She who knows what and how is likely to get a good job. She who knows why is likely to be her boss."

Paraphrase in your own words. Paraphrasing helps you understand information using a familiar language (your own).

Compare and contrast. This forces you to look closely at the *parts* of something as well as the *whole*, helping you get more familiar with both things you're comparing. For example, if I ask you to compare two different kinds of apples, you have to look closely at both of them. As a result of comparing them, you are more likely to know and remember each type of apple better.

Organize and reorganize information. Organizing information helps you see certain patterns, but it may make you *miss* others. Reorganizing it helps you see some of those other patterns. For example, compare the following groups of numbers (each group contains the same numbers, organized differently). What patterns do you see and which is easier to remember?

36345643   34343 656   333 44 566

Develop good habits of inquiry. Develop habits that aid in the search for the truth, such as keeping an open mind, verifying information, and taking enough time.

Revisit information. When you give something "a second pass"—coming back and studying it afresh period of time—you'll probably view it differently.

Replace the phrases "I don't know" or "I'm not sure" with "I need to find out" or "Let's find out." This shows you have the confidence and ability to find answers and mobilizes you to locate resources.

Share your mistakes, and turn them into learning opportunities. We all make mistakes, and we need to work together to find ways to prevent them. Mistakes are often stepping-stones to maturity and new ideas. If you aren't making any mistakes, maybe you aren't trying enough new things.

CTIs for Knowledge and Intellectual Skills

Chapter 1 addressed CTIs that demonstrate attitudes of critical thinkers (page 10). This section addresses CTIs that demonstrate *knowledge* and *intellectual skills*.

Study the *knowledge* CTIs (listed on page 49) and the *intellectual skill* CTIs (page 50). Keep in mind that developing *intellectual skills* requires you to be able to *apply knowledge*. For example, *distinguishing normal from abnormal* (listed under *intellectual skills* CTIs) requires you to apply knowledge of *normal and abnormal function* (listed under *knowledge* CTIs).

CRITICAL THINKING INDICATORS (CTIs): Behaviors Demonstrating Knowledge

Note: Knowledge requirements vary, depending on context of specialty practice (e.g., pediatrics vs. adult health care).

Clarifies Nursing Knowledge

- ❏ Nursing and medical terminology
- ❏ Nursing vs. medical and other models, roles, and responsibilities
- ❏ Signs and symptoms of common problems and complications
- ❏ Related anatomy, physiology, pathophysiology, microbiology
- ❏ Normal and abnormal function (bio-psycho-social-cultural-spiritual)
- ❏ Factors that promote or inhibit normal function (bio-psycho-social-cultural-spiritual)
- ❏ Related pharmacology (actions, indications, contraindications, side effects, nursing implications)
- ❏ Reasons behind interventions and diagnostic studies
- ❏ Normal and abnormal growth and development
- ❏ Nursing process, nursing theories, and research principles
- ❏ Applicable standards, laws, practice acts
- ❏ Policies and procedures and the reasons behind them
- ❏ Ethical and legal principles
- ❏ Spiritual, social, and cultural concepts
- ❏ Where information resources can be found

Demonstrates

- ❏ Focused nursing assessment skills (e.g., breath sounds, IV assessment)
- ❏ Mathematical problem solving for drug calculations
- ❏ Related technical skills (e.g., n/g tube, IV pumps, or other equipment management)

Clarifies

- ❏ Personal values, beliefs, and needs
- ❏ How own thinking, personality, and learning style preferences may differ from others' preferences
- ❏ Level of commitment to organizational mission and values

Source: Alfaro-LeFevre, R. (2008). *Critical thinking indicators: Evidence-based version.* Available at www.AlfaroTeachSmart. com. No copying without permission.

To assess your abilities related to *knowledge* and *intellectual skills* CTIs, consider each indicator above and on the next page. Rate your ability to demonstrate the behavior using the following 0-10 scale:

0	=	This indicator is very difficult for me
10	=	This indicator is pretty much a habit for me, therefore easy

CRITICAL THINKING INDICATORS (CTIs): Behaviors Demonstrating Intellectual Skills and Competencies

Nursing Process and Decision-Making Skills

- ❑ Applies standards, principles, and ethical codes when planning, giving, and adapting care
- ❑ Assesses systematically and comprehensively; uses a nursing framework to identify nursing concerns, uses a body systems framework to identify medical concerns
- ❑ Detects bias; determines credibility of information sources
- ❑ Distinguishes normal from abnormal; identifies risks for abnormal
- ❑ Determines significance of data; distinguishes relevant from irrelevant; clusters relevant data together.
- ❑ Identifies assumptions and inconsistencies; checks accuracy and reliability; recognizes missing information; focuses assessment as indicated
- ❑ Concludes what's known and unknown; makes reasonable inferences (conclusions) and judgments—gives evidence to support them
- ❑ Identifies both problems and their underlying cause(s) and related factors; includes patient and family perspectives
- ❑ Considers multiple explanations and solutions
- ❑ Determines individualized outcomes; focuses on results
- ❑ Manages risks, predicts complications, promotes health, function, and well-being; anticipates consequences and implications—plans ahead accordingly
- ❑ Sets priorities and makes decisions in a timely way; includes key stakeholders in making decisions
- ❑ Weighs risks and benefits; individualizes interventions
- ❑ Reassesses to check responses and monitor results (outcomes)
- ❑ Prevents accidents, mistakes, and microbial transmission
- ❑ Communicates effectively orally and in writing
- ❑ Identifies ethical issues and takes appropriate action
- ❑ Identifies and uses technologic, information, and human resources; critiques and applies research

Additional Related Skills

- ❑ Establishes empowered partnerships with patients, families, peers, and co-workers
- ❑ Teaches patients, self, and others
- ❑ Addresses conflicts fairly; fosters positive interpersonal relationships
- ❑ Facilitates and navigates change
- ❑ Organizes and manages environment
- ❑ Manages stress, time, and energy
- ❑ Facilitates teamwork (focuses on common goals; helps and encourages others to contribute in their own way)
- ❑ Gives and takes feedback (constructive criticism)
- ❑ Delegates appropriately; leads, inspires, and motivates others
- ❑ Advocates for patient, family, community and staff needs
- ❑ Demonstrates systems thinking (shows awareness of the interrelationships existing within and across health care systems)

Source: Alfaro-LeFevre, R. (2008). *Critical thinking indicators: Evidence-based version.* Available at www.AlfaroTeachSmart. com. No copying without permission.

If you're a beginner, don't be concerned about low scores when comparing yourself to the CTIs. As you get practice in real situations, you soon find that these behaviors become habit. You also get to practice and develop these skills as you complete the exercises throughout the book. What's key is that you start to get a picture of *what behaviors promote critical thinking.*

Box 2-4 shows the results of two studies that aimed to describe critical thinking skills. This information was incorporated into the CTIs.

Developing Character and Acquiring Knowledge and Skills

Becoming a critical thinker requires a commitment to develop character and acquire the necessary knowledge and skills. Study the four circles of the 4-circle CT model on the inside front cover. Identify some things you can do to develop your abilities in each of the four circles.

BOX 2-4	RESULTS OF TWO STUDIES DESCRIBING CRITICAL THINKING SKILLS

Scheffer and Rubenfeld*

Analyzing: Separating or breaking down a whole into parts to discover their nature, function, and relationships

Applying standards: Judging according to established personal, professional, or social rules or criteria

Discriminating: Recognizing differences and similarities among things or situations and distinguishing carefully as to category or rank

Information seeking: Searching for evidence, facts, or knowledge by identifying relevant sources and gathering objective, subjective, historical, and current data from those sources

Logical reasoning: Drawing inferences or conclusions that are supported in or justified by evidence

Predicting: Envisioning a plan and its consequences

Transforming knowledge: Changing or converting the condition, nature, form, or function of concepts and contexts

The American Philosophical Association Delphi Report†

Interpretation: Categorizing, decoding sentences, clarifying meaning

Analysis: Examining ideas, identifying arguments, analyzing arguments

Evaluation: Assessing claims, assessing arguments

Inference: Querying evidence, conjecturing alternatives, drawing conclusions

Explanation: Stating results, justifying procedures, presenting arguments

Self-regulation: Self-examination, self-correction

---

*Scheffer, B., & Rubenfeld, M. (2000). A consensus statement on critical thinking in nursing. *Journal of Nursing Education,* 39(8), 353.

†Table I, Critical thinking: A statement of expert consensus for purposes of educational assessment and instruction. "The APA Delphi Report" (1990). ERIC Document Reproduction Service No. ED 315423.

Assessing and Evaluating Thinking

Let's end this chapter by addressing issues related to assessing and evaluating thinking. In context of trying to determine how someone thinks, the terms *assess* and *evaluate* are often used interchangeably, as I will use them.

Evaluating critical thinking is important for two reasons:
1. You need to know what you are doing well, and what you need to work on.
2. Your teachers and employers need to know whether you're competent to practice in the clinical setting.

Unlike *Star Trek's* Dr. Spock, we humans can't read minds—it's a challenge to assess what goes on in someone else's head. We are all unique, with various personalities and thinking styles. What may seem like good thinking to *you* may seem disorganized and inefficient to someone *else*. We're still in the early stages of learning how to evaluate thinking. To help you prepare for when you're involved in either giving an evaluation or getting one, this section briefly addresses issues related to evaluating thinking.

Basic Principles of Evaluating Thinking

It takes a knowledgeable, experienced, critical thinker who is familiar with key elements of assessing reasoning to evaluate thinking. Drawing valid conclusions about someone's thinking abilities requires focusing on *patterns over time*, not *single incidences.* For example, anyone can make a mistake, but if the person makes the same mistake several times, it's a problem.

Your ability to think critically and your clinical performance are closely linked.[5,6] For this reason, critical thinking abilities are often discussed during clinical performance evaluations. To evaluate thinking, consider the following, using "Pat" as an example.

1. **Outcomes (results): Does the person usually get respectable outcomes?** In the clinical setting, it means assessing Pat's patients directly to determine level of care (e.g., Are the patients safe, comfortable, and satisfied with care?). In class, evaluating outcomes means analyzing completed projects (e.g., papers and presentations).
2. **Process: How does the person usually go about achieving desired outcomes?** On the whole, does Pat usually seem organized and prepared? Be sure to consider style differences that may affect your opinion. For example, if Pat usually gets respectable results, but seems disorganized to you, consider whether this is simply a style difference between you and Pat.
3. **Behavior: What patterns of behavior and communication do you and others observe in the person *over time*?** Does Pat's usual behavior send messages of CTIs such as *being inquisitive, persistent, confident, and proactive*? If you're not sure about behavior, ask for an explanation of the *reasoning behind behavior.* For example: *Help me understand what you're trying to accomplish and why it's important… Tell me what's going on in your head… I realize I'm putting you on the*

spot, but take your time and try to explain your thinking… Can we talk later so that I can understand what was going on here? To understand whether opinions and decisions are based on evidence, ask questions like *What information do you have to support this?* To determine whether someone is proactive, ask questions like *What do you expect to happen when you do this? What if _____ happens… how will you handle it?* and *What alternatives have you thought about?*

Valid assessment of someone else's thinking depends on the level of trust in the relationship and having many ways of looking at the person's thinking. For example, consider all of the following: observation of behavior, dialogue, assessment of patient outcomes, and analysis of written information.

Self-Assessment

Assessing your own progress is one of the most important things you can do to improve. What are you doing well? What areas do you target for improvement? What knowledge, skills, and experiences do you need to gain? Be honest. Remember that "self-deception" is a human habit that impedes thinking. Share your target areas for improvement with your instructors, peers, and supervisors. We all learn together—ask for help when you need it. This shows that you are confident and committed to improvement and keeping patients safe.

Peer Review

Because of the importance of getting others' perspectives to increasing the likelihood of valid evaluations, many schools and hospitals have a *peer review* process to get input from peers and colleagues.[7] With peer review, nurses (or students) assess and judge the performance of their peers against predetermined standards (for example, against the behaviors listed in the CTIs on pages 10, 49, and 50). By comparing what they observe in their colleagues with the predetermined standards, they form opinions about performance. Keep in mind that personal style differences sometimes make understanding others' thinking difficult. For example, someone who's a logical, step-by-step thinker may have trouble understanding a creative person who's great at multitasking. Peer review is an important, yet complex, process. Ask your school or hospital for policies related to peer review, and think about how they affect your progress. Don't be afraid to discuss concerns about peer review with your teacher or supervisors. Resolving these concerns often improves the peer review process.

Using Tests and Instruments

It's common to use tests or instruments (tests that aim to determine where someone stands in relation to critical thinking abilities) to measure (evaluate) thinking. Realize, however, that the results of these sorts of tests don't *always* predict ability to think critically *in real situations*. They indicate your ability to think critically *in context of that particular test*. If you do poorly on tests or instruments, think about how you do in real situations. For example, I often do poorly on timed tests because I am indecisive and like to mull over the questions. This doesn't, however, translate to my being indecisive *when it matters:* I was charge nurse in the intensive care unit (ICU) and an evening supervisor of a 300-bed hospital—I can make timely decisions in the clinical setting as well as anyone. If you have a track record of success in handling real situations, it's quite likely that you're one of those creative, complex thinkers who struggles with test taking and needs lots of practice to develop test-taking skills (see pages 138-142).

There are many standard tests that aim to measure critical thinking. When these types of tests are used, the best-qualified people (e.g., educators) should carefully examine the test plan and, personally, answer at least some of the questions themselves. This gives first-hand knowledge of the test and prevents the use of tests that aren't really suited to the purpose they want. From a priority perspective with students, the best standard tests to use to assess critical thinking are those that have questions that are formatted in the same way as the national state board exams (e.g., NCLEX). This increases the likelihood of being able to predict students' ability to pass tests like NCLEX and gives opportunities to practice "thinking in the way the test requires you to." When students have lots of practice, they gain both the knowledge and test-taking skills needed to do well when "it really counts."

To summarize, evaluating thinking is a complex issue, and it is best accomplished using as many methods as possible—observing behavior, asking the person to share self-assessment, peer review, considering test scores, considering written work, and directly assessing patient care. Using several approaches to evaluating thinking increases the likelihood of drawing valid conclusions. Evaluation helps you validate your knowledge and identify areas that have to be developed. Ultimately, the aim of evaluation is to improve your ability to think critically and make a positive impact on your patients' lives.

CRITICAL MOMENTS

MOTIVATION: WHAT'S IN IT FOR THEM?
Connecting with others' motivations sparks critical thinking. When trying to motivate others, use the human instinct to self-focus to your advantage. Ask yourself questions like *What's in it for them?* and *How can I make this relevant and worth their while?*

CONSIDERING ALTERNATIVES GETS RESULTS
People aren't successful because they come up with one right answer or explanation. Rather, it's because they come up with many answers or explanations. To get results, make it a habit to look for alternative explanations, problems, or solutions.

NAME EMOTIONS TO TAME THEM
To deal constructively with negative emotions like fear and anger, take the time to "name them to tame them." Work to understand the main issues involved, so that you can do something about them.

FOCUSING ON OUTCOMES: IMAGINE THE FUTURE

Focusing on outcomes—the end products or results—helps you think things through and avoid "best-laid plans" problems. To think critically, put your mind in the future and imagine what things will be like on the day you reach the outcomes. For example, once I was on a program planning committee. One of our goals was to keep costs down, so we decided to skip refreshments for the afternoon break. This seemed to make sense until someone put her mind in the future and said, "I don't want to be the one who has to stand up in front of 100 tired, thirsty people and announce, 'There will be no refreshments during this break.'" When determining outcomes, "think future." Imagine consequences: Exactly how will things be on the day you reach your outcome?

OTHER PERSPECTIVES

HOW LITERATE ARE YOU?

"The illiterate of the twenty-first century will not be those who cannot read and write, but those who cannot learn, unlearn, and relearn."[10]

—*Alvin Toffler, author of* Future Shock

LOVE YOUR BRAIN

"I have a very weird brain. But I like it: it is the only one I have."[11]

—*Ruth Hansten, FACHE, PhD, MBA, BSN*

LEARNING PROVERB

"I hear: I forget. I see: I remember. I do: I understand."

—*Quoted by astronaut John Glenn*

SWEATING SILENCE

"As part of my teaching strategies class, I had to practice student questioning. One strategy required that I ask a question, and then remain silent until someone responded. My instructor videotaped the class and told me that under no circumstances was I to answer my own question. Soon into the class, I asked why a certain clinical activity was done. No one answered. I waited. Then waited some more. I began to sweat, but I refused to say anything. Finally, after what seemed like 2 full minutes of staring, someone spoke up. The next day I watched the video and timed the pause after my question. It was only 9 seconds! Like anyone in front of a group, teachers are uncomfortable with silence. We need to let learners think through the answer and take a chance by speaking up. Students' often let the teacher answer so they then find out the 'right' answer. This lesson can be applied to all important communication. Whether we're dealing with patients, colleagues, or peers, silence is often golden."[12]

—*Brent Thompson, DNSc, RN*

"CONFIDENT VULNERABILITY" PROMOTES CRITICAL THINKING
"Developing *confident vulnerability*—showing that you're vulnerable and open to suggestions, yet confident in who you are—promotes critical thinking. If you're too confident, you don't have an open mind to different opinions or new ideas. *Confident vulnerability* is the opposite of 'the God complex' often seen in 'prima donnas' who believe they can do no wrong."[13]
—*Cheryl Herndon, ARNP, MSN, CNM*

A 4-YEAR-OLD CRITICAL THINKER
Susie (age 4) was helping her mother pour medications. As she struggled with the lid of one of the bottles, her mother said, "You can't get that off because little children like you shouldn't get medications on their own." Susie responded, "How does it know it's me?"

CRITICAL THINKING EXERCISES

Note: Exercises followed by asterisks(*) have example responses listed in the Response Key *beginning on page 250.*

1. Using your own words and giving an example, explain the relationship between *goals* and *outcomes*.
2. Think of an outcome that you'd like to achieve 6 months from now; then apply the 10 critical thinking questions listed on the inside back cover to determine your approach to achieving your outcome.
3. How would your approach to critical thinking change in the following two situations?*
   a. You want your committee to brainstorm about ways to improve satisfaction with surgical experiences.
   b. You want your committee to develop a policy for managing postoperative complications.
4. a. **Arranging data into related patterns helps you remember better.** Rearrange the following numbers into a pattern that helps you remember them: 992887656780898
   b. **Using spatial intelligence (e.g., using shading, boxes, and circles to highlight information) enhances learning.** Draw a square around the numbers "765" above, then notice how they stand out from the rest of the numbers.
5. **Identifying assumptions—recognizing things you've taken for granted without realizing it—is essential for critical thinking.** Answer the following riddle, and then check the response on page 250 to see what assumptions you made. Think of a question you could have asked that may have helped you avoid making the assumptions.*

RIDDLE

Jack and Jill were found dead on the floor, surrounded by water and pieces of broken glass. There was no blood. What happened?

6. One of the first steps to developing CTIs is to observe *others'* behaviors. Compare the behavior of those around you with the behaviors listed in the CTIs on page 49. You can find a guide for observing behaviors in the clinical stetting at www.AlfaroTeachSmart.com (click on "Publications" and then "Handouts," and then choose "Clinical Cards" under "Faculty Handouts").
7. Decide where you stand in relation to being able to achieve the *Learning Outcomes* listed on page 25.

STRATEGIES FOR LEARNING PREFERENCES

Learning Preference	Strategies to Maximize Learning
Observers (visual learners) Learn best by watching. For example, you'd rather watch someone give an injection before reading the procedure.	Sit in the front of the room, so you stay focused on the teacher, not on what's going on around you. Visualize procedures in your mind's eye, rather than trying to follow individual steps. In skills labs, don't go first. Rather, watch your classmates and take a later turn. Ask for observational experiences. Take lots of notes and use a highlighter. Recopy your notes when you're studying. When learning new terms or concepts or trying to remember something, write them on "sticky notes" and put them where you'll see them frequently (e.g., the bathroom mirror, the computer). Preview chapters by scanning headings and illustrations.
Doers (kinesthetic learners) Learn best by moving, doing, experiencing, or experimenting. For example, you'd rather play with a syringe and inject a dummy before reading the procedure.	Start by doing (e.g., play with equipment before reading about how to use it) because it will make observing, reading, and listening more meaningful. Be sure you know the risks of doing without much knowledge and find ways to minimize them (e.g., if you're playing on the computer, make sure you can't inadvertently erase a file). When taking notes, use arrows to show relationships. Draw boxes and circles around key concepts; make diagrams. Pace up and down while reciting information to yourself; ride a bicycle while listening to an instructional tape. Make tapes with the information you're trying to learn and play them while exercising (e.g., riding a bike), or read while riding a stationary bike. Write key words in the air; use your fingers to help you remember (bend the forefinger as you memorize a concept, then bend the next for the next concept, and so on). Change positions frequently while studying; take frequent short breaks involving activity. Study in a rocking chair; play background music. Ask if you can do assignments in an active way (e.g., create a poster, be part of a discussion group).
Listeners (auditory learners) Learn best by hearing. For example, you learn best when you can listen without worrying about taking notes.	Whisper as you read, listening to your words (especially important when reading test questions). Listen in class without taking notes, focusing on understanding what the teacher says, and then copy someone else's notes. Tape classes and listen to the tapes 2 or 3 times before exams. Ask if you can give an oral report or hand in an audiotape for extra credit. Memorize by making up songs or rhymes. Study with a friend, so you talk about the information. Tape yourself as you read key information out loud, and then listen to the tapes.

KEY POINTS / SUMMARY

- Improving thinking requires three main steps: (1) Gain insight and self-awareness; (2) get agreement on what critical thinking entails; and (3) make the choice to practice and develop the attitudes, knowledge, and skills that promote critical thinking.
- Becoming aware of your personal style—how and why you think and learn the way you do—is a key starting point for improving thinking.
- Each of us is responsible for connecting with our preferred styles and learning strategies to help us think and learn effectively in our own way. Connecting with your own particular personality type helps you gain insight into how and why you think the way you do. Understanding personality types different from your own helps you realize how and why *others* think the way *they* do.
- Birth order, upbringing, and the culture you embrace greatly impacts on your thinking.
- Without trust in relationships, you're unlikely to have meaningful dialogue, as people are afraid to speak their minds. Page 27 shows a code of conduct that promotes critical thinking.
- Human habits can either promote or impede critical thinking (pages 38-40).
- Using simulated learning experiences, and drawing maps, diagrams, and decision trees are all useful strategies to develop critical thinking skills. Goals, because they focus on *intent,* may be vague and unrealistic. Identifying observable, measurable outcomes (results) helps you be realistic and focused from the start.
- Logic—sound reasoning based on evidence—provides the foundation for critical thinking. Using intuition as a guide to look for evidence is an effective strategy that should be nurtured. Before acting on intuition alone, however, be sure you consider the possible risks of harm.
- Trial and error (trying several solutions until you find one that works) is sometimes risky, but sometimes a necessary and useful approach to problem solving.
- CTIs that demonstrate the knowledge and intellectual skills required to think critically in nursing are listed on pages 48 and 49.
- The 4-circle CT model on the inside front cover shows how critical thinking requires a blend of critical thinking characteristics, knowledge, intellectual skills, interpersonal skills, and technical skills.
- The inside back cover summarize 10 questions to promote critical thinking in context of evidence-based practice.
- Evaluating someone else's thinking is a difficult task for both educators and employers. Studying results, processes (how those results were achieved), and patterns of behavior and communication helps you evaluate someone else's thinking. Self assessment and peer review are key strategies to evaluating thinking.

REFERENCES

1. Alessandra, T. The platinum rule. Retrieved April 5, 2007, from www.alessandra. com/abouttony/aboutpr.asp.
2. Thompson, P. (2000). Mentoring power. *Reflections on Nursing LEADERSHIP,* *26*(1), 7.
3. Ecklund, M. (January 2001). Reach out and touch: Making the mentoring connection. Retrieved April 5, 2007, from www.aacn.org.
4. Dracup, K., & Bryan-Brown, C. (2004). From novice to expert to mentor: Shaping the future. *American Journal of Critical Care, 4*(13), 448-450.
5. Di Vito-Thomas, P. A. (2002). *The Relationship between nursing student performance and critical thinking in clinical judgment.* Unpublished doctoral dissertation, University of Oklahoma, Norman, OK.
6. Di Vito-Thomas, P. A. (2005). Nursing student stories on learning to think like a nurse. *Nurse Educator, 30*(3), 133-136.
7. Elliott, N., & Higgins, A. (2005). Self and peer assessment—does it make a difference to student group work? *Nurse Education in Practice, 5*(1), 40-48.
8. Alessandra, T. op cit
9. Anthony, A. (February 2007). e-Mail communication.
10. Toffler, A. In S. Thorpe (2000), *How to think like Einstein* (p. 26). Naperville, IL: Sourcebooks.
11. Hansten, R. (March 2007). e-Mail communication.
12. Thompson, B. (January 2007). e-Mail communication.
13. Herndon, C. (February 2007). e-Mail communication.

Critical Thinking and Clinical Judgment in Nursing

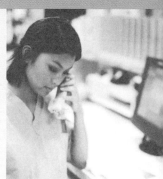

This chapter at a glance...

- Critical Thinking and Clinical Judgment
    - Applied Definition
    - What Other Nurses Say
- Mapping Critical Thinking
- Improving Practice and Performance
- Critical Thinking Indicators and 4-Circle Model
- Goals and Outcomes of Nursing
- Novice Versus Expert Thinking
- Paying Attention to Context
- Changes in Health Care Impacting on Thinking
    - Institute of Medicine (IOM) Competencies
    - Empowering Patients and Families: Nurses as Stewards for Safe Passage
    - *Diagnose and Treat* Versus *Predict, Prevent, Manage, and Promote*
    - Disease Management
- Outcome-Focused, Evidence-Based Care
    - Clinical, Functional, and Other Outcomes
    - Dynamic Relationship of Problems and Outcomes
- Critical Thinking Exercises
- A Changing Nursing Process
    - Proactive, Dynamic, and Outcome-Focused
    - Interplay of Intuition and Logic
    - Using Standard Tools to Improve Thinking
    - Computerized Decision-Support Tools
    - Is the Care Plan Dead?
- Expanding Roles Related to Diagnosis and Management
    - Growing Responsibilities
    - Legal Implications of Diagnosis
    - Defining Nursing Diagnosis
    - Accountability for Diagnosis

    Frequently Encountered Diagnoses and Complications
    Using Standard or Recognized Terms
- Developing Clinical Reasoning Skills
    Activating the Chain of Command
    Scope of Practice Decisions
    Decision Making and Nursing Standards and Guidelines
    Applying Delegation Principles
    How to Develop Effective Clinical Judgment
    10 Strategies for Developing Clinical Judgment
- Charting That Shows Critical Thinking
- Critical Thinking Exercises
- Key Points / Summary

PRECHAPTER SELF-TEST

Decide where you stand in relation to each of the following learning outcomes:

Learning Outcomes

After completing this chapter, you should be able to:

1. Describe what critical thinking and clinical judgment means to you.
2. Explain the relationship between managing your personal life and critical thinking.
3. Address the implications of the major goals and the outcomes of nursing.
4. Describe *outcome-focused, evidence-based care* using your own words.
5. Explain the difference between clinical, functional, and quality of life outcomes.
6. Compare and contrast the diagnose-and-treat (DT) and the predict, prevent, manage, promote (PPMP) approaches.
7. Clarify the purpose of each phase of the nursing process.
8. Discuss the interplay of intuition and logic in novice and expert thinking.
9. Explain the legal implications of the terms *diagnose* and *diagnosis.*
10. Clarify your responsibilities related to diagnosis and management of medical and nursing problems.
11. Explain the role of ethics codes, standards, guidelines, and laws in making decisions.
12. Explain how to use standard tools to promote critical thinking.

OTHER PERSPECTIVES

CARING NO SUBSTITUTE FOR COMPETENCE

"Compassion is no substitute for competence. In superficial, short-term medical encounters, a smiling face and a gentle hand impress. In the long term, it's competence that you begin to value. You find that kindness is a relatively abundant commodity. It's confidence, borne of knowing, that's too often in short supply. Does this mean I found myself disinterested in compassion? Not at all. But I also found it didn't count for much unless it was bundled with competence."[34]

—Daniel Beckman, parent of an acutely ill child

Caring and compassion—important parts of nursing—means *caring enough* to make the commitment to develop the knowledge and skills required to deal with the complex issues facing patients, families, nurses, and health care organizations today. This chapter and the next one are designed to help you meet the challenges of acquiring the knowledge, confidence, and thinking skills you need to succeed in six common nursing situations: reasoning in the clinical setting (clinical judgment), moral and ethical reasoning, evidence-based practice, teaching others, teaching ourselves, and test taking. To keep the length of the chapters manageable—to avoid asking you to do too much at one time—content is divided into two chapters. This chapter focuses on how to use critical thinking to promote clinical reasoning (clinical judgment). Chapter 4 focuses on moral and ethical reasoning, evidence-based practice, teaching others, teaching ourselves, and test taking.

Critical Thinking and Clinical Judgment

As explained in Chapter one, nurses use the terms *critical thinking, clinical judgment*, and *clinical reasoning* interchangeably. Remember, though, that *critical thinking* and *clinical reasoning* are a process. *Clinical judgment* is the *result* of the process (the conclusion you come to, the decision you make, or the opinion you form).

Applied Definition

To begin this section, let's review the applied definition from Chapter 1 on page 7.[1,2]

What Other Nurses Say

To get a deeper understanding of the importance of nurturing critical thinking, think about the following quotes:

"Fostering, supporting, and rewarding critical thinking is key to recruitment and retention. If we don't encourage nurses to grow in these skills, they become task-oriented and frustrated, thinking, 'I'll just do as I'm told, try not to think too much, and not say a word"[3]

—Donna D. Ignatavicius, MS, RN, ANEF

"Improving thinking allows nurses to develop the most important tool they have in their toolbox: themselves. This means being clear about who you are as a person, and how your attitudes, assumptions, frames of reference, and tendencies to stereotype affect problem solving—how your personal choices and behaviors affect communication and interpersonal relationships."[4]

—Ruth Hansten, RN, PhD, FACHE, MBA, BSN

"To think critically, you have to look at each situation objectively, uncovering layers to get a deep understanding of what's happening. This often requires playing devil's advocate and looking at the circumstances from all angles, even those you'd rather not consider."[5]

—Karen Elechko, RN, MSN

"Critical thinking involves using our brainpower to view and interact with the world and to act in a reflective, discerning way. It includes having intellectual curiosity, being creative, being open to new ideas, examining underlying assumptions, and considering alternative ways of thinking to make reasoned judgments that are sensitive to context."[6]

—Theresa M. Valiga, EdD, RN, FAAN

Mapping Critical Thinking

Mapping critical thinking gives you another perspective of what critical thinking and clinical judgment entail. Figure 3-1 (on the next page) maps the relationships among key features of critical thinking in nursing. All of the features in the map are integrated throughout this book. However, there are some points that are worth discussing here:

- **In the circle at the top:** Remember that critical thinking is an "umbrella term" that includes reasoning both *inside and outside* of the clinical setting. The arrow pointing from "outside the clinical setting" to "inside the clinical setting" indicates that who you are as a person, and how you manage things *outside* of the clinical setting, impacts on your ability to think critically *in* the clinical setting. For example, your knowledge and experience, your ability to learn, how you manage stress, and whether you maintain a healthy lifestyle impact on your ability to think critically in the clinical setting. *Nursing process* is placed at the

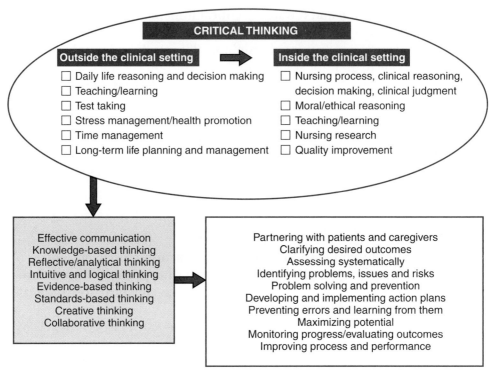

Figure 3-1 The above shows a map of key aspects of critical thinking in nursing. Notice that the circled section at the top illustrates that critical thinking is an "umbrella term" that includes reasoning both *inside and outside* of the clinical setting. The arrow pointing from "outside the clinical setting" to "inside the clinical setting" indicates that who you are as a person, and how you manage things *outside* of the clinical setting, impacts on your ability to think critically *in* the clinical setting. For example, your ability to learn in class, manage stress, and maintain a healthy lifestyle greatly affects your clinical performance. (Source: Copyright 2006. www.AlfaroTeachSmart.com. No copying without permission.)

top of the left column in the circle, because American Nurses Association (ANA) standards stress that the nursing process (1) underpins all care models and decisions nurses make, and (2) is the model that nurses use to promote critical thinking and provide competent care.[7] Deep understanding of nursing process *principles*, such as *assessing systematically* and *individualizing interventions*, gives you the foundation you need to learn other critical thinking models.

■ **In the box on the above left:** *Effective communication* is placed at the top to stress that all thinking depends on the quality of communication (verbal, non-verbal, written). *Knowledge-based, evidence-based,* and *standards-based thinking,* also in this box, point out that critical thinking requires the ability to apply (1) relevant theoretical and experiential knowledge, (2) the best available evidence, and (3) professional practice standards (e.g., ANA standards, ethics codes, and national and organizational standards). Evidence-based practice is discussed in depth in the next chapter.

■ **In the box on the right on page 66:** *Partnering with patients and families* and *clarifying outcomes* is at the top to stress the importance of getting patients involved *early in the care process.* From getting mutual agreement on desired outcomes to identifying care approaches, apply the saying, "Nothing about me, without me."* Keep patients involved in all decision-making. *Maximizing potential* stresses the need to use human, professional, community, and technological resources to promote independence and get the best results.

Box 3-1 summarizes conclusion drawn by Christine Tanner, a clinical judgment expert, after she reviewed almost 200 articles on clinical judgment.[8]

BOX 3-1	CRITICAL THINKING AND CLINICAL JUDGMENT: WHAT RESEARCH SUGGESTS*

After a review of almost 200 studies, author Christine Tanner came to the following conclusions:

1. Clinical judgments are more influenced by what nurses bring to the situation than by the objective data about the situation at hand.
2. Sound clinical judgment rests to some degree on knowing the patient and his or her typical pattern of responses, as well as an engagement with the patient and his or her concerns.
3. Clinical judgments are influenced by the context in which the situation occurs and the culture of the nursing care unit.
4. Nurses use a variety of reasoning patterns alone or in combination.
5. Reflection on practice is often triggered by a breakdown in clinical judgment and is critical for development of clinical reasoning.

*Tanner, C. (2006). Thinking like a nurse: A research-based model of clinical judgment in nursing. *Journal of Nursing Education, 45*(6), 204.

Improving Practice and Performance

To many nurses, critical thinking simply means good problem solving. Although problem-solving skills are required, you need a broader view of critical thinking to succeed in today's competitive health care setting. If you don't have a sincere desire to improve—to find ways to broaden your knowledge and skills and to make current practices more efficient and effective—you aren't thinking critically.

Another way to describe critical thinking is a commitment to look for the best way, based on the most current research and practice findings (e.g., the best way to manage pain in a specific person or for a specific health problem). The following diagram shows how critical thinking in nursing constantly strives to improve.

---

*The South African disability movement began the slogan "Nothing about me, without me" in the 1990s. Search for this slogan on Google and you will find multiple citations.

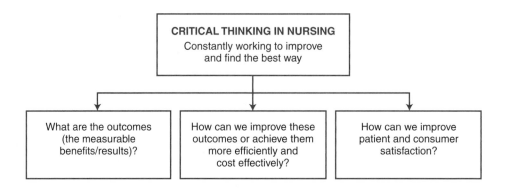

Critical Thinking Indicators and 4-Circle Model

Being familiar with critical thinking indicators (CTIs)—short descriptions of behaviors that demonstrate the knowledge, characteristics, and skills that promote critical thinking—is central to learning to think critically. If you're not familiar with CTIs, take time now to review pages 10, 48 and 49. Keep in mind that no one is perfect or able to demonstrate all of the behaviors perfectly all the time. If you use the CTIs as a checklist, you can compare yourself with the listed indicators and decide what you do well and what needs improving. You can also use the CTIs to jog your mind about what you have to do to think critically when you're in a new or complex situation. For example, when you know that a key CTI is *assessing systematically and comprehensively*, it's likely that one of your first thoughts will be, *I need to figure out a way to assess this patient in a systematic, comprehensive way.*

Also remember that the 4-circle CT model on the inside front cover also helps you assess and improve your ability to think critically. Asking questions like *What parts of the circles do I need to work on most?* helps you prioritize what knowledge and experience you need to gain.

Goals and Outcomes of Nursing

To better understand nursing's critical thinking, let's consider the question *What are the major goals and outcomes of nursing?*

Major Goals of Nursing

Broadly speaking, nurses aim to achieve the following goals in a humanistic way:
1.   To help people avoid illness and its complications
2.   To help people—whether they are ill, injured, disabled, or well—gain the best possible function, independence, and sense of well-being (in cases of terminal illness, the goal of dying peacefully is also appropriate)
3.   To continually improve care practices aimed at improving patient outcomes

Major Outcomes of Nursing

Broadly speaking, the following shows the major outcomes that demonstrate the benefits of nursing care.

After receiving individualized, evidence-based care, people will demonstrate improved physical, mental, and spiritual health, as evidenced by the following:

- Absence of (or reduction in) signs, symptoms, and risk factors of illness, disability, or injury
- Use of behaviors and strategies that evidence shows promote health, function, and quality of life
- Documentation of individualized, evidence-based, state-of-the-art care

What Are the Implications?

There are three main implications of the goals and outcomes of nursing:

1. Because the conclusions and decisions we as nurses make affect people's lives, our thinking must be guided by sound reasoning—precise, disciplined thinking that promotes accurate data collection that's as complete and in depth as the situation warrants.
2. Since our ultimate goal is for people to be able to manage their own health care to the best of their ability, we must stay focused on *patient perceptions, needs, desires, and capabilities.*
3. Because we're committed to achieving quality outcomes in a cost-effective, timely way, we must constantly seek to improve both our personal ability to give nursing care and the overall quality of health care delivery. We must continue to work to find answers to questions like *How can we achieve better outcomes? How can we improve satisfaction with our services? How can we contain costs, yet maintain high standards?* and *How can we ensure competent nursing practice?*

Novice Versus Expert Thinking

Consider the following scenario.

Case Scenario

A car hits a young man riding his bicycle in the park. Thrown 60 feet, he lies motionless. Within minutes, two park rangers arrive. They put on latex gloves and begin to assess his injuries. An ambulance pulls up and one ranger yells, "We'll need intubation equipment!" A woman, out for a walk, looks on from a distance. A second woman, riding a bicycle, comes upon the scene. Here's how the conversation goes:

First woman: This is terrible. I wish the ambulance had gotten here sooner.
Second woman: Oh?

First woman: Yes. He was thrown at least 50 feet. If the ambulance had arrived sooner, they could have done more. I can't believe these two rangers didn't start resuscitation right away. They waited for this ambulance ... they should have been breathing for him.

Second woman: These rangers look like they know what they're doing. They would have started resuscitation if he needed it. This young man has been thrown so far, I'm sure they're concerned about spinal cord injuries. If they tilt his head back to start respirations, they risk severing his spinal cord—they don't want to do that unless it's absolutely necessary.

The above is a true story. I was the second woman on the bicycle. As I talked more with the first woman, I learned she was a student nurse. She thanked me for pointing out something she hadn't thought about. After it was all over, I realized our conversation demonstrated a common difference between expert and novice thinking: The student nurse felt a need to *act* immediately. As an experienced nurse, I knew the importance of *assessing before acting*.

We're all novices at one time or another. We all know what it's like to be new at something and watch an experienced professional and wonder, *Will I ever know this much?* And almost always, with time and commitment, we soon find ourselves helping someone else who looks at us and thinks, *Will I ever know this much?*

To gain insight into the difference between novice and expert thinking, think about where you stand in relation to being a novice or expert by studying Benner's descriptions in Box 3-2.[9] Then study Table 3-1 (page 72), which shows the differences between novice and expert thinking.

If you're a novice, determine some things you can do to enhance your ability to think critically; if you're an expert, decide how you can help a novice.

Paying Attention to Context

Paying attention to context (circumstances) is a major part of critical thinking. What works in one situation may not work in another with different circumstances. For example, think about the difference between working in pediatrics versus working with adults. Growth and development issues and differences in anatomy and physiology affect many aspects of care. Always remember that critical thinking is contextual—thinking changes according to circumstances. Realize that you may be an expert nurse, but if the circumstances change and you're unfamiliar with giving care under those circumstances, you're like a novice. Don't be afraid to say, "I'm unfamiliar with dealing with these circumstances and need help."

BOX 3-2	PATRICIA BENNER: HOW NOVICES BECOME EXPERTS

Patricia Benner, who since 1984 has studied how nurses move from novice to expert, determined that nurses go through the following levels of knowledge and expertise acquisition.*

1. **Novices:** Beginners who lack experience in specific situations (e.g., a new graduate with no experience in nursing or an experienced psychiatric nurse who is beginning to work in obstetric nursing)
2. **Advanced beginners:** Those with marginally acceptable performance based on a foundation of experience with real situations (e.g., a nurse who is in the first year of employment or the first year of a new clinical specialty)
3. **Competent:** Those with 2 or 3 years of experience in similar situations (e.g., a nurse who has practiced emergency and intensive care nursing for 2 or 3 years)
4. **Proficient:** Those with broad experience that allows meaning to be understood in terms of the big picture rather than isolated observations (e.g., a nurse who is in charge of making patient assignments)
5. **Expert:** Those with extensive experiences that enable an intuitive grasp of situations and problems (e.g., an experienced nurse who serves as charge nurse, preceptor, or member of committee)

*Summarized from Benner, P. (2001). *From novice to expert.* Upper Saddle River, NJ: Prentice Hall. For more on Benner's work, go to www.bennerassociates.com.

Remember that patients are *individuals* who may have similar problems, but different attitudes and responses. Each person and each situation has its own "unique story." Look for differences in patient responses or changes in circumstances—for example cultural, physical, or emotional differences—and adjust care as needed. When you have a deep understanding of patients' individual circumstances, you can avoid making assumptions and tailor care to achieve the best outcomes.

Changes in Health Care Impacting on Thinking

Health care is changing more quickly than you can say the word *computer*. Pardon the word play, but computers are one of the main reasons for rapid change. From diagnostic technology to information management and decision support, computers are at the core of many changes in health care. This section describes major changes that affect how you think and work today.

Institute of Medicine (IOM) Competencies

The 2000s brought a "wake-up call" for health care consumers and providers. We experienced terrorism, hurricanes, and new diseases that damaged or threatened large populations on unprecedented scales. IOM studies revealed that because of reliance on outmoded systems, there were many safety and quality problems in health care.[10-13]

TABLE 3-1 NOVICE THINKING VERSUS EXPERT THINKING	
Novice Nurses	**Expert Nurses**
▪ Knowledge is organized as separate facts. Rely heavily on resources (e.g., texts, notes, preceptors). Lack knowledge gained from experience (e.g., listening to breath sounds).	▪ Knowledge is organized and structured, making recall of information easier. Have a lot of experiential knowledge (e.g., what abnormal breath sounds are like, what subtle changes look like).
▪ Focus so much on actions that they tend to forget to assess before acting	▪ Assess and think things through before acting
▪ Need clear-cut rules	▪ Know when to bend the rules
▪ Hampered by unawareness of resources	▪ Are aware of resources and how to use them
▪ Hindered by the brain-drains of anxiety and lack of self-confidence	▪ More self-confident, less anxious, and more focused
▪ Have limited knowledge of suspected problems; therefore, they question and collect data more superficially	▪ Have a better idea of suspected problems, allowing them to question more deeply and collect more relevant and in-depth data
▪ Rely on step-by-step procedures. Tend to focus more on procedures than on the patient response to the procedure	▪ Know when it's safe to skip steps or do two steps together. Are able to focus on both the parts (the procedures) and the whole (the patient response)
▪ Become uncomfortable if patient needs preclude performing procedures exactly as they were learned	▪ Comfortable with rethinking procedure if patient needs necessitate modification of the procedure
▪ Follow standards and policies by rote	▪ Analyze standards and policies, looking for ways to improve them
▪ Learn more readily when matched with a supportive, knowledgeable preceptor or mentor.	▪ Are challenged by novices' questions, clarifying their own thinking when teaching novices

The IOM came to the conclusion that poorly designed systems set staff up to fail—regardless of how hard they tried. The IOM cited four underlying reasons for inadequate care quality:[14]
1. The growing complexity of medical science and technology
2. Increase in the number of people with chronic conditions
3. Poorly organized health care delivery systems
4. Lack of the application of informatics (the use of computers to manage information)

IOM core competencies require that all health care providers be able to do the following:[15]

- **Provide patient-centered care:** Stay focused on patients' desires, keeping them informed and encouraging them to be involved in all aspects of their care, including taking responsibility for health promotion.
- **Work in interdisciplinary teams:** Collaborate with others to use the best resources, apply broad knowledge, and promote continuity of care.
- **Employ evidence-based practice:** Integrate the best up-to-date knowledge from research and clinical experts to achieve the best outcomes.
- **Apply quality improvement methods:** Identify risks for safety, develop ways to prevent errors, learn from near-misses, and address issues to improve care.
- **Use informatics:** Find ways to use computers to improve communication, manage knowledge, reduce errors, and support decision making.

If the above sounds familiar to you, it's probably because we've already addressed many of these issues. Content related to IOM competencies is integrated throughout this book. For example, patient-centered care is stressed throughout, as is the use of practice guidelines and evidence-based practice. Quality improvement is addressed in the next chapter. Chapter 6 addresses *transforming a group into a team, accessing and using information, preventing and dealing with mistakes constructively*, and other skills you need to achieve the IOM competencies.

Empowering Patients and Families: Nurses as Stewards for Safe Passage

All too often, economic reality requires that we work to give better care with fewer resources. To achieve respectable outcomes, empowering patients and encouraging them to take control of their own health care is key. Much like a ship's steward—who has the job of protecting passengers on a journey—your job as a nurse is to protect patients and help them navigate safe passage through the health care system. As a steward, you hold *patients' lives* in your hands, but *they* should be "at the helm," directing where they want to go. Involve patients and families early in health care decisions, respecting individual needs and desires and asking questions like *What are the main things you want to accomplish?* Help patients understand the concept of *stewardship* by saying things like "I'm here to take care of you, but even more importantly, I'm here to make sure you know how to take care of yourself when I'm not here" "Let me know when you have questions or concerns" and "Stay involved in your care—you know yourself best and will do better if you let us know what you need and want."

If you're unfamiliar with the process of establishing empowered partnerships, review *Developing Empowered Partnerships* on pages 209-212. Also review the *Speak Up* initiatives on the next page (Box 3-3) and *Patients' Rights* on page 266.

BOX 3-3	IMPROVE SAFETY: URGE YOUR PATIENTS TO SPEAK UP*

The Joint Commission* *encourages patients to become active, involved, and informed participants on the health care team. The following simple steps are based on research that shows that patients who take part in decisions about their health care are more likely to have better outcomes.*

Speak up if you have questions or concerns, and if you don't understand, ask again. It's your body, and you have a right to know.

Pay attention to the care you are receiving. Make sure you're getting the right treatments and medications by the right health care professionals. Don't assume anything.

Educate yourself about your diagnosis, the medical tests you are undergoing, and your treatment plan.

Ask a trusted family member or friend to be your advocate.

Know your medications and why you take them. Medication errors are the most common health care errors.

Use a hospital, clinic, surgery center, or other type of health care organization that has undergone a rigorous on-site evaluation against established state-of-the-art quality and safety standards, such as that provided by The Joint Commission.

Participate in all decisions about your treatment. You are the center of the health care team.

*Courtesy of The Joint Commission.

Diagnose and Treat Versus Predict, Prevent, Manage and Promote

Care has shifted from a *diagnose and treat* (DT) approach, which implies that we wait for evidence of problems to start treatment, to a predictive model: *predict, prevent, manage, and promote* (PPMP). Today, we *predict, prevent, and manage* problems. We also *promote* health and manage risks, even when no problems exist.

PPMP is considered a *predictive model* because it focuses on predicting and managing risk factors *before* problems arise. PPMP is based on evidence. Thanks to research and clinical expert consensus, we can often predict which people are at risk for certain problems and, if needed, begin an aggressive prevention plan. Sometimes prevention requires "treatment." For example:

- We may give an influenza vaccine to someone with chronic lung disease and also vaccinate the entire family. This reduces the person's risk of contracting the virus from a family member.
- In hip surgery, we routinely "treat to prevent" the potential complication of embolus (clot) formation. We apply pulsating antiemboli stockings and give anticoagulants to high-risk patients.
- For those with significant exposure to the human immunodeficiency virus (HIV), treatment begins immediately, before there's evidence of the virus in the blood.

- Sometimes taking an antihistamine for a week *before* allergy season can reduce allergic response.

This PPMP model is based on the fact that evidence shows that recovery often follows an orderly pattern along predictable milestones. We know the importance of recognizing early when patients aren't progressing as expected and intervening to get the patient back on track to recovery. When patients fail to achieve specific milestones (for example, if someone who has had open-heart surgery isn't off the ventilator and breathing on his own within 24 hours of surgery), a multidisciplinary team evaluates whether there are problems to be solved or resources needed to get him back on track. (The milestone in this case is that the person should be able to breathe on his own within 24 hours of surgery.)

The PPMP approach requires you to do the following:

1. **Predict common problems and complications, and then develop a plan to monitor and prevent them.** For example, if you're caring for someone with a heart problem, you
   - Monitor closely for early signs and symptoms that indicate increasing problems (e.g., monitor for irregular pulse, fluid in the lungs, ankle swelling, and chest discomfort).
   - Initiate actions to prevent complications (e.g., prevent fluid overload by ensuring that intake doesn't significantly exceed urine output).
   - Be prepared to manage complications in case they can't be prevented (e.g., have a fully prepared emergency cart near by and know to use it).

2. **Focus on risk management:** Screen for the presence of risk factors and identify ways to eliminate or manage them. For example, you make a home visit to assess an infant. As part of the assessment, you look for risks to the infant's safety (check where the baby sleeps, and find out if the parents are aware of possible infant hazards). If you identify risks to the baby's safety, you're responsible for making a plan to correct the situation. Failing to make a plan may be considered negligence.

3. **Encourage behaviors that promote health, optimum function, independence, and sense of well-being.** For example, explain to asthmatics that a walking or exercise program is key to promoting optimum lung function, encourage all smokers to stop, and stress the need for colonoscopy after age 50. For more information on health screening and risk management, see *Healthy People 2010 Initiatives* at www.healthypeople.gov.

4. **Use technology to reduce errors and improve accuracy and efficiency.** Ask, *What technologic advances are there to monitor this patient and prevent complications?* For example, for many years, to ensure proper placement of central venous lines, we did chest x-rays to be sure the lines were in the vein, not in the chest cavity. Now we know the importance of preventing this complication by using live ultrasound *as the line is inserted.*

The PPMP approach—predict, prevent, manage, promote—helps prevent problems, prioritize care, improve satisfaction, and contain costs.

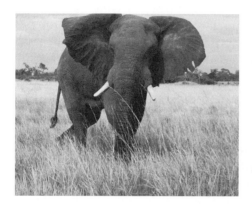

What does this elephant have to do with clinical judgment and the PPMP model?
When we were in Africa, this elephant gave us a menacing look. As our guide quickly put the jeep into reverse, someone asked, "Do they teach you how to use that gun on the dashboard?" The guide replied, "Yes. But, even more important—they teach us how not to get in the position that we need it." Be proactive. Predict and prevent complications. Be ready to manage unavoidable complications. Promote health through patient teaching. (Copyright 2007 by R. Alfaro-LeFevre.)

Disease Management

Disease management—a model of care that focuses on keeping people with chronic diseases such as *diabetes, kidney disease,* and *hypertension* healthy—is an important part of the PPMP approach. We now know the importance of *managing,* not just *treating,* chronic conditions. For example, with asthma, you don't just keep *treating* asthma attacks. You *manage* the asthma by monitoring asthmatics when healthy—fine-tuning medications and inhalers to keep them symptom-free. Make sure they receive the most current, effective drugs with the fewest side effects.

Today, many people live with chronic diseases and disabilities. We can expect nursing roles related to disease management to grow. For example, telehealth nurses—nurses whose job it is to help patients to manage chronic conditions such as kidney disease, diabetes, and congestive heart failure—improve the quality of people's lives and save millions of dollars. They reduce the number of emergency room visits and hospitalizations by helping patients manage their diseases at home, calling them periodically and asking very specific questions. For example, with diabetics, they may ask questions like "How are you feeling?" "What are your blood-sugars running?" "How much insulin are you taking?" and "How's it going with your exercise plan?" They also say things like "I see that you're overdue for a doctor's appointment. Can I make an appointment with the doctor for you?"

The following scenario shows the importance of risk management and being proactive when promoting health and managing health problems.

Living in Florida, where we have heat, humidity, and a lot of elderly people, I learned the need to manage—rather than treat—dehydration first-hand. Many health care providers tell people to walk to gain strength. Sometimes these instructions backfire, and people faint in the heat. If you or someone else is going to exercise, improve performance by pacing yourself and ensuring adequate hydration. On hot days, predict the risk of salt depletion and dehydration from sweating. Prevent dehydration and heat stroke by teaching about risk factors (obesity, alcohol or caffeine use, use of some medications like diuretics, and being very young or old put you at risk). Teach signs of heatstroke (weakness, nausea, vomiting, chills, confusion, disorientation, hallucinations). Stress the importance of improving ability to exercise by drinking water *before* exercising (so you start out well hydrated), wearing loose-fitting clothes, avoiding the hotter parts of the day, avoiding tea or caffeine (they act as diuretics), and replacing fluids during exercise (water is usually best). If you suspect heatstroke, manage it by cooling down the person immediately (place the person near an air conditioner or place damp towels all over the body, especially to the temples and wrists, where blood vessels are near the skin). If the person can tolerate liquids, offer cool drinks. If the person becomes dazed, confused, or has stopped sweating, head for the emergency room because dehydration is severe, requiring immediate medical management.

Box 3-4 on the next page summarizes additional health care trends that impact on critical thinking.

Outcome-Focused, Evidence-Based Care

From professional and economic perspectives, the care we give must be driven by the best available evidence. As we move toward highly-refined evidence-based approaches, to think critically, you must be able to answer questions like the following:
1. Exactly what does the patient, family, client, or group want to achieve?
2. Have the best-qualified professionals considered the above and decided what, realistically—based on circumstances—can be achieved?
3. Have the key stakeholders—those with a vested interest in how care is given and what results are achieved (e.g., patient, family, care providers)—agreed to the expected outcomes of care (specifically, *what benefits will be observed* in the patient, client, or group after care is given)?
4. Have the key stakeholders agreed to deadlines for achieving these outcomes?
5. What is the evidence that indicates that the outcomes are likely to be achieved in this particular situation?

BOX 3-4   TRENDS INFLUENCING THINKING

- **Nurses at all levels take on more responsibilities.** Licensed practical nurses, registered nurses, and advanced-practice nurses (APNs) continue to gain responsibilities, making it important to know how to decide whether you are qualified to accept new responsibilities.
- **Nurses must prove value.** Regulatory requirements stress that nurses must prove their value to consumers and their employers, showing how they impact on outcomes.
- **Use of simulation,** with highly sophisticated patient simulators, becomes a valuable source of learning. Allowing for "hands-on" practice and "learning by doing," simulators provide a safe alternative to practicing on real patients.
- **HIPAA (Health Insurance Portability and Accountability Act) rules**—required by law—guard private personal health information. The "portability" part of the act minimizes barriers to health coverage for workers, including (a) limits on excluding coverage for preexisting conditions, (b) special enrollment rights for those who lose other health coverage, and (c) elimination of medical underwriting in group health plans. For up-to-date information and frequently asked questions on HIPAA rules, go to www.hhs.gov/ocr/hipaa and www.healthprivacy.org/.
- **Creating a healthy workplace and focusing on patient safety** continue to be major goals.
- **Informatics**—the use of computers to keep health records, manage data, provide decision support, and improve outcomes—continues to grow.
- **More documentation is done directly on the computer**, often at patients' bedsides. Computerized patient records (CPR) —sometimes called computerized medical records (CMR) or online patient records (OLPR)—are common.
- **New threats emerge.** Resistant bacteria bring new infections that are difficult to treat. International travel brings threats of pandemics (epidemics over a wide geographic area and affecting a large part of the population). Terrorism, including bioterrorism, is a constant threat, requiring new levels of preparedness and responsiveness.
- **Concerns for care of the elderly and the chronically ill grow.** Many people are living longer with illnesses and disabilities, which creates new challenges to keep them as healthy and independent as possible. When these people get sick, the problems are often complex because of preexisting problems.
- **New diagnostic and treatment modalities change approaches to care.** Researchers study new diagnostic and treatment modalities such as vaccine use and genetic manipulation to prevent illness and find new cures.
- **Ethical dilemmas grow.** Ethical issues (e.g., end-of-life care, assisted suicide, fertility issues, cloning, and stem-cell research) require in-depth thinking that's clearly grounded in ethical principles (see Chapter 4).
- **Technology moves into homes.** Nurses must be able to give "high tech" care in homes, and must have excellent assessment and interpersonal skills. Being flexible, resourceful, and practical in the home is key.
- **Case management**—the use of collaborative approaches to ensure that the best available resources are used to reach outcomes efficiently—promotes quality. This approach is grounded in prevention and early intervention. Today all nurses are expected to be "case managers," closely monitoring progress toward outcomes to detect variances in care (a variance in care is when a patient isn't progressing toward outcomes in the expected time frame—for example, if someone has surgery and is expected to get out of bed on the first day after surgery but is unable to do so, it's considered a variance in care, which requires further evaluation).

BOX 3-4	TRENDS INFLUENCING THINKING—cont'd

- *Healthy People 2010* **initiatives** guide organizations, businesses and communities to come together to achieve two major goals: (1) to help people of all ages improve life expectancy and quality of life, and (2) to eliminate health disparities among different segments of the population. (See www.healthypeople.gov/.)
- **Affordable health insurance and access to health care are major concerns. Services are driven by consumer and community needs.** Health care organizations aiming to succeed recognize that they must compete for their clients' dollars—services must be driven by consumer needs and customer satisfaction. Insurance companies and consumers alike want to know that they are getting the best value for their dollar.
- **Managed care.** Managed care organizations aim to furnish services within a group of providers who network to provide quality care in the most cost-effective manner. Nurses, physicians, and therapists working in a managed care environment are challenged to deliver the highest standard of care with the best value.
- **Wellness centers and holistic and alternative therapies gain respect.** More people recognize the value of keeping people healthy and triggering the body's natural healing powers through holistic and alternative therapies (for example, diet, exercise, acupuncture, and stress reduction through meditation and aroma therapy).
- **Cultural and spiritual needs matter.** Nursing and health care standards make it necessary that we identify and address cultural and spiritual needs.

Evidence-based care is discussed in depth in the next chapter (pages 123-127). For now, just remember that it's important to evaluate the strength of the evidence that supports your plan of care.

Clinical, Functional, and Other Outcomes

Because determining *overall* quality of care requires you to examine outcomes from *several* perspectives, this section explains clinical, functional, and other outcomes. Study the following types of outcomes listed in the context of a surgical repair of a fractured hip. Think about the importance of considering all the outcomes to determine overall care quality.

- **Clinical outcomes:** To what degree are the patient's health problems resolved? For example, is the hip healed?
- **Functional outcomes:** To what degree is the patient able to function independently, physically, cognitively, and socially? For example, is the person able to do required daily activities without help? Are there problems with cognitive function?
- **Symptom severity and quality of life outcomes:** To what degree is the patient free of symptoms and able to do desired, as well as required, activities? For example, is there any hip pain, and is the person able to meet physical work requirements and do favorite activities?
- **Risk reduction outcomes:** To what degree is the patient able to demonstrate ways to reduce health risks? For example, is he able to explain ways of improving

safety, such as using a cane when fatigued? Does he keep his home free from hazards that may cause falls?

- **Protective factor outcomes:** To what degree does the patient's environment protect him from deteriorating health? For example, when bedridden, are bedrails up as needed and skin care protocols followed?
- **Therapeutic alliance outcomes:** To what degree does the patient express a positive relationship between himself and health care professionals? For example, when asked, does he state that he feels free to ask questions?
- **Satisfaction outcomes:** To what degree do the patient and family express satisfaction with care given? For example, when asked, do they state that they had competent, efficient treatment? Were services convenient?
- **Use of services outcomes:** To what degree were appropriate nursing services used? For example, was a case manager used, if needed?

    Remember the following rule.

RULE

Outcome-focused thinking means not just "fixing the problems;" it means fixing the problems in ways that you get the best results, from a cost, time, and patient satisfaction perspective.

In formal care plans and important situations, outcomes must be stated in very specific ways, as addressed in Chapter 5 (pages 184-187). At the bedside talking with patients, you can be more general. Begin patient care by asking questions like *What are the most important things you want to accomplish today?*

Dynamic Relationship of Problems and Outcomes

There's a close, dynamic relationship between problems and outcomes. For example, you have a certain problem, and your desired outcome is that you *don't have that problem*. Sometimes you will find yourself focusing on *problems* and sometimes on *outcomes*, depending on the situation. Think about the following examples:

- You're familiar with a patient and the desired outcomes. Things aren't going well, so you say to the patient, "Things aren't going well today. I need to understand the problems you're experiencing."
- You're working with a patient with multiple problems. Knowing the overall outcomes of care (like when and where the patient will be discharged) helps you decide which problems *must* be addressed and by *when*.
- You're working with a patient on a respirator and your desired outcome is that the patient has *adequate ventilation*. You see that the patient seems to be

struggling for air. You check the tubing and see a lot of water from condensation. You empty the water. If the patient is still struggling, you continue to look for other problems that might be interfering with the desired outcome of *adequate ventilation*. For example, you assess breath sounds and help the patient to get in a position to cough and clear mucus. You continue looking for problems until you reach your desired outcome.

- You're working with a group with many complex issues. Instead of getting bogged down in the problems, you say: "It's going to take us forever if we stay mired in long-standing, complicated issues. Let's focus on *results*, rather than *problems*. Let's decide together the major things we want to achieve and then get agreement on what we need to do to achieve them."

You'll get practice in identifying relationships between problems and outcomes in Chapter 5. For now, just remember that with critical thinking, you shift back and forth between focusing on outcomes and focusing on problems, issues, and risks.

CRITICAL THINKING EXERCISES

Note: Exercises followed by asterisks (*) have example responses listed in the Response Key *beginning on page 251.*

1. Get a piece of paper and make two columns. On the left, list the key points of the applied critical thinking definition on page 7. On the right, write your own interpretation of what each key point implies about what you need to do to think critically in nursing.
2. Write two or three paragraphs describing where you stand in relation to the description in *Novice Thinking Compared with Expert Thinking* (Table 3-1, page 72) and *Moving from Novice to Expert* (Box 3-2, page 71).
3. Study Box 3-3 on page 74 (*Speak Up*), then decide how you would handle a drug addict who insists that he or she must have more medication.*
4. Decide what's "wrong with the picture" in the following scenario.

Mr. Duncan, an elderly diabetic, is seen at home every other day by a nurse, who checks a healing incision. Mr. Duncan has been looking for an assistive device that he can attach to the toilet to help him get up and down. When he asks the visiting nurse if she knows where she can find such a device, the nurse replies, "I'm sorry. I know what you mean, but I don't know where you get them."

Scenario
WHAT'S WRONG WITH THIS PICTURE?

---

5. Write two to four paragraphs explaining the relationships in the map on page 66.*

6. a.   Using your own words and giving examples, or drawing a map, explain how you use a PPMP approach to health care delivery.*

   b.   In a group, or with some friends, share personal stories about people who are living with chronic diseases and disabilities. Keep the person's names private. Think about how the PPMP model applies to keeping them healthy. Share their struggles and successes and the factors that help or hinder their ability to stay as healthy as possible.

7. Critical thinking is guided by laws and standards. Find out more about your state practice act. Read and discuss the following article by Nancy Brent: *Protect yourself: Know your nurse practice act* (www.nurse.com/ce/syllabus.html?CCID=2813).

8. Decide where you stand in relationship to being able to achieve the following learning outcomes, lifted from prechapter self test on page 63.

   a.   Describe what critical thinking and clinical judgment means to you in relation to the descriptions in this chapter.*

   b.   Explain the relationship between managing your personal life and critical thinking.*

   c.   Address the implications of the major goals and outcomes of nursing.*

   d.   Describe *outcome-focused, evidence-based care* using your own words.*

   e.   Explain the difference between clinical, functional, and quality of life outcomes.*

   f.   Compare and contrast the *DT* and the *PPMP* approaches.*

A Changing Nursing Process

As evidence-based approaches continue to evolve, you can expect that the nursing process won't be the *only* model you will learn to promote critical thinking. Learning several models improves your ability to think critically for two reasons: (1) Each model brings new insights, and (2) some models work better in one context than another. Understanding nursing process *principles* is the key to learning new models; once you have a good foundation in nursing process, you readily grasp how to use other models. For this reason, and because you need to know the nursing process to pass NCLEX and other certification tests, this section addresses how to use the nursing process in dynamic ways.

Take a few moments to study the next few pages, which summarize the phases of the nursing process when used as tool for critical thinking. Keep in mind that it's important to remember the *purpose* of each phase, and that the phases are interrelated. What happens in one phase affects the others.

NURSING PROCESS SUMMARY: A CRITICAL THINKING TOOL

Assessment
Collect and record data to provide the information needed to:
- Predict, prevent, detect, manage, and resolve problems, issues, and risks.
- Clarify expected outcomes—observable desired results and benefits—of care.
- Identify individualized interventions to achieve outcomes, promote health, and attain optimum function and independence

Diagnosis / Outcome Identification
Analyze data to (1) clarify realistic expected outcomes (benefits of care), and (2) identify the problems, risks, or issues that must be managed to achieve the outcomes. *Diagnosis* and *outcome identification* often happen almost simultaneously (a "chicken or egg" situation) with thinking going back and forth between questions like *What are the major problems, issues, and risks? What does the patient want to achieve? What, realistically, must be achieved?* During this phase, in addition to clarifying outcomes, you:
- Identify signs and symptoms that may indicate the need for referral to a more qualified professional (report these immediately).
- Rule in and rule out suspected problems.
- Decide what problems, issues, and risks must be managed in order to achieve the outcomes.
- Identify risk factors that must be managed.
- Determine the patient's resources, strengths, and use of healthy behaviors.
- Recognize health states that are satisfactory but could be improved.
- **Reflect on thinking** to determine whether **(1)** Patient participation in the process has been at an optimum level; **(2)** data are accurate and complete; **(3)** assumptions have been identified, and thinking tailored to individual patient and circumstances; **(4)** conclusions are based on facts (evidence), rather than guesswork; and **(5)** alternate conclusions, ideas, and solutions were considered. **(Reflecting on thinking applies to all the phases, but is placed here because it requires analysis, which is the focus of this phase.)**

Planning
Ensure that there's a comprehensive, recorded, outcome-focused plan that's tailored to the individual patient and circumstances. The plan should be designed to do the following:
- Specify short-term and long-term outcomes.
- Monitor and manage *priority* problems, issues, and risks.
- Promote optimum comfort, function, independence, and health.
- Coordinate care and include patients as partners in decision making and care.
- Achieve the desired outcomes safely, efficiently, and cost-effectively.
- Include teaching to help patients make informed decisions and become independent.
- Provide a record that can be used to monitor progress and communicate care.

Implementation
Put the plan into action:
- Assess the patient to determine whether interventions are still appropriate and patient is ready
- Prioritize, delegate, and coordinate care as indicated, including patients as partners in decision making and care
- Prepare the environment and equipment for safety, comfort, and convenience
- Perform interventions, then reassess to determine initial responses

NURSING PROCESS SUMMARY: A CRITICAL THINKING TOOL—cont'd

❑ Make immediate changes as needed—update the recorded plan if required
❑ Chart as needed to monitor progress and communicate care

Evaluation
Carefully determine outcome achievement and how the process can be improved:
❑ Assess patient status to determine whether expected outcomes have been met and what factors promoted or inhibited the success of the plan.
❑ Plan for ongoing assessment, improvement, and patient independence.
❑ Discharge the patient, or modify the plan as indicated.

Proactive, Dynamic, and Outcome-Focused

Today we stress that the nursing process must be proactive and focused on outcomes, risk management, and health promotion—as well as dealing with problems.

In the clinical setting, the nursing process is dynamic, unlike how it's described in books or classrooms. If you jump around in books or classrooms trying to explain how things happen in real life, you confuse people—you have to present content in a logical, step-by-step way.

In real life, the nursing process is fluid and changing. You apply principles of nursing process, but move back and forth within various phases. Think about the following scenario showing the thinking that's likely to go on in a nurse's head as he applies the nursing process at the bedside.

Scenario
DYNAMIC THINKING AT THE BEDSIDE

Bob, a medical-surgical nurse, walks into a patient's room. A picture flashes in his mind—his brain assesses the room in an instant. The picture he sees is that of bed linens in disarray, trash on the floor, and someone who is restless and has a distressed look. Bob's mind jumps to phase 2 (diagnosis), thinking, *there's a problem here*. Automatically, he goes back to basics—phase 1 (assessment)— and assesses closely to find out exactly what's going on. He may start thinking, "Something bad is happening here and I need to get help," or he may simply intervene with a lot of little things, which resolves the *overall problem*. Either way, he is so busy *doing* that he's unaware that his brain is assessing, correlating, and forming opinions, as he goes along.

In the above scenario, Bob is experienced and comfortable in his role. If Bob were a novice, his thinking would be slower—hampered by lack of experience and lack of confidence. He would see a picture of the room, but he'd probably miss key details. He may also lose brainpower from dealing with his doubts about his own capabilities.

Remember the following rule:

Experts use the nursing process in dynamic ways because they quickly assess situations and correlate information in their heads. They know what steps can be safely skipped, combined, or delayed. They also know when situations warrant a rigorous, comprehensive, step-by-step approach. If you're inexperienced, you need to follow the steps more rigidly, carefully reflecting on each step. You take risks when you skip or delay steps.

Students need to learn nursing process principles in a step-by-step way, completing detailed maps and papers. These assignments promote development of clinical reasoning skills by teaching the skills of "thinking out loud," explaining reasoning, identifying relationships, and applying *principles*.

Interplay of Intuition and Logic

Much has been written about the role of intuition in nursing.[16-19] This section addresses the question: What roles do *both* intuition (knowing without evidence) and logic (rational thinking that's based on evidence) play in clinical judgment?

Most agree that intuition—an important part of thinking—is often seen in experts, as a result of years of experience and in-depth knowledge of patients. However, there's a concern that encouraging the use of intuition sends the message that it's okay to act on gut feelings without evidence, which is *risky*. To clarify the use of intuition and logic in clinical judgment, it's important to answer two questions:

1. Is the rapid thinking that goes on in experts' heads simply the use of intuition—what many describe as "knowing in your gut"?
2. If you can't explain your thinking, does it mean that you're thinking intuitively?

To the outsider, many experts' actions seem to be based on intuition alone. But, as in the example of Bob's thinking in the scenario on page 84, this rapid thinking is usually the result of "thinking in pictures"—like watching a video—and using intuition and logic *together*. In experts' minds, there's a dynamic interplay between intuition and logic. Experts make leaps in thinking with intuitive hunches, then almost at the same time draw on logic and past experience to make well-reasoned conclusions.

Experts who juggle several priorities at once often have trouble explaining their thinking at the very moment it's happening. But, if it's really important—for example, if decisions are later challenged in court—they can readily reconstruct the logic of their thinking (and if they can't, they're in trouble). Remember the following rule:

> **RULE**
>
> **Intuitive thinking is fostered by two things:** (1) In-depth knowledge and experience related to the clinical situations at hand, and (2) deep understanding of the patient's normal patterns, circumstances, needs, and desires.

Clinical judgment requires using your whole brain—both the intuitive-right and logical-left sides. Use intuitive hunches as guides to search for evidence. Use logic to formulate and double-check your thinking, ensuring that your conclusions are based on the best available facts. In important situations, be careful about acting on intuition alone. Ask questions like *Does this make logical sense? How do I know I'm right? Could this situation actually be counter-intuitive?* and *What could go wrong if I act on intuition alone?*

Ready, Fire, Aim

Ready, fire, aim—instead of *ready, aim, fire*— is a phrase that describes the risks of working in today's fast-paced world.[20] Critical thinking means not jumping to conclusions or acting on impulse. Time constraints today sometimes push you to make diagnoses before you have all the data. If you're not *sure* of the diagnosis or problem, however, it's best to say something like "there seems to be some issue with (whatever), but we don't know enough yet to completely understand what's going on." Remember that ANA standards support this approach by saying that nurses deal with "diagnoses or *issues*."[21] *Issues* are problems that are still muddy and not clearly defined.

What about Creativity?

Every so often, I'm asked whether the use of creativity is acceptable in clinical judgment. This question surprised me at first. I wondered, Why not? Then nurses gave me two examples of dangerous or problematic creativity. The first example was of a nurse who was going to administer blood, but found that the blood warmer was broken. She used a "creative" (and dangerous) approach: she heated the blood in the microwave. The other example is that of nurses who continually reinvent the wheel, creating new approaches that aren't really better, or coming up with ideas that aren't practical or user-friendly. Creativity has an important place in clinical nursing. Be sure to use *principle-centered* creativity and be sure that your ideas are useful to the end users. Learn ways to facilitate brainstorming both individually and in a group (e.g., try the *DEAD ON!!* game on page 267). Don't be happy with the status quo. Think outside the box. Ask questions like *Are there new evidence-based approaches we should be using? Is there something creative we can do? How can technology help? What human resources might be willing to give their time?* and *How can we involve patients and families to get better results?*

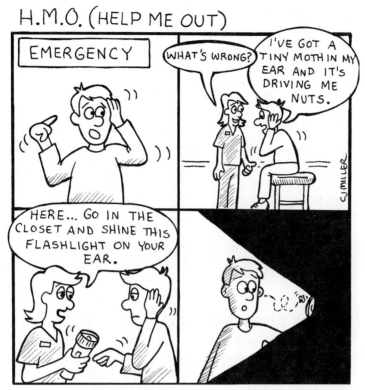

Using principle-centered creativity.

Using Standard Tools to Improve Thinking

Using standard tools to improve thinking is now a part of everyday practice. Clinical pathways, practice guidelines, and treatment protocols—tools that are used as guides to standardize care, improve quality, and ensure effective use of resources—are commonplace. Algorithms—tools that describe an ordered sequence of steps to take under specific circumstances—are also common. (See an example of a critical pathway on pages 268-271 and an example of an algorithm for clinical decision making on page 90.)

Using structured tools to guide and record phases of nursing process promotes critical thinking for several reasons:

1. We can't rely on memory, since our brains are prone to error. Completing computerized or printed tools—for example, assessment tools like the ones on pages 157 and 272-275—helps you avoid omission errors and be focused, systematic, and comprehensive.
2. Using structured tools frees your brain to focus on other important aspects of care. For example, you can really listen to patients when you're not wracking your brain trying to be sure you remember all the things you need to assess.

3. When you use a standard tool, two things happen: (1) Because you use the tool over and over again in various situations, your brain "creates a mental file" of what's most important (e.g., what to assess *first*). (2) The recorded tool gives you and the rest of the team a document you can reflect on to look for omissions, patterns, and relationships.

    Remember the following rule.

RULE

There are three things to remember about using standard tools: (1) Recording data *in a standard way* reduces omission errors and promotes safety, consistency, and efficiency. (2) Tools must be designed for specific purposes—one size doesn't fit all. (3) Tools do not *think* for you. *You* are accountable for making judgments such as what information needs to be reported immediately, what problems are indicated by the data you recorded, and what problems must be dealt with first.

Collecting Versus Analyzing Data

Virtually all facilities have tools to guide data collection. However, *collecting and recording information* is not the same as *analyzing* it. After you *record* data, you have to do a lot of *analysis* to clarify priority problems and risks.

Patients don't often have just *one* problem. They usually have several problems that contribute to one another, requiring you to decide which problems must be dealt with *first*. (See *Setting Priorities* on pages 180-184.)

Computerized Decision-Support Tools

Computerized decision-support tools are becoming an important part of nursing care. For example, you enter into a computer that a patient is diabetic, and the computer prompts you to decide whether diabetic teaching or a nutritionist referral must be made. You learn from computerized decision-support tools, and they help reduce errors. But don't depend on the computer to think for you. You're the *human*. You're the one who has the most up-to-date knowledge of the patient and can decide whether what the computer suggests is appropriate in each particular situation.

RULE

Computers can jog memory and guide decision making, but they don't transform decision making. You are accountable for ensuring that you have the most up-to-date information, for applying critical thinking, and for considering the context (big picture) to make ultimate decisions.

Is the Care Plan Dead?

As we continue to use critical pathways and standard plans, some nurses have begun to wonder, *"Is the care plan dead?"* The answer is that the care plan is alive and well—it's just changed. Standards in virtually all health care organizations—from hospitals to nursing homes—mandate that patients have an individualized plan of care that demonstrates that specific needs and problems are being addressed.

You may not find the care plan all in one place. Rather, parts of the plan may be addressed in different places of the chart (e.g., the nursing assessment may be in one place, routine interventions may be covered in critical paths or protocols and an individual plan covered in another, and so on). To be able to determine whether the plan of care is sufficiently documented, you must be familiar with nursing process and care planning principles. Whether you're developing a plan yourself or using standard plans, use the memory-jog **EASE** to remember the major care plan components.

MAJOR CARE PLAN COMPONENTS

Expected outcomes
Actual/potential problems that must be addressed to reach overall outcomes
Specific interventions designed to achieve the outcomes
Evaluation statements (progress notes)

Expanding Roles Related to Diagnosis and Management

Another change in the nursing process is that nurses have greater accountability for various aspects of diagnosis and care management. We have moved from *"nurses diagnose and treat only nursing diagnoses* to *nurses diagnose and manage various issues and problems, depending on their knowledge, expertise, and qualifications.* For example, advanced-practice nurses (APNs) may diagnose or manage problems that used to be managed only by physicians (e.g., they manage stable hypertension and common infections).

So then, how do you know when you're accountable for diagnosing and managng a problem? This question is especially difficult for beginners. Study the clinical decision-making map on the next page (Figure 3-2), which is central to helping you answer questions related to accountability. Then go on to read the following section, which gives specifics on growing nursing responsibilities.

Growing Responsibilities

Nursing responsibilities for all aspects of care continue to grow, requiring nurses to have strong diagnosis, management, and interpersonal skills, as noted in the following quotes.

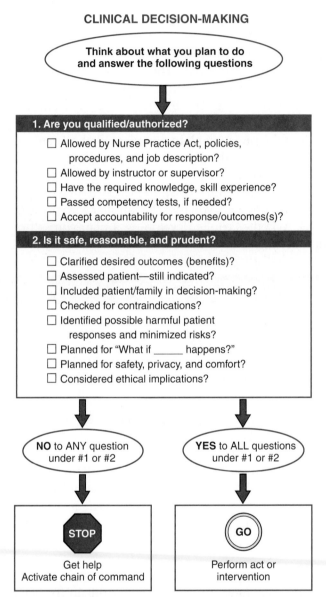

Figure 3-2 Clinical decision making. (Copyright 2006 by R. Alfaro-LeFevre. www.AlfaroTeachSmart.com. No copying without permission.)

"As you know, your doctor's job is to diagnose your medical problem and prescribe the necessary treatment. My job, as your nurse, is to monitor your body's response to treatment, help prevent complications before they begin, keep you as comfortable as possible, and help you adjust to the outcomes of your medical problems"

—Phyllis G. Cooper, MN, RN[22]

"The public needs to know that nurses—regular, ordinary bedside nurses, not just nurse practitioners or advanced practice nurses—are constantly participating in the act of medical diagnosis, prescription, and treatment and thus make a real difference in medical outcomes. Nurses can help the public understand that nursing is a package of medical, technical, caring, nursing know-how—that nurses save lives, prevent suffering, and save money. If nurses wear not only their hearts, but also their brains on their sleeves, perhaps the public ... will finally understand what nurses know and do."[23]

—Journalist Susan Gordon

The following BLOG also gives insight into the complexity of nursing today.

ICU BLOG

Last night I took care of a man who was hypoxic and needed oxygen via mask. Most people tolerate masks fine, but there are a few that just can't handle having something on their face. He was one of those few. Even though the nasal prongs were doing the trick, the pulmonologist wanted us to use a mask because "he will probably take a turn for the worse eventually." (Side rant: This is the same pulmonologist who, upon walking onto the unit, said, "Geena, when you have a critically ill patient, wouldn't it be at the forefront of your mind to have the chart available?" I replied, "Dr. B, the very fact that I have a critically ill patient who is hypoxemic and trying to climb out of bed actually explains why I don't have the faintest idea where the chart is.") Anyway, owing to other circumstances, I didn't immediately connect that the patient became severely agitated when we applied the oxygen mask. I had to give him an antipsychotic shot and spent as much time as I could at his bedside to avoid having to restrain his arms (which I correctly assumed would make him worse and wouldn't work anyway...when another nurse watching him for me went ahead and restrained him, he just bent over and put his face to his hand to take the mask off). I tried to chat with him about other things to help take his mind off the bothersome mask, and he finally stopped struggling against the restraints and lay back on the pillow. After a few moments, he looked at me and asked, "How long have you been working here?"

"Three years," I replied. "Before that, did you get your bachelor's, or your master's...?" Before I could answer him, he finished, *"IN TORTURE???"*

I'm sure it's not good nursing etiquette, but I laughed quite hard at that—which made him laugh. I eventually decided that the amount of energy he was exerting to remove the mask far outweighed the benefits of it, so I switched him to the nasal prongs again. After a few minutes of low oxygen saturation (O_2 sats) readings, he calmed down considerably and actually drifted off to sleep. His O_2 sats came up perfectly, and the rest of the night was fabulous.

Adapted with permission from www.codeblog.com.

Legal Implications of Diagnosis

As nursing responsibilities continue to grow, remember the following rule.

RULE
_____

> **The terms *diagnose* and *diagnosis* have legal implications**. They imply
> that there's a specific problem that requires management *by a qualified
> professional*. If you make a diagnosis, it means that you accept account-
> ability for accurately naming and managing it. If you treat a problem or
> allow a problem to persist without ensuring that the *definitive diagnosis
> —the most specific, correct diagnosis—has been made*, you may cause
> harm and be accused of malpractice. For example, if you deal with the
> problem of *chronic constipation* without determining whether the con-
> stipation has been evaluated by a physician, you may be missing a
> *major symptom* of *colon or ovarian cancer*.

Because of the importance of keeping patients safe and remembering the legal
implications associated with diagnosis, this section addresses definitions of nursing
diagnosis, the use of standard terms, and your roles and responsibilities related to
medical and nursing diagnosis.

Defining Nursing Diagnosis

The definition of *nursing diagnosis* continues to evolve, as nurses take on increased
accountability for preventing and managing health problems. The following
is the definition of nursing diagnosis developed by North American Nursing
Diagnosis Association-International (NANDA-I):

> **Nursing diagnosis:** *A clinical judgment about an individual, family, or commu-
> nity response to actual or potential health problems and life processes. Nursing di-
> agnoses provide the basis for selection of nursing interventions to achieve outcomes
> for which the nurse is accountable.*[24]

   This definition stresses that nurses are accountable for identifying issues related
to *how health problems influence each unique person's ability to function independently as
a bio-psychosocial human being.* This definition is an important one, since it is similar
to the definitions addressed in most nurse state practice acts. But, as acknowledged
by NANDA-I, this definition is limited (nurses do more than focus on *responses*).[25]
This definition is likely to evolve. For example, a broader definition of nursing diagnosis is "any problem that a nurse is accountable for managing, based on individual state practice acts, qualifications, and policies and procedures."
   In the clinical setting—as the ANA's *Nursing Scope and Standards of Performance
and Standards of Clinical Practice* states—nurses have accountability for *various problems and issues.*[26] Diagnosis and accountability is a complex issue—read on to
clarify your responsibilities in relation to diagnosis and management.

Accountability for Diagnosis

As a nurse, you have accountability for *both* human responses and medical problems. For example, suppose that you're caring for Mrs. Hernandez, who has a cardiac problem. Her *response* to the cardiac problem is *Activity Intolerance.* You must assess the status of the *cardiac problem* before you can determine how to deal with the *Activity Intolerance* (her response). If her vital signs are *unstable,* you're accountable for notifying the physician or APN, before dealing with the *Activity Intolerance.* If her vital signs *are* stable, you must ensure that the cardiac problem is being managed effectively by a qualified professional and that you follow the medical treatment plan for activity, before you design a plan to promote activity tolerance.

You're accountable for detecting signs and symptoms of problems that are within your expertise to manage independently. For example, all nurses are accountable for managing *Risk for Impaired Skin Integrity.*

With common medical diagnoses and complications, you're accountable for certain aspects of care management. For example, as a nurse, you *aren't* qualified to diagnose and manage a medical diagnosis such as *pneumonia* independently. But, you *are* accountable for the following:

1. **Detecting and reporting signs and symptoms that may suggest a medical diagnosis or complication** (e.g., you must notify the physician if a patient has fever, productive cough, fatigue, and malaise—all symptoms of *pneumonia*)
2. **Preventing common complications by recognizing when your patient is at risk, and monitoring closely and performing preventative nursing interventions** (e.g., elderly postoperative patients are at risk for *pneumonia*—a key priority is to monitor respiratory and hydration status and help them cough and breathe deeply)
3. **Ensuring that medical problems are monitored and treated according to the physician's treatment plan** (e.g., with *pneumonia,* you monitor lung sounds, oxygen administration, IV management, and vital signs)
4. **Diagnosing and managing *human responses to pneumonia*** (e.g., humans often respond to having pneumonia by experiencing fatigue, lack of appetite, dehydration, and difficulty clearing mucus)
5. **Diagnosing problems with independence** (e.g., if the person with pneumonia lives alone, he is likely to need assistance with shopping and preparing meals)
6. **Monitoring treatment and medication regimens for adverse reactions and individualizing the regimens within prescribed parameters**: Nurses are intimately involved in ensuring that overall regimens are as safe, effective, cost-effective, and convenient as possible, considering the age, culture, religion, roles, occupation, and lifestyles of those involved (e.g., with *pneumonia,* ask whether prescribed antibiotics are the best available, considering cost, convenience, and results).

Remember the following rule:

> **RULE**
>
> **Nurses play a key role in preventing complications related to medication and treatment regimens.** Use TACIT to remember the key things you must monitor when caring for patients on various treatment and medication regimens.
> Therapeutic effect (Is there a therapeutic effect?)
> Allergic or Adverse reactions (Are there allergic or adverse reaction signs?)
> Contraindications (Are there contraindications to giving this drug?)
> Interactions? (Are there possible drug interactions?)
> Toxicity or overdose (Are there signs of toxicity or overdose?)

The following are additional key nursing roles and responsibilities related to managing various health problems:

- **Promoting comfort and managing pain:** Nurses are accountable for promoting comfort and managing pain through both prescribed medications and holistic therapies.
- **Promoting safety and preventing infection; detecting and managing risks**: At every patient encounter, you' re accountable for keeping patients safe and preventing injury and complications. For example, you must detect, record, and manage patients at risk for falls, skin breakdown, infection, violence, or self-harm. You are also responsible for *surveillance of overall systems*. *Surveillance* means that you must be vigilant in observing for problems within health care systems that may put patients at risk (e.g., if a new drug is ordered and no one seems to be very informed about it, you report this to your manager).
- **Monitoring for changes in health status**: Because nurses spend the most time with patients—the ones in the "front line"—they are responsible for detecting signs and symptoms of possible problems requiring medical (or other multidisciplinary) management. For example, in the case of surgery, nurses are accountable for monitoring for signs of potential complications, such as bleeding.
- **Identifying and meeting learning needs**: Nurses must ensure that patients or their caregivers have the knowledge and ability to manage their own health. For example, ensuring that parents know how to care for their newborn at home is a nursing responsibility.
- **Promoting optimum health, sense of well-being, and quality of life:** Nurses promote health by teaching about healthy behaviors and detecting and managing risk factors. They "raise the bar" of care by focusing on *what each individual patient wants to do in life* (e.g., horseback riding may be important to one patient and sewing may be important to another).

Frequently Encountered Diagnoses and Complications

Box 3-5 shows nursing diagnoses frequently encountered in medical-surgical nursing. Boxes 3-6 and 3-7 (pages 96 and 97) show common potential complications of medical diagnoses and medical management. You should become familiar with the problems in each of these boxes, and learn to answer all of the following questions.

What You Must Know About Common Health Problems
- What are the signs, symptoms, and risk factors of each problem?
- What is the related pathophysiology?
- What are the common issues with independence and quality of life related to these problems?
- How do you monitor (assess) for the status or onset of each problem?
- What interventions are commonly used to prevent and manage each problem?
- What are common complications of each problem?
- Who is ultimately accountable for developing and recording a plan to monitor, prevent, and manage each problem? (Accountability changes, depending on severity or complexity of the problem.)
- How do you find out what your responsibilities are in relation to each problem, in various situations?

As you can see, nurses are accountable for managing care related to a *variety* of issues, depending on their education, qualifications, and clinical setting.

BOX 3-5	NURSING DIAGNOSES FREQUENTLY ENCOUNTERED IN MEDICAL-SURGICAL NURSING

High Priority at Every Patient Encounter:
- Acute and Chronic Pain
- Risk for Falls/Injury
- Risk for Infection
- Risk for Impaired Skin Integrity
- Impaired Communication
- Ineffective Airway Clearance
- Risk for Aspiration
- Impaired Swallowing
- Ineffective Breathing Pattern
- Impaired Mobility
- Risk for Violence
- Knowledge Deficit
- Self-Care Deficit (Feeding, Bathing, Dressing, Toileting)

Additional Priority Diagnoses
- Activity Intolerance
- Altered Comfort
- Altered Nutrition
- Altered Bowel Elimination
- Altered Urinary Elimination
- Anxiety / Fear / Coping Problems
- Constipation
- Dehydration*
- Latex Allergy Response
- Risk for Impaired Oral Mucous Membrane
- Ineffective Therapeutic Management
- Spiritual Distress

*Terms vary slightly from North American Nursing Diagnosis Association—International and from one hospital to another. For example, *Dehydration* is listed instead of *Fluid Volume Deficit* because it is well studied and used more frequently in the clinical setting. Use the terms commonly used by your school or clinical facility.

BOX 3-6	COMMON MEDICAL DIAGNOSES AND RELATED POTENTIAL COMPLICATIONS

Angina/Myocardial Infarction

Dysrhythmias
Congestive heart failure / Pulmonary edema
Shock (cardiogenic, hypovolemic)
Infarction, infarction extension
Thrombi/emboli formation (pulmonary emboli, stroke)
Hypoxemia
Electrolyte imbalance
Acid-base imbalance
Pericarditis
Cardiac tamponade
Cardiac arrest
See also Kidney Disease

Lung Diseases (asthma, chronic obstructive pulmonary disease [COPD], etc.)

Hypoxemia
Acid-base and electrolyte imbalance
Respiratory failure
Infection
See also Pneumonia and Angina / Myocardial Infarction

Pneumonia

Respiratory failure
Sepsis / septic shock
Pulmonary embolus
See also Angina / Myocardial Infarction

Diabetes

Hyper- and hypoglycemia
Coma, shock
Skin ulcers
Delayed wound healing
Hypertension
Eye problems (retinal hemorrhage)
Infection
See also Angina / Myocardial Infarction and Kidney Failure

Hypertension

Stroke (cerebrovascular accident [CVA])
Transient ischemic attacks (TIAs)
Hypertensive crisis
See also Angina / Myocardial Infarction and Kidney Failure

Kidney Disease

Congestive heart failure
Kidney failure
Edema
Hyperkalemia
Electrolyte / acid-base imbalance
Anemia
See also Hypertension

Urinary Tract Infection

Septic shock
Kidney failure

Fractures

Bleeding (internal or external)
Bone fragment displacement
Edema / pressure points
Compromised circulation
Nerve compression
Thrombus or embolus formation
Infection

Head Trauma

Respiratory depression
Airway occlusion
Aspiration
Bleeding (internal or external)
Shock
Brain swelling
Increased intracranial pressure
Seizures, coma
Hyper- or hypothermia
Infection

Other Trauma

See Anesthesia / Surgical Procedures in Box 3-7

Depression / Psychiatric Disorders

Reality distortion
Dehydration, malnutrition
Suicide
Violence (against self or others)
Self-protection problems
Trauma, death

BOX 3-7 | COMMON COMPLICATIONS RELATED TO TREATMENTS AND INVASIVE PROCEDURES

Anesthesia/Surgical Procedures
Respiratory depression
Airway management problems
Aspiration
Atelectasis, pneumonia
Bleeding (internal or external)
Hypovolemia, shock
Infection, septic shock
Fluid or electrolyte imbalance
Thrombus, embolus
Paralytic ileus
Urinary retention
Incision complications (infection, poor healing, dehiscence, or evisceration)
See also Angina / Myocardial Infarction in Box 3-6

Cardiac Catheterization—Invasive Monitoring
Bleeding (internal or at insertion site)
Hemo-pneumothorax
Thrombus or embolus formation
Stroke
Infection, sepsis
See also Angina / Myocardial Infarction in Box 3-6

Chest tubes—Thoracocentesis
Bleeding (internal or at insertion site)
Hemo-pneumothorax
Atelectasis
Chest tube malfunction or blockage
Infection, sepsis

Foley Catheter
Infection, sepsis
Catheter malfunction or blockage
Bladder spasms

Intravenous Therapy
Bleeding (internal or at insertion site)
Air embolus
Phlebitis, thrombophlebitis
Infiltration, extravasation, tissue necrosis
Fluid overload
Infection, sepsis

Medications
Adverse reactions (allergic response, exaggerated response, side effects, drug interactions)
Overdose or toxicity

Nasogastric Suction
Electrolyte imbalance
Tube malfunction or blockage
Aspiration
Bleeding

Paracentesis
Bleeding (internal or at insertion site)
Paralytic ileus
Infection, sepsis

Skeletal Traction or Casts
See Fractures in Box 3-6

What's most important is that you remember the legal implications of the terms *diagnosis* and *definitive diagnosis* as noted in the Rule on page 92, and that you determine your responsibilities related to risk management, diagnosis, interventions, and outcomes in each particular clinical setting.

Using Standard or Recognized Terms

A major requirement of National Practice Safety Goals (NPSG) is that of improving communication and documentation by using standard or recognized terms.[27-28] For this reason, you'll see increasing attention given to what terminology to use and what terminology to *avoid*.[29] For example, the Joint Commission* requires organizations to keep a *Do Not Use* list of terms, and ANA standards stress the need to use standard, recognized terms.[30-31]

As you move from one facility to another, use the terminology recommended by your school or the facility where you work. Recognize that there may be two terms for similar problems, and you may be required to use the most commonly used term. For example, you may find that the well-studied term *dehydration* may be used more often than *Fluid Volume Deficit*. Ultimately, you will need to learn whatever terminology is used by documentation systems and staff of the facility where you work.

The following box lists the organizations that continue to develop new knowledge and terms for nursing diagnoses, interventions, and outcomes. Keep in mind that some of the terms are commonly used (e.g., *Risk for Injury, Risk for Infection, Constipation*), but many of them are still at the creative level, with much work needed to be done before evidence will support their clinical use. Also realize that specialty practice organizations such as the American Association of Critical Care Nurses (AACN), the Association of Rehabilitation Nursing (ARN), and others have a significant impact on knowledge development and terminology used.

ORGANIZATIONS WORKING TO STANDARDIZE NURSING TERMS

North American Nursing Diagnosis Association—International (NANDA-I)
   www.nanda.org/html/about.html
Nursing Interventions Classification (NIC)*
   http://coninfo.nursing.uiowa.edu/nic/overview.htm
Nursing-Sensitive Outcomes Classification (NOC)*
   http://coninfo.nursing.uiowa.edu/noc/index.htm
Omaha Nursing Classification System for Community Health
   http://con.ufl.edu/omaha/omahas.htm
Perioperative Nursing Data Set (PNDS)
   www.aorn.org/research/pnds.htm
Home Health Care Classification (HHCC)
   www.sabacare.com
International Classification for Nursing Practice (ICNP)
   www.icn.ch/icnp.htm

*Page 276 gives examples of NIC and NOC terms.

---

*Formerly the Joint Commission of Accreditation of Hospital Organizations (JCAHO)

Developing Clinical Reasoning Skills

Developing clinical judgment—clinical reasoning skills—is one of the most important and challenging aspects of becoming a nurse. It's important because people's lives depend on it. It's challenging because thinking in the clinical setting is often fraught with more anxiety and risks than any other situation.

Clinical judgment entails things like knowing what to look for, how to recognize when a patient's status is changing, and what to do about it. For beginners, this is particularly taxing because it requires an ability to recall facts, put them together into a meaningful whole, and apply the information to current clinical situation (a situation which is often fluid and changing). For example, you note that someone is pale and sweaty and has a rapid pulse. To use good clinical judgment, you must be able to *recall* that these are symptoms of shock and that an immediate priority is to take a complete set of vital signs to further evaluate the patient's condition. Remember the following rule.

RULE

Using "sound clinical judgment" means *drawing valid conclusions and acting appropriately* **based on those conclusions** (e.g., monitor more closely, begin independent treatment, or contact a more experienced professional to activate the chain of command).

Activating the Chain of Command

As noted in the preceding rule, when a patient's status indicates the need for more qualified help, you are responsible *activating the chain of command*. Activating the chain of command means following communication guidelines, and *staying with the problem* until the appropriate qualified professional has responded. Think about the following example.

Example: Activating the Chain of Command. You give medication for incisional pain, but the patient has no relief. You try repositioning and other holistic measures, but the person still has no relief. You leave two messages for the doctor to call you about this problem. One hour later, you haven't heard from the doctor, and the patient is still in distress. You are accountable for activating the chain of command and notifying your supervisor about this problem and finding out what to do next.

Because *chain of command problems* have resulted in patient harm and subsequent law suits, most facilities have chain of command policies that guide you through the proper lines of communication. You should become familiar with these policies. For now, just remember: In important situations, leaving a message isn't enough. Stay with the problem until you get the results you need.

Scope of Practice Decisions

Learning to make decisions about what actions are within your scope of practice is an important part of developing sound clinical judgment. How do you know when you're qualified to give a professional opinion or perform a nursing action? For beginners especially, this is a tough question to answer. The clinical decision-making map on page 90 helps you answer this question. The following section gives additional details you need to know when making decisions about care management.

Decision Making and Nursing Standards and Guidelines

Critical thinking and clinical judgment in nursing is guided by professional standards. National practice standards give broad standards that address how nurses are expected to plan and give care (see the ANA Standards for Practice on pages 277-278). Each specialty organization (e.g., American Association of Critical Care Nurses, Association of Rehabilitation Nurses) develops its own unique standards. Each hospital or health care organization develops standards to guide decision making in specific situations (e.g., standards of care, policies, protocols, procedures, care plans, and critical paths).

When determining care management, there are three main questions to answer related to standards:

1. Has this facility developed specific standards, guidelines, or policies for the care of this specific situation? For example, if you're caring for someone with a mastectomy, ask, Has this facility developed guidelines or pathways for someone undergoing a mastectomy?
2. Are there national or local evidenced-based practice guidelines relating to this particular problem?
3. To what degree do these standards and guidelines apply to my patient's particular situation?

Practice standards and guidelines are valuable tools to help you make care decisions. However, don't follow guidelines blindly. Decide whether they are appropriate by carefully comparing your patient's situation with the information in the guidelines. For example, suppose that you're looking after an elderly man after prostate surgery, and the critical path for this problem states that on the first postoperative day, the patient gets out of bed twice. On the first postoperative day, you assess the man and find he has chest pain. This finding is significant enough for you to question whether he should indeed get out of bed. Could this man be suffering a complication such as myocardial infarction or pulmonary embolus? In this case, it's your responsibility to report the symptoms and keep the man in bed until a physician or more qualified nurse evaluates him.

Applying Delegation Principles

Knowing when and how to delegate care is an important part of managing time and resources. It's also important for passing NCLEX, since the exam tests your knowledge of delegation principles. The ANA's *Principles for Delegation* stresses that you are accountable for making the decision to delegate, and for the results (outcomes) of your delegation.[32] You can find guidelines and principles of delegation in Box 5-4 (page 182), where delegation is addressed in context of setting priorities. Most importantly, remember the following rule.

RULE

You are accountable for the outcomes of your decision to delegate—when you delegate a task, follow up after the task is done by *assessing the patient response yourself.* This does two things: (1) You have first-hand knowledge of how the patient responded to care, and (2) when the person you delegated to knows that you check results *directly with the patient*, he or she is more likely to do a good job.

How to Develop Effective Clinical Judgment

Developing clinical judgment comes with *clinical experience*. It requires a commitment to study common health problems, seek out clinical experiences, and come prepared to the clinical setting. The following strategies help you plan ahead and make the most of clinical learning opportunities.

10 Strategies for Developing Clinical Judgment

1. Keep references—texts, hand-held computers, pocket guides, and personal "cheat sheets"—handy, and be sure that you
   - **Learn terminology and concepts.** If you encounter words like *embolus, thrombus,* or *phlebitis* and you don't know what they mean, look them up as you encounter them, so that they become part of your long-term memory. Learning terms *in context* helps your brain to store information in related groups, rather than as isolated facts.
   - **Become familiar with normal findings** (e.g., normal lab values, assessment findings, disease progression, growth and development) before being concerned with abnormal findings. Once you know what's normal, you'll readily recognize when you encounter information that's *outside the norm* (abnormal).
   - **Ask** why? Find out what principles explain why normal and abnormal findings occur (e.g., Why is there edema in heart failure?).
   - **Learn problem-specific facts.** You need to know how problems usually present themselves (their signs and symptoms), what usually causes them, and how they're managed. Box 3-8 on the next page lists questions you need to answer to be prepared for going to the clinical setting.

BOX 3-8	QUESTIONS TO ANSWER BEFORE GOING TO THE CLINICAL AREA

1. Based on this particular clinical setting, what common problems are seen, and what problems do I know or suspect my patients have?
2. What are the signs and symptoms of these problems?
3. What risk factors do I know or suspect my patients have?
4. What must I assess to determine the status of these signs, symptoms, and risk factors?
5. What are the usual causes of these problems?
6. What must I assess to determine the status of the causes of the problems?
7. How do these problems usually progress, and how are they managed?
8. How can these problems be prevented?
9. What are the signs and symptoms of potential complications of these problems, and how will I monitor for these signs and symptoms?
10. How can I be prepared to manage potential complications if they should occur?
11. What medications and treatments are likely to be used, and why?
12. What medication-related or treatment-related problems might I encounter, how will I monitor to detect them, and how are they usually managed?
13. What cultural factors, values, or beliefs might have a bearing on health practices in relation to these health problems?
14. What are the key things people need to know to manage these problems independently, and what will I do to ensure that this knowledge is gained?

■ **Apply principles of the nursing process.** For example, assess before acting, stay focused on outcomes, anticipate, and change approaches as needed. Make judgments based on evidence rather than guesswork. Remember the following rule:

RULE

Always consider your *direct assessment* of the patient to be the *primary source* of information (e.g., if someone tells you a patient has pain, assess the pain *yourself* before giving a medication).

2. Ask your instructor or manager whether there are standard tools to guide your thinking and documentation in various situations.
   ■ You'll find *comprehensive assessment tools* and *focused assessment tools*. Comprehensive tools are usually used for patient admissions (see pages 272-275). Focus assessment tools are usually used to monitor a specific problem (see page 157 for a focus assessment tool for monitoring neurologic status).
   ■ Be sure you understand the reasoning behind the tools you use. Finding out *why* you collect each piece of data on the tool helps you learn what's *relevant* to each situation.

- Don't just record the data. *Think* about what you recorded, looking for patterns and omissions.
- Realize that the tool you use affects how you *think* about the data. For example, Box 3-9 shows *Gordon's Functional Health Patterns*, a framework that's often used to organize data collection to identify problems with *human functioning*. Figure 3-3 on the next page shows the *Body Systems* approach to collecting data, which helps identify medical problems. Realize that you should use *both* ways of organizing data—*Functional Health Patterns* and *Body Systems*—to identify possible nursing and medical problems.

3. **Learn to think ahead, think-in-action, and think back** (reflect on your thinking), as addressed on page 16.
4. **Follow policies, procedures, and standards of care carefully, with a good understanding of the reasons behind them.** Policies, procedures, and standards of care are designed to help you use good judgment, but you must know the *reasons behind them* to know when and how to adapt them.
5. **Determine a system that helps you make decisions about what must be done now and what can wait until later** (see *Setting Priorities*, pages 180-184).
6. **Never perform actions (interventions) if you don't know why** they're indicated, why they work (the rationale), and what the risks of harm are in the context of the current patient situation.
7. **Learn from human resources** (e.g., educators, preceptors, classmates, other nurses). When in doubt about your responsibilities, activate the chain of

---

BOX 3-9	GORDON'S FUNCTIONAL HEALTH PATTERNS

1. **Health perception–health management pattern:** The person's perception of health and well-being; knowledge of, and adherence to, health promotion regimens
2. **Nutritional-metabolic pattern:** Usual food and fluid intake; height, weight, age
3. **Elimination pattern:** Usual bowel and bladder elimination patterns
4. **Activity-exercise pattern:** Usual activity and exercise tolerance
5. **Sleep-rest pattern:** usual hours' sleep and rest.
6. **Cognitive-perception pattern:** Ability to use all senses to perceive environment; usual way of perceiving environment
7. **Self-perception or self-concept pattern:** The person's perception of capabilities and self-worth
8. **Role-relationship pattern:** Usual responsibilities and ways of relating to others
9. **Sexuality-reproductive pattern:** Knowledge and perception of sex and reproduction
10. **Coping-stress tolerance pattern:** Ability to manage and tolerate stress
11. **Value-belief pattern:** Values, beliefs, and goals in life; spiritual practices

Summarized from Gordon, M. (2002). *Manual of nursing diagnosis* (10th ed.). St. Louis: Mosby.

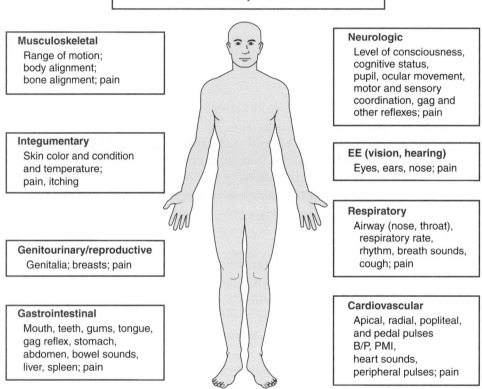

Figure 3-3. Body systems assessment.

command—get help from a qualified professional. Your patients' right to timely care takes precedence over your need to learn independently. Other professionals can help you decide whether you have time to look up your concerns in a reference. Also learn from your peers' experiences. Collaborating with classmates is a win-win situation: Asking questions like *What did you look for in that patient? How did you know?* and *What was the biggest thing you learned?* helps your classmates clarify their knowledge and helps you learn from being involved in real situations. However, don't use names or talk about patients in public places where others might overhear (e.g., cafeteria, elevators)—you may be violating Health Insurance Portability and Accountability Act (HIPAA) privacy laws.

8. **Reduce the "brain drain" of learning new technology**: become familiar with the technology you'll use (e.g., IV pumps, computers, heart monitors) *before* you go to the clinical setting.

9. **Remember the importance of caring**. Patients describe caring as *vigilance* (attentiveness, highly skilled practice, basic care, nurturing, and going the extra mile); *mutuality* (building relationships among nurses, patients, and families); and *healing* (lifesaving behaviors and freeing the patient from anxiety and concerns).[33]

10. **When planning time for nursing care,** consider the time required for (a) direct care interventions (things you do directly for or with the patient, such as helping someone walk), and (b) indirect care interventions (things you do away from the patient, such as consulting with the pharmacist or analyzing lab study results).

Charting That Shows Critical Thinking

Finally, let's end this chapter with a few words of caution: Be sure your charting shows critical thinking. Your charting is used by others to make patient care decisions. It also reflects whether or not you're a critical thinker. If your supervisor or instructor reads your charts and sees nothing but rote repetition of what the person ahead of you charted, a flag goes up that says, *This person never seems to have an original thought*. Follow policies and procedures for charting—these may include using a system of flow charts and check marks—but always ask yourself whether there is something *different* today that you should add.

When entering individualized notes, use standard terms and good handwriting. Whether you're using a computer or a pen, make sure your charting reflects crucial thinking by including the following as appropriate:

1. **Assessment:** What you assessed in the patient
2. **Conclusion:** What you concluded about your patient—state the facts to support your conclusions
3. **Interventions**: What you did, and how the patient responded (assess, intervene, reassess)
4. **Safety measures:** Anything you did to correct or prevent adverse responses

    Example: Rates incisional pain at 7. Dressing clean and dry. Vital signs normal. Appears stable. Pain med given. Bedrails raised. Call bell given and told to call for help if needed. Reassessed 30 min later and rates pain at 2.

RULE

Charting influences thinking: Follow charting policies and procedures closely. To improve accuracy, identify trends early, and pick up things you may have forgotten to do, chart *as soon as you can. Think* about what you record. If you use a computer, don't just dump the data into it; find a way to *reflect* on your charting and patient care.

CRITICAL THINKING EXERCISES

Note: Exercises followed by asterisks (*) have example responses listed in the Response Key *beginning on page 252.*

1. Discuss the how the situations in *a* and *b* relate to *novice* and *expert thinking* as described in this chapter.
   a. Compare how your brain thinks when encountering familiar situations with what happens when you encounter unfamiliar situations: For example, think of the difference between what you see and understand the minute you walk into your own home, compared to what it's like when you are visiting someone you don't know very well for the first time.*
   b. Think about the following analogy: When you go to a new clinical setting or have a patient for the first time, it's like watching a movie for the first time. Each time you see the same movie over and over, you understand it better and see new things. The same thing happens when you are familiar with patients, staff, and routines in a particular clinical setting.
   c. What are some things you can do to increase your ability to function in unfamiliar situations?*
2. Use the clinical decision model on page 90 to decide whether you're allowed to irrigate a nasogastric tube in the clinical setting.*
3. An important aspect of developing clinical judgment is being willing to place great importance on the wants and needs of patients and their significant others. Keeping this in mind, how would you interpret the statements made by the off-going nurse below?*
   On-coming nurse: "How is the family doing?"
   Off-going nurse: "They seem to be fine. They don't say much, but they're sticking to visiting hours and have been here 15 minutes this morning and 15 minutes this afternoon."
4. Pick a situation you need to think critically about—a patient, a presentation, a dilemma, or a problem you have. Together with someone else, use the *DEAD ON!!* game on page 267 to make some decisions.
5. With a peer or in a group, and using additional references as needed, discuss the following in relation to the BLOG on page 91.
   a. Risks of applying restraints
   b. Independent thinking on the part of the nurse
   c. The value of the human relationship between the nurse and the patient
   d. The many things that influence hypoxia
6. How you manage stress affects your ability to think critically. Go to www. teachhealth.com and take the stress scale test. What are the stressful things in your life, and how are you handling them? What healthy behaviors might help?

7. Suppose that you have a postoperative patient whose blood pressure is abnormally high. You call the doctor twice, but there is no response. How will you know what to do to activate the chain of command?*

8. Suppose your neighbor asks you whether it's okay to give an aspirin to her normally healthy 5-year-old who is alert, but has a fever of 100°, orally. Apply the 10 critical thinking questions on the inside back cover to this situation, and decide how you will respond.

9. How can you use the memory jog **m & m** on page 109 to prioritize your thinking when making diagnoses?

10. Decide where you stand in relation to being able to achieve the following learning outcomes from page 63.
    a. Clarify the purpose of each phase of the nursing process.*
    b. Discuss the interplay of intuition and logic in novice and expert thinking.*
    c. Explain the legal implications of the terms *diagnose* and *diagnosis*.*
    d. Clarify your responsibilities related to diagnosis and management of medical and nursing problems.*
    e. Explain the role of ethics codes, standards, guidelines, and laws in making decisions.*
    f. Explain how to use standard tools to promote critical thinking.

OTHER PERSPECTIVES

CRITICAL THINKING: A SIXTH SENSE?

"Critical thinking is a 'sixth sense' that's developed over time from an accumulation of years of knowledge and experience—both personal and what you've learned from others. When you do a job for years, you learn what to look for and what to do. In almost a split second, you evaluate what you see, correlate it with what you've learned, and take appropriate action."—*Doris Alfaro, SRN, class of 1944, Chesterfield Royal Hospital, Derbyshire, UK*

THE DIFFERENCE BETWEEN NOVICES AND EXPERTS

"There is an accumulation of evidence that expert problem solving... is dependent on (1) a wealth of prior specific experiences that can be usaved in routine solution of problems by pattern recognition... and (2) elaborate conceptual knowledge applicable to the occasional problematic situation.... The main difference between expert clinicians and students is that experts generate better hypotheses (from the beginning, they have better hunches about what the problems may be)."[35]—*Dr. Geoffrey Norman*

USING INTUITION AND LOGIC: DO A LITTLE DANCE

"I agree that nurses must focus on evidence. I'm told I 'do a dance' when I know something's wrong with my patient but I can't quite figure it out. First, I get quiet (this usually gets attention since I am not really a loud person, just not really silent).

Second, I gather all my information—the bedside notes, medication record, etc. Then, I take another set of vital signs, and then sort of pace back and forth, assessing the patient, and thinking while standing in the doorway. I reassess the patient and review the trends for the day. Then I reassess again, checking the lab results, the urine output, etc. Then, when I 'get it,' I get verbal again. I page the doctor or consult a more experienced nurse or colleague in the unit. Patricia Benner calls this 'thinking in action.' My group calls it my 'intuitive dance.' Once I get the hunch something's up, I keep going until it makes sense."[36]—*Elizabeth E. Hand, MS, CCRN*

DEALING WITH HIPAA PRIVACY LAWS

"I give high priority to maintaining privacy of patient information. But, when it's clear to me that families are involved in care and need information on what may happen with their loved one, I say something like, 'Because of privacy laws, I can't tell you what's going on with your family member. I can tell you what typically happens in a situation like this is, but I can't be sure that this is what will happen with your family member.'"—*Matthew Riley*[37]

DECISION MAKING: A SKILL THAT'S LEARNED

"It's important to remember that clinical decision making is a skill. Like any other skill, it can be improved with practice—by seeking out (and reflecting on) decision making in various situations (e.g., clinical setting, simulations, postclinical conferences). Nurses aren't born good decision makers. They develop their skills through constant reflection on their practice. One thing you can do to develop your skills is always ask yourself, 'What could happen next?' Thinking ahead for potential outcomes and considering the likely progression of a patient's condition helps you consider solutions in advance. This 'what if' mentality is a characteristic of expert decision-makers."[38]—*Bernie Garrett, author of* Student Nurses' Perceptions of Clinical Decision-Making in Their Final Year of Adult Nursing Studies[39]

GETTING LEARNERS AND MENTORS ON THE SAME PAGE

"Understanding personality and learning style differences, and getting 'on the same page' about what behaviors demonstrate critical thinking is key to mentor-learner success. For example, when both mentors and learners use CTIs in the form of a checklist, they have a 'language' to talk about critical thinking. They can reflect on the ideal behaviors, compare them with current status, and develop a plan to improve."[40]—*Kathie Kulikowski, MSN, RN, BC*

MOMENTUM LEADERSHIP: PREPARE FOR TOMORROW

"Momentum leadership—the idea that you need some type of sustained drive or force to get where you want to be—is a tool that helps you choose paths to future career goals. For example, if you want to be a nurse anesthetist, position yourself for program acceptance by seeking out education and clinical experiences in critical care. Momentum leadership is proactive and requires in-depth critical thinking."[41]—*Kathleen D. Pagana, PhD, RN*

CRITICAL MOMENTS

OUR BRAINS NEED HELP

To grasp the importance of helping our brains to remember by using standard tools, answer this question: The next time you're on an airplane, do you want the pilot to rely on his memory to check that "all systems are go"? Do you want him to use his own tool? Or, do you want him to use a tool designed by the FAA (Federal Aviation Administration)? In the clinical setting, whenever possible, use approved tools. If you need additional memory jogs, make your own tool to help you remember in your own way.

WHEN MAKING DIAGNOSES, REMEMBER M & M

Always ask, *Could these signs and symptoms be related to medical or medication problems that are undiagnosed?*

CRITICAL PATHWAYS: NOT LIKE IN THE LAND OF OZ

Critical pathways, protocols, and standard plans aren't meant to be like the yellow brick road in the land of Oz, which allowed Dorothy to find the wizard without much thought. Use critical pathways as maps, carefully considering how they apply to your particular patient situation. Think about this analogy: Imagine you're driving down the road, and you come to a temporary roadblock. Even though the map says you have to go straight, you clearly have to figure out another way. Whether talking about care maps or road maps, *you* are the one who has to "assess the actual road conditions, change speed, and make detours" as needed. When using standard plans, don't be a task-oriented thinker. Think about the difference between the following approaches:

Task-Oriented Thinking

"I have a critical path for this patient's problem…This will be easy and straightforward because I already know what the problems are going to be."

Critical Thinking

"I'm familiar with the critical path for my patient's problem…I wonder how he's doing in relation to the predicted care on the path."

ELDERLY AND CHRONICALLY ILL: BE CAREFUL OF ASSUMPTIONS

When dealing with aging and chronically ill clients, be especially careful of the human tendency to make assumptions. The complexity of their health status often hides problems that might otherwise be quite obvious. For example, we had a 70-year-old man with chronic back pain. He complained of increasing pain for weeks before someone said, "Maybe it's not his back. Has anyone checked his kidneys?" Only then were kidney stones diagnosed. Getting results requires you to examine alternative explanations, problems, or solutions. The more alternative solutions, explanations, and problems you consider, the more likely it is that you're thinking critically.

LEARN MORE ABOUT RISK MANAGEMENT
Go online to the Harvard Center For Risk Analysis at www.hcra.harvard.edu/. The center is dedicated to promoting reasoned public responses to health, safety, and environmental hazards. It also addresses statistics and approaches for problems like stroke, heart disease, suicide, cancer, and drowning and other accidents. The Centers for Disease Control and Prevention Web page (www.cdc.gov/) also has a wealth of information on disease and disability prevention.

IMPROVE OUTCOMES AND JOB SATISFACTION—GET INVOLVED IN SHARED GOVERNANCE
Shared governance—an organizational innovation that gives nurses control over their practice and some areas previously controlled only by managers—can improve patient outcomes and job satisfaction. Learn how to get staff and leaders to work together by visiting http://sharedgovernance.org.

KEY POINTS / SUMMARY

- The terms *clinical judgment, clinical reasoning,* and *critical thinking* are often used interchangeably. Figure 3-1 (page 66) maps key features of critical thinking that are integrated throughout this book.
- Problem-solving skills are crucial to critical thinking—but critical thinking requires more than problem solving. It requires creativity, risk management skills, and constantly striving to improve.
- Being familiar with CTIs—short descriptions of behaviors that demonstrate the knowledge, characteristics, and skills that promote critical thinking—is central to learning to think critically (see pages 10, 48, and 49).
- The 4-circle CT model on the inside *front* cover helps you assess your ability to think critically and target areas to develop.
- The questions on the inside *back* cover can be used as a guide to critical thinking.
- Pages 68-69 address the major goals and outcomes of nursing.
- Box 3-2 (page 71) shows Benner's descriptions of *novice to expert* stages. Table 3-1

(page 72) shows the differences between the novice and expert thinking.
- Paying attention to context (circumstances) is a major part of critical thinking. Patients are *individuals* who may have similar problems, but different attitudes, responses, and "stories."
- Institute of Medicine (IOM) competencies require nurses to be able to provide patient-centered care, work in interdisciplinary teams, employ evidence-based practice, apply quality improvement methods, and use informatics.
- The concept of *stewardship* stresses that your job is to protect patients and *empower them* to navigate safely through the health care system.
- Care has shifted from a *diagnose and treat* (DT) approach, which implies that we wait for evidence of problems to start treatment, to a predictive model: *predict, prevent, manage and promote* (PPMP).
- Disease management is a model of care that focuses on keeping those with chronic diseases as healthy as possible by

managing risks and illnesses, even when symptoms aren't obvious (e.g., determining whether an asthmatic who has no asthma attacks is on the best prevention regimen with lowest side effects).

- From professional and economic perspectives, the care we give must be driven by the best available evidence. Evaluate the strength of the evidence that supports your approaches and the expected outcomes.

- Page 79 explains the importance of looking at clinical, functional, and other outcomes.

- Outcome-focused thinking requires fixing problems in ways that you get the *best results*, from cost, time, and patient satisfaction perspectives.

- Understanding nursing process *principles* is the key to learning other models of critical thinking and also to think your way through NCLEX and other certification tests. Pages 83-84 summarize the phases of the nursing process when used as tool for critical thinking.

- Experts use the nursing process in dynamic ways because they quickly assess situations and correlate information in their heads. Novices need to learn nursing process principles and techniques in a step-by-step way, doing detailed maps and papers that explain their thinking.

- *Ready, fire, aim* is a phrase that describes the risks of working in today's fast paced world—critical thinking means not jumping to conclusions or acting on impulse.

- Intuitive thinking is fostered by (1) in-depth knowledge and experience related to the clinical situations at hand, and (2) deep understanding of the patient's normal patterns, circumstances, needs, and desires.

- Use intuitive hunches to search for evidence. Use logic to formulate and double-check your thinking.

- Using principle-centered creativity and ensuring that ideas are useful to the end users are important parts of critical thinking.

- Remember three things about using standard tools: (1) Recording data *in a standard way* reduces omission errors and promotes safety, consistency, and efficiency. (2) Tools must be designed for specific purposes: One size doesn't fit all. (3) Tools don't *think* for you—*you* are accountable for making independent judgments.

- Computers can jog memory and guide decision making, but they don't transform decision making. You're accountable for ensuring up-to-date data, using critical thinking, and considering the context (big picture) to make ultimate decisions.

- While standards mandate that patients have individualized plans of care, you may not find the care plan all in one place. Use the memory-jog EASE (page 89) to remember the major care plan components.

- The terms *diagnose* and *diagnosis* have legal implications. They imply that there's a specific problem that requires management *by a qualified professional*. If you make a diagnosis, you accept accountability for accurately naming and managing the problem. If you treat a problem or allow a problem to *persist* without ensuring that the definitive diagnosis (the most specific correct diagnosis) has been made, you may cause harm and be accused of negligence.

- Definitions of nursing diagnosis continue to evolve, since nurses have varied responsibilities related to diagnoses, interventions, risk management, and outcomes. Pages 93-95 summarize these responsibilities. Box 3-5 (page 95) shows nursing diagnoses frequently encountered in medical-surgical nursing. Boxes 3-6 and 3-7 (pages 96 and 97) show common potential complications.

- Using sound clinical judgment means *drawing valid conclusions* and *acting appropriately* on those conclusions (e.g., monitor more closely, begin independent treatment, or contact a more qualified professional to activate the chain of command).

- Because standards mandate that you use recognized terms, be sure to use the terminology recommended by your school or the facility where you work. Recognize that there may be two terms for similar problems, and you may be required to use the most commonly used term.

- Critical thinking and clinical judgment in nursing is guided by laws, ethics codes, and standards. National practice standards provide broad standards that address how nurses are expected to plan and give care. The facility where you work has detailed standards, policies, and procedures—become familiar with them.

- Knowing when and how to delegate care is an important part of managing time and resources. It's also important for passing NCLEX. Box 5-4 (page 182), summarizes delegation principles and addresses when it's safe and *not* safe to delegate.

- You're accountable for the outcomes of your decision to delegate. After you delegate a task, follow up *with your direct assessment* of the patient.

- Developing clinical judgment comes with *clinical experience*. It requires a commitment to study common health problems, seek out clinical experiences, and come prepared to the clinical setting.

- Thinking ahead, thinking-in-action, and thinking back (reflecting on thinking) are important parts of using sound clinical judgment.

- Documentation tools influence how you *think* about the data. Box 3-9 (page 103) shows *Gordon's Functional Health Patterns*, a framework that's often used to organize data to identify problems with *human functioning*. Figure 3-3 (page 104) shows the *Body Systems* approach to organizing data, which helps identify *medical problems*. Consider *both* ways of organizing data—*Functional Health Patterns* and *Body Systems*—to identify both nursing and medical problems.

- Charting influences thinking: follow charting policies and procedures closely. To improve accuracy, identify trends early, and pick up things you may have forgotten to do, chart *as soon as you can*, and reflect on what you record.

REFERENCES

1. Alfaro-LeFevre, R. (2006). *Applying nursing process: A tool for critical thinking* (6th ed.). Philadelphia, PA: Lippincott Williams & Wilkins.
2. Alfaro-LeFevre, R. (2007). Evidence-based critical thinking indicators. Retrieved January 17, 2007, from www.alfaroteachsmart.com/cti.htm.
3. Ignatavicius, D. (2007). e-Mail communication.

4. Hansten, R. (2007). e-Mail communication.
5. Elechko, K. (2007). e-Mail communication.
6. Valiga, T. (2007). e-Mail communication.
7. American Nurses Association. (2004). *Nursing scope and standards of performance and standards of clinical practice.* Washington, DC: American Nurses Publishing.
8. Tanner, C. (2006). Thinking like a nurse: A research-based model of clinical judgment in nursing. *Journal of Nursing Education, 45*(6), 204-211.
9. Benner, P. (2001). *From novice to expert.* Upper Saddle River, NJ: Prentice Hall.
10. Institute of Medicine. (2001). *Crossing the quality chasm: A new health system for the 21st century.* Washington, DC: National Academies Press.
11. Institute of Medicine. (2004). *Keeping patients safe: Transforming the work environment of nurses.* Washington, DC: National Academies Press.
12. Institute of Medicine. (2000). *To err is human: Building a safer health system.* Washington, DC: National Academies Press.
13. Institute of Medicine. (2003). *Health professions education: A bridge to quality.* Washington, DC: National Academies Press.
14. Institute of Medicine. (2001). op cit.
15. Institute of Medicine, (2003). op cit.
16. Benner, P., Tanner, C., & Chesla, C. (1996). *Experience in nursing practice: Caring, clinical judgment and ethics.* New York: Springer.
17. Lamond, D., & Thompson, C. (2000). Intuition and analysis in decision making and choice. *Journal of Nursing Scholarship, 32*(3), 411-414.
18. Hansten, R., & Washburn, M. (2001). Intuition in professional practice: Executive and staff perceptions. *Journal of Nursing Administration, 30*(4), 185-188.
19. Scheffer, B., & Rubenfeld, M. (2000). A consensus statement on critical thinking in nursing. *Journal of Nursing Education, 39*(8), 352-359.
20. Levinson, H. *Ready, fire, aim: Avoiding management by impulse.* Accessed March 2, 2007, from www.levinsoninst.com/.
21. American Nurses Association. (2004). *Nursing scope and standards of performance and standards of clinical practice.* Washington, DC: nursesbooks.org.
22. Cooper, P. G. (2007). Professionalism means clarity about what we do. *Nursing Forum, 39*(1), 3-4.
23. Gordon, S. (2006). What do nurses really do? *Topics in Advanced Nursing eJournal, 6*(1). Retrieved July 24, 2006, from www.medscape.com/viewarticle/520714?src=mp.
24. North American Nursing Diagnosis Association-International. (2007). *Nursing diagnosis: Definitions and classifications 2007-2008.* Philadelphia: Author.
25. Herdman, H. (2007). President's message. *NANDA E-news.* Retrieved March 22, 2007, from www.fernley.com/nanda-enews/winter07/content.html#1.
26. American Nurses Association. (2004). op cit.

27.   Smith, L. Charting tips: How to use focus charting. Retrieved March 17, 2007, from www.findarticles.com/p/articles/mi_qa3689/is_200005/ai_n8880050.

28.   The Joint Commission. The official do not use list. Retrieved March 6, 2007, from www.jointcommission.org/PatientSafety/DoNotUseList/.

29.   Ibid.

30.   Ibid.

31.   American Nurses Association. (2004). op cit.

32.   American Nurses Association. (2005). *Principles for delegation.* Washington, DC: nursesbooks.org.

33.   Burfitt, S., Greiner, D., & Miers, L. (1993). Professional nurse caring as perceived by critically ill patients: A phenomenologic study. *American Journal of Critical Care, 2*(6), 489-499.

34.   Beckman, D. (1993). Andrew's not-so-excellent adventure. *Healthcare Forum Journal*, May/June, 90-96.

35.   Norman, G. (1988). Problem-solving skills, solving problems and problem-based learning. *Medical Education, 22,* 280.

36.   Hand, E. (February 2007). e-Mail communication.

37.   Riley, M. (January 2007). e-Mail communication.

38.   Garrett, B. (January 2007). e-Mail communication.

39.   Garrett B. (2005). Student nurses perceptions of clinical decision-making in their final year of adult nursing studies. *Nurse Education in Practice, 5*(1), 30-39.

40.   Kulikowski, K. (January 2007). e-Mail communication.

41.   Pagana, K. (January, 2007). e-Mail communication.

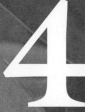

4

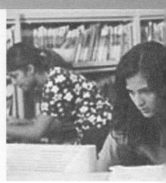

Critical Thinking in Nursing: Beyond Clinical Judgment

This chapter at a glance...

- Moral and Ethical Reasoning
    - Clarifying Values
    - Moral Versus Ethical Reasoning
    - How Do You Decide?
    - Seven Ethical Principles
    - Standards, Ethics Codes, and Patients' Rights
    - Steps for Moral and Ethical Reasoning
- Evidence-Based Practice (EBP)
    - Relationship of Research to EBP
    - Transforming Knowledge to EBP
    - Clinical Summaries
    - ACE Star Model of Knowledge Transformation
    - Nursing Research, EBP, and Critical Thinking
        - Frequently Asked Questions about Staff Nurses' Role
    - Scanning before Reading Research Articles
- Questioning Care Practices: Promoting Inquiry and Creativity
- Surveillance and Quality Improvement
- Critical Thinking Exercises
- Teaching Others: Promoting Independence
    - 10 Steps for Teaching Others
- Teaching Yourself: Grab the Spoon
    - Memorizing Effectively
    - Learning and Memorization Strategies
- Test Taking: Improving Grades and Passing the First Time
    - Strategies for Successful Test Taking
        - Preparing For Tests
        - Taking Tests
        - After the Test
    - Strategies for NCLEX and Other Standard Tests
        - Fast Facts on NCLEX
        - Preparing for NCLEX

- Critical Thinking Exercises
- Key Points / Summary

Decide where you stand in relation to each of the following learning outcomes:

Learning Outcomes

After completing this chapter, you should be able to:

1. Develop or adopt a personal code of conduct based on your personal values and content in this chapter.
2. Compare and contrast the terms *moral reasoning* and *ethical reasoning*.
3. Make prudent decisions based on ethical principles, codes, and practice standards.
4. Explain the relationship between nursing research and evidence-based practice (EBP).
5. Describe your responsibilities for research, EBP, surveillance, and quality improvement (QI).
6. Explain why it's important to choose refereed (peer-reviewed) journals when looking for research articles.
7. Use critical thinking to create individualized teaching plans.
8. Address the roles of memorizing and reasoning in teaching ourselves.
9. Describe at least five strategies that help you improve your test scores and pass NCLEX on the first try.

Having examined how to promote critical thinking in clinical judgment in Chapter 3, let's go on to examine reasoning in the five other major nursing situations: (1) moral and ethical reasoning, (2) research and evidence-based practice, (3) teaching others (4) teaching ourselves, and (5) test taking. Learning to think critically in each of these situations is central to your success as a nurse. In the clinical setting, you must be able to reason about ethical issues, apply evidence-based practice, and teach others and yourself. In school and clinical practice, test-taking skills—your ability to reason your way through tests such as NCLEX, competency exams, and advance certification exams—can make the difference between passing on the first try and having to retake the test or failing completely.

This chapter helps you gain the knowledge and skills you need to succeed in context of all the above situations. Let's start with moral and ethical reasoning. In this complex, multicultural world, how can you learn to make ethical decisions that are in *your patients' best interests?*

Moral and Ethical Reasoning

Treatment advances, longer life spans, and more emphasis on partnering with patients to improve outcomes continue to create new challenges. Questions related to end-of-life care, genetic advances, quality of life, and the distribution of resources are common. Knowing how to reason your way through moral and ethical issues is a cornerstone of competent nursing practice.

Clarifying Values

Because your values and beliefs deeply affect your thinking, *clarifying values* is a major starting point for moral and ethical reasoning. Values are often considered in two ways:

- **Personal values:** These are the beliefs, qualities, and standards that you're passionate about—things you hold "near and dear." You have significant emotional investment in your personal values, but it takes "serious thinking" to really get in touch with them. Once you clarify what you believe, why you believe it, and how it affects your ability to be objective in various situations, you improve your ability to deal with moral and ethical issues.
- **Organizational values:** These are deeply held beliefs within an organization (e.g., a school or hospital). These values are expected to be demonstrated through the day-to-day behaviors of all organizational members. Examples of common organizational values are leadership, collaboration, honesty, integrity, dedication to customer service, and respect for diversity.

Think about what's important to you as a person, learner, and nurse. For example, what are your beliefs about how terminal illnesses should be managed, how people should treat one another, and how much autonomy and responsibility students and patients should have? Reflect on the values of your school or hospital. Are they compatible with your own values? Review the *Code of Conduct* on page 27 and decide whether you value the listed behaviors. You may not have the answers to all these questions now, but keep these in mind as you read this section. For starters, think about where you stand in relation to the following *Other Perspectives*.

OTHER PERSPECTIVES

WHAT ETHICS GUIDE YOUR CONDUCT?

"An ethic of care respects individual uniqueness, personal relationships, and the dynamic nature of life. Essential to an ethic of care are compassion, collaboration, accountability, and trust."[16]—*The American Association of Critical Care Nurses*

"Everyone has an ethical framework—the question is how aware of it are they? We all need to clarify our ethical frameworks before we're faced with dilemmas. Just as we're too late if we're flipping through our advanced life support book during a code, we can make some regrettable decisions if we haven't given thought to how we'll respond to difficult situations."[17]—*Michael Riley, LMSW, LPC, EMT, paramedic*

Moral Versus Ethical Reasoning

Moral reasoning and *ethical reasoning* are often used interchangeably. There is, however, a difference between these two terms:

- **Moral reasoning:** Refers to judgments made based *on personal standards of right and wrong* (e.g., I personally believe it's okay to tell little white lies now and then)
- **Ethical reasoning:** Refers to professional judgments made based *on standards derived from the formal study of what criteria should to be used to determine whether actions are justified and therefore ethically right or wrong* (e.g., I, personally, don't think that there's anything wrong with little white lies now and then, but most ethicists will tell you it's wrong to lie to patients).

To better grasp the difference between *moral* and *ethical reasoning*, imagine that you're caring for a woman who is freely and knowledgeably asking for her tubes to be tied to prevent pregnancy. *Morally* (according to your personal standards), you believe sterilization is wrong. However, you know that professional standards and ethics codes stress that people have the right to make their *own choices*, based on their own beliefs. It's *unethical* for you, as a nurse, to tell her that sterilization is wrong.

How Do You Decide?

So how do you make decisions about moral and ethical issues? The answer is that *it's not easy*. These types of issues are rarely simple. Let's look at how to handle situations that have no clear "right" answers—when each answer has its own merits and drawbacks, and it's hard to say that one is better than another.

Moral and ethical problems may be divided into three categories:

- **Moral uncertainty:** You aren't sure which moral or ethical principles apply. Example: A patient asks you whether you think his doctor is a good doctor. You don't think the doctor is very competent. Do you tell him?
- **Moral dilemma:** You're faced with a situation in which you have two (or more) choices available, but neither (or none) of them seems satisfactory. Example: A doctor takes you aside and tells you she's sure your friend Susan has cancer, but she tells Susan, "I won't know anything until the diagnosis is made by the lab next week." When Susan begs you to tell her what the doctor knows, what do you do? If you tell her you don't know, you're lying. If you tell her what the doctor told you, you risk breaking Susan's trust in her doctor.
- **Moral distress:** You know the right thing to do, but institutional constraints make it nearly impossible to do what is right. Example: You think a patient isn't ready for discharge because his wife is unprepared to care for him. When you report this problem to the physician, you're told the hospital has "no choice" but to discharge him. What do you do?

Did you know what to do in the above examples? If so, on what did you base your decisions? Gut feelings? Personal values? Professional standards?

Making moral and ethical decisions requires knowledge of personal values, ethical principles, and codes, as discussed in the next section. As a nurse, you must know the standards and principles that guide moral and ethical reasoning—and be able to justify your actions to others in a professional way.

Seven Ethical Principles

There are seven ethical principles you should apply when making ethical decisions.

1. **Autonomy.** People have the right to self-determination and to make legally acceptable decisions based on (a) their own values and beliefs, (b) adequate information that is given free from coercion, and (c) sound reasoning that considers all the alternatives.
2. **Beneficence.** Aim to benefit others and avoid harm.
3. **Justice.** Treat all people fairly, and give what is due or owed.
4. **Fidelity.** Keep promises, and don't make promises you can't keep.
5. **Veracity (truth telling).** Be honest and tell the truth.
6. **Confidentiality.** Keep information private. This is now *law* according to Health Insurance Portability and Accountability Act (HIPAA) privacy rules.
7. **Accountability.** Accept responsibility for the consequences of your actions.

Standards, Ethics Codes, and Patients' Rights

Standards, ethics codes, and statements of patients' rights also influence how you conduct yourself as a nurse. For example, the American Nurses Association's (ANA's) *Code of Ethics* stresses that nurses must do the following:[1-2]

- **Practice with compassion and respect for each person's dignity, worth, and unique individuality.** This applies to co-workers, families, and patients, regardless of the nature of health problems present, socio-economic status, or culture.
- **Keep your primary commitment to consumers (patients, families, and communities).** It's your responsibility to promote, advocate, and protect the health, safety, privacy, and rights of consumers.
- **Maintain professional relationships.** Although nursing is inherently personal—often requiring a friendly attitude—maintain professional boundaries. You're the professional. The patient isn't your friend.
- **Ensure safe, effective, efficient, ethical care by collaborating with others, seeking professional opinions and delegating tasks appropriately, when needed.** Involve consumers and care providers to make shared decisions and goals. Recognize when you have an ethical dilemma that requires input from qualified ethicists. Get informed consent from patients involved in research studies.
- **Respect your own worth and dignity.** Maintain a healthy lifestyle. Strive to grow personally and professionally. Broaden your knowledge, and seek out learning experiences. Help advance the profession by contributing to practice, education, administration, and knowledge development (this improves patient care and your own worth and employability).
- **Participate in establishing, maintaining, and improving the health care environment.** Work to ensure that the physical environment and conditions of employment are conducive to providing quality health care.
- **Get involved in professional organizations.** Help clarify nursing values, shape policies, and maintain and improve the integrity of the profession and its practice.

Page 266 gives an example of a *patients' bill of rights*. Other bills of rights (e.g., pregnant patient's bill of rights, Indian patients' bill of rights, nursing home residents' bill of rights, and Veteran's Administration code of patient concern) also guide how nurses respond to ethical issues.[3] Advance Directives (Box 4-1) help us make decisions about cardiac resuscitation and other end-of-life treatments.

| **BOX 4-1** | **WHAT ARE ADVANCE DIRECTIVES?** |

Advance directives include two documents*:

1. **Living will:** Designates the types of medical treatments you would or wouldn't want in specific instances (e.g., whether you want to continue ventilator support if you become permanently unconscious).
2. **Durable power of attorney for health care (DPAHC):** Identifies who you want to make treatment decisions if there comes a time when you aren't able to do so for yourself.

Don't wait too late: Too many people wait until it's too late to address advance directives. Encourage people to talk with loved ones about what they would want if they were unable to speak for themselves. This eases the burden of making tough decisions about whether to refuse aggressive treatment that merely prolongs dying.

---

*These two documents may be combined into one document called a *combination directive.*

Steps for Moral and Ethical Reasoning

The following steps help you develop an in-depth approach to moral and ethical reasoning.*

1. **Clearly identify the ethical issues** based on the perspectives of the *key stakeholders.* Stakeholders are those who are most affected by the results of the decision. The patient's perspectives should be considered first, but families and caregivers must also be considered. For example, Mrs. Morris, an elderly woman who lives alone, tells you she doesn't want her leg amputated and that she'd rather die than live as an amputee. Mrs. Morris's daughter tells you her mother is incompetent to make this decision. Who has the right to make this decision? Is Mrs. Morris competent? Does she have the right to refuse surgery? Does the daughter have the right to overrule her mother?

2. **Clarify your personal values and how they influence your ability to participate in decision making.** For example, in Mrs. Morris's case, do you believe that no one has the right to refuse lifesaving surgery? If so, how would this affect your ability to help Mrs. Morris with this decision? If you can't be objective, let your supervisor know so that another caregiver can assist with decision making.

3. **Decide what your role will be.** Does this family rely heavily on your judgment? Do you just need to listen and help them sort out their thoughts? Who else will be involved in helping make decisions (e.g., chaplain or case manager)?

4. **Determine some possible courses of action (go "out of the box"—think about as many alternatives as you can).** Would it be possible to have the daughter come in to discuss caring for her mother? Could social services help? Should you request an ethics consult?

5. **Determine the outcomes (consequences) of each of the courses of actions you thought about.** For example, what would happen if the daughter is incapable of caring for her mother—what role could the daughter have in this case?

6. **List the courses of action, and rate them according to which choice is most likely to produce an outcome that gives greatest balance of benefits over possible harm.** To do so, don't consider "good" versus "bad." Instead, ask where each choice fits on the following scale.

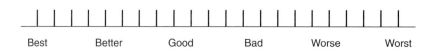

Best   Better   Good   Bad   Worse   Worst

*The author acknowledges the help of Carol Taylor, RN, PhD, Director, Center for Clinical Bioethics, Georgetown University, Washington, DC.

7. **Together with key stakeholders (patients, families, and caregivers),** develop a plan of action aimed at achieving the best outcomes based on the circumstances.
8. **Put the plan into action, and monitor patient and family responses closely.** Modify the plan if needed. The following are great Internet resources to learn more about moral and ethical reasoning.
   - American Nurses Association, Center for Ethics and Human Rights: www.nursingworld.org/ethics/
   - National Reference Center for Bioethics Literature: http://georgetown.edu/research/nrcbl/
   - American Society of Law and Ethics: www.aslme.org
   - American Society of Bioethics and Humanities: www.asbh.org
   - Nursing Ethics of Canada: www.nursingethics.ca
   - Markkula Center for Applied Ethics, Santa Clara University: www.scu.edu/SCU/Centers/Ethics/

OTHER PERSPECTIVES

TWO WOLVES IN EACH OF US

An old Indian told his grandson about a battle that goes on inside people. He said, "My son, there is a battle between two 'wolves' inside all of us. One is *Evil*. It is anger, envy, jealousy, sorrow, regret, greed, arrogance, self-pity, guilt, resentment, inferiority, lies, false pride, superiority, and ego. The other is *Good.* It is joy, peace, love, hope, serenity, humility, kindness, benevolence, empathy, generosity, truth, compassion, and faith." The boy thought about it for a minute and then asked his grandfather: "Which wolf wins?" The old Indian replied simply, "The one you feed."

Evidence-Based Practice (EBP)

Thanks to informatics (the use of computers to manage information) and hard work on the part of committed experts and researchers, care has shifted from approaches based in tradition ("we do it this way because that's the way it's always been done") to evidence-based approaches ("we do it this way because the most current evidence shows we get the best outcomes when we do it this way").

Relationship of Research to EBP

To understand the relationship between research and evidence-based practice, study the following definitions:

- **Research:** An orderly, systematic, and objective approach to creating new knowledge (and refining current knowledge) under rigorous testing conditions.[4]
- **Evidence-based practice (EBP):** Decisions and care practices that are based on the most current research *and expertise.* EBP bridges the gap between *scientific*

evidence and its *practical use* in the clinical setting. EBP integrates (1) the best research evidence, (2) knowledge from clinical experts, and (3) patient preferences into clinical practice.[5] It aims to give the most consistent and best possible care by creating clinical guidelines that are based on current evidence.[6]

Transforming Knowledge to EBP

EBP requires that knowledge be transformed by the systematic study of how evidence from research can best be *applied in practice*. Transforming knowledge from research to practice is something you don't do alone. The volume of scientific information is such that no one can do it all. You need the collaborative knowledge of a team of experts to interpret the data and decide how it can best be applied to practice.

Clinical Summaries

Many research articles can be too in-depth and scholarly for "everyday nurses" to understand. For this reason, there is more use of clinical summaries to make research more useable.[7] This section explains the work that goes into transforming knowledge from research into useful clinical information that is integrated into actual care practices.

ACE Star Model of Knowledge Transformation

Figure 4-1 on the next page shows the ACE (Academic Center for Evidence-Based Practice) Star Model of Knowledge Transformation. In this model, research evidence moves through the following cycles and then is combined with other knowledge and integrated into practice.[8]

1. **Discovery:** New knowledge is discovered through traditional research and scientific inquiry.
2. **Evidence Summary:** A single, meaningful statement of the state of the science is developed (this is a complex task that takes a lot of critical thinking on the part of knowledgeable experts).
3. **Translation:** Evidence summaries are translated into practice recommendations and integrated into practice. Recommendations are made in clinical practice guidelines, care standards, clinical pathways, protocols, and algorithms.
4. **Integration:** Individual and organizational practices are changed through formal and informal channels.
5. **Evaluation:** The impact on patient health outcomes, provider and patient satisfaction, efficacy, efficiency, and economic costs is continually examined.

The ACE Star model helps ensure that care is driven by evidence, rather than tradition: It combines the best of what we know from research with the best of what we know from clinical practice to give current information that's clinically relevant.

Box 4-2 on page 126 addresses where you can find the most up to date information on clinical practice guidelines and evidenced-based practice.

ACE STAR MODEL® OF KNOWLEDGE TRANSFORMATION

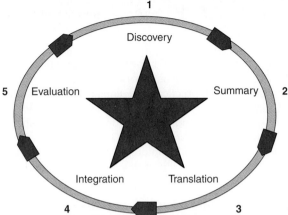

Figure 4-1 The star shows the process for developing Evidence-Based Practice (EBP)—how evidence from research moves through several cycles (discovery, summary, translation, integration, and evaluation). (Reprinted with permission from Stevens, K. R. [2004]. *ACE star model of EBP: Knowledge transformation.* Academic Center for Evidence-Based Practice. The University of Texas Health Science Center at San Antonio. Retrieved August 10, 2007, from www.acestar.uthscsa.edu.)

Nursing Research, EBP, and Critical Thinking

To give nursing care that's based on the best available knowledge, we must continue to question current practices and develop new knowledge through nursing research. Yet many nurses don't understand or value research. Often, they feel this way because they had little or no research training, the courses they took were overwhelming, or they don't have enough time and resources.[6,8]

One way to get excited about research is to start by looking at some of the significant findings from research in the past few years. For example, think about the importance of the results from following studies:

- **Traditionally, we have taught that mouth care must be done for hygiene and to prevent problems in the mouth.** Research shows that poor mouth care can result in microbes colonizing the oropharynx. This colonization is a critical factor in the development of nosocomial (hospital-acquired) pneumonia. We now know that if we don't have evidence-based guidelines for giving oral hygiene, we put patients at risk for deadly *pneumonia.*[9]
- **Nurses are concerned about inadequate registered nurse (RN) staffing.** Research shows that having more RN staff reduces the number of infections, pressure ulcers, falls, and other adverse events such as failure to rescue (deaths after complications). It reduces the length of hospital stays and promotes early detection of complications and patient and nurse satisfaction.[10-12] This type of data is very persuasive when justifying the need to hire more nurses.

BOX 4-2	CLINICAL PRACTICE GUIDELINES AND EVIDENCE-BASED PRACTICE*

What are clinical practice guidelines (CPGs)?
CPGs are recommendations for how to manage care in specific diseases, problems, or situations (for example, how to best manage smoking cessation or neonate umbilical cord care). CPGs are developed for specific use and are designed by a collaborative panel of clinical and scientific experts. When scientific evidence is sufficient, practice guidelines are obvious and clear. When scientific evidence is insufficient, other sources of knowledge—for example, wisdom gained from clinical experts or specific cases—must be brought to bear on the recommendations to fill in the gaps in the research evidence. Evidence summaries and CPGs are the essence of evidence-based practice (EBP). EBP provides mechanisms for fulfilling our social responsibility to provide the best care in the most effective and affordable way. Find many helpful links and resources at www.acestar.uthscsa.edu/.

What are the best EBP websites for updating practice standards?
For evidence summaries, the two best resources are the Agency for Healthcare Research and Quality (AHRQ), found at www.ahrq.gov/, and the Cochrane Library, found at www.cochrane.org/resources/brochure.htm and www.update-software.com/publications/cochrane/. For CPGs, the most definitive source is the National Guideline Clearinghouse (NGC), found at www.guideline.gov/. The NGC is a publicly available electronic repository of clinical practice guidelines, easily searchable by clinical topic.

How do you best use the information on these websites?
AHRQ offers free access to evidence summaries and reports (on its home page, click on Evidence-Based Practice, then see listings under Evidence Reports). They also archive CPGs developed from 1992-1996. If you access archived CPGs, use the information only after updating them with the latest research on the topic. The Cochrane Library produces systematic reviews, which give a single statement that summarizes the state of the science and draws on all research on a given topic. A systematic review is the strongest level of evidence for clinical decisions. You can find evidence summaries through bibliographic databases (such as CINAHL) by limiting results of the search to "publication type: systematic review." Full-text summaries are available only through subscription. Using online data bases takes a lot of critical thinking—you need to have a knowledgeable, analytical, creative mind to apply the content in the context of each specific person and situation.

---

*The terms *clinical practice guideline, practice standard,* and *protocol* are sometimes used interchangeably. All three terms address how care should be managed in certain situations. Answers to questions provided by Kathleen R. Stevens, RN, EdD, FAAN, Director, Academic Center for Evidence-based Practice (ACE), The University of Texas Health Science Center at San Antonio (www.acestar.uthscsa.edu).

■ **Restraining patients may create the very problems we're trying to avoid.** Many assume that restraining patients protects them from injury. One study shows that restrained patients are more likely to (1) sustain serious injury when they fall, (2) be hospitalized twice as long as those who aren't restrained, and (3) die during hospitalization than patients who are not restrained. It also shows that restraints contribute to depression, anger, nosocomial (hospital-acquired) infection, pressure ulcers, and deconditioning—all of which leave patients in a worse condition than before they were admitted.[13]

Studies like this one have resulted in major revisions to standards that aim to increase safety by reducing the use of restraints and seclusion. Standards now restrict the use of restraints and seclusion to emergency situations in which there's imminent risk that the individual may physically harm himself or others. Even then, restraints are to be used only as a last resort.[14]

Nursing research is a rigorous, disciplined use of critical thinking. Researchers need highly developed critical thinking skills—from knowing how to clearly identify the issue to be studied to determining the best way to collect meaningful data, to analyzing and interpreting statistical data.[15] Although it's beyond the scope of this book to address how to actually *conduct research studies*, this section addresses staff nurses' roles in research and EBP. Let's start by addressing frequently asked questions.

Frequently Asked Questions about Staff Nurses' Role

Q. If I'm a student or staff nurse, what are my responsibilities related to research and EBP?

A. As a staff nurse, you have five main responsibilities:

1. **Think analytically about the situations you encounter** and seek out evidence of findings that might improve nursing care. For example, if you frequently care for people with postoperative leg edema after heart bypass surgery, you should be asking, *I wonder if there are any new studies explaining why this happens and what can be done about it?*

2. **Know the rationale behind your actions:** How strong is the evidence that supports what you do? For example, are the rationales behind your actions supported by clinical practice guidelines? A textbook? Your instructor? You may not always have "hard clinical evidence" to support your actions, but you should be completely aware of the strength of the evidence. There are various rating systems for determining strength of evidence. The following ABC scale, adapted from www.aafp.org, is an example of a useful scale.

   - **Level A:** Actions are supported by a high-quality randomized controlled trial (RCT) that considers all important outcomes.
   - **Level B:** Actions are supported by other evidence (e.g., well-designed clinical trials; lower quality RCTs; case-controlled studies with nonbiased selection of study participants and consistent findings; other evidence).
   - **Level C:** Actions **are** supported by consensus/expert opinion (consensus viewpoint or expert opinion).

3. **Raise questions** that might prompt a researcher to formulate a question to guide a study. For example, you could ask your manager, "Since we seem to be having an increase in infections, should we study our procedure for hand sanitizing. Is it convenient? Are we applying EBP?"

4. **Help researchers collect data.** If you're asked to complete a questionnaire or to chart specific data for research purposes, it's your professional

responsibility to do so, diligently and accurately, as long as it doesn't interfere with nursing care.

5. **Acquire and share knowledge** related to research and EBP. We must constantly ask ourselves questions like *Am I making time to become familiar with EBP related to the clinical situations in which I'm involved?* and *Do I interact with others (peers, educators) to learn more about research and EBP?* If you find reading research articles tedious, get started by talking with peers and educators or perhaps joining a journal club. This helps you to learn in a dynamic, stimulating environment. Once you learn the basics, reading research articles becomes easier, more interesting, and even an enjoyable challenge!

Q. If I have limited knowledge of research, how do I know whether there are results from research studies that I should be using in my practice?

A. As a student or staff nurse, it's important that you ask your leaders and educators for help with finding and using research articles. However, be sure that you understand the following basic facts about choosing useful research articles and information:

- Decide whether the studies are valid and reliable (i.e., whether it was conducted in such a way that you can trust that the results are accurate). Consider whether there's vested interest on the part of the researchers or publishers. For example, how often have you heard a commercial that proclaims, "In a recent research study, our product was proven to be more effective than the other leading products"? Do you believe every one of these commercials? Probably not. Think independently, and ask questions.

- Choose refereed or peer-reviewed journals (journals that publish articles only after they've been reviewed by peer experts). Whether or not a journal is peer-reviewed is usually found in the front of the journal where you find information like who's on the editorial board, who's the publisher, and so on. These journals are more likely to have reliable information.

- Use the following Web pages to keep up to date on new research:
  - Nursing Spectrum National Institute of Nursing Research News: http://nsweb.nursingspectrum.com/NurseNewsEzine/NINR/index.cfm
  - The National Institute of Nursing Research: www.nih.gov/about/almanac/organization/NINR.htm
  - Also see the websites in Box 4-2 *(Clinical Practice Guidelines and Evidence-Based Practice)* on page 126

- You can find a self-paced tutorial and refresher for research for beginners at http://library.nyu.edu/research/health/tutorial/beginners.htm.

Scanning before Reading Research Articles

Knowing how to scan research articles saves you time. You can quickly eliminate irrelevant articles, giving you more time to focus on ones that *are* relevant. Here are some steps to systematically scan articles so you can choose the ones most relevant to your needs.

1. **Read the abstract first:** This summarizes the issues, the methods, and the results. If the abstract isn't applicable to your clinical problem, you might choose to read no further.

2. **If the abstract seems applicable, skip to the end of the article,** and then scan the article by reading the content under the following headings, in the order listed here:
    - Summary (may also be listed as Conclusions)
    - Discussion
    - Nursing Implications
    - Suggestions for Further Research

    You may be able to eliminate articles just by reading the content under any of the above headings.

3. **If what you scanned is relevant, go on to read the entire study.** Give yourself plenty of time, and don't be discouraged if you find sections you don't understand. Instead, take notes on what you do understand. Come back to the more difficult sections at another time, after getting help from an expert or textbook (or both).

4. **After you read the article,** ask yourself whether you understand the following:
    - What's already known about the topic?
    - What did the researchers study, and why and how did they study it?
    - What did they find out, and are the results valid?
    - What do results imply, and how do they apply to my particular clinical situation?
    - Might the study be biased (for example, when drug companies fund a study, there may be a vested interest)?
    - How do the results of the study compare with the results of other, similar studies? (If other studies produced similar findings, the probability that the results are reliable increases.)

Questioning Care Practices: Promoting Inquiry and Creativity

Too many nurses continue to do things based on tradition without going "out of the box" and questioning care practices. Don't settle for the status quo. Question what you do, why you do it, what your patients' experiences are, and how patient care and nurses' jobs can be improved. Use the following strategies to promote inquiry and creativity:

1. On a bulletin board, post a blank paper with "What Do You Want to Know?" at the top. For example, someone might write, "Does anyone know the most recent information on managing wound infections?"
2. Make reading research articles convenient. If you find a good article, post it on the bulletin board, and ask people to initial that they've read it. Reward nurses who bring in useful literature.
3. Encourage nurses to critique practice protocols, and make suggestions for improvement.
4. Join an Internet listserv where nurses with common interests share questions and information.
5. Keep a real or virtual suggestion box: Reward nurses who raise questions or come up with creative, practical solutions.

Surveillance and Quality Improvement

Most facilities have risk managers and quality improvement (QI) nurses who are in charge of surveillance and improving care quality. Surveillance, in the context of QI, is defined as "monitoring patients and systems for the presence of factors that cause delays in treatment or increase the likelihood of illness or harm."

Bedside nurses are in the unique position of being able to identify overall system problems that affect patient care. They bring important insights into deciding whether care practices are practical, uniform, and timely. For example, in one case, nurses noted that medications were always arriving late from the pharmacy. They did a study that showed that delays in medication administration increased the length of hospital stays. As a result, policies and procedures changed to ensure that medications came to the units in a timely way, ultimately shortening patients' length of stay.

QI studies seek to improve health care delivery by evaluating three different aspects of care:

1. **Outcomes** evaluation (studies *results*). *Example:* Studying the number of respiratory complications in postoperative patients
2. **Process** evaluation (studies *how* care was given). *Example:* Studying how frequently the respiratory status of patients was assessed and whether care was managed by a registered nurse
3. **Structure** evaluation (studies *the setting* in which care was given). *Example:* Studying the locations of the rooms of patients who had respiratory complications in relation to closeness to the nurses' station

Studying *all three* of these aspects gives you a comprehensive analysis that helps you improve practice. If you only examine outcomes (results), you won't be able to improve efficiency. You could be getting great outcomes, but there may be more efficient, cost-effective ways to achieve them.

Your responsibilities related to surveillance and QI are the same as the previously listed responsibilities for research and EBP. You can find ready-to-use tools for measuring and improving the quality of health care in the Agency for Healthcare Research and Quality's (AHRQ's) Quality Tools website (www.qualitytools. ahrq.gov).

CRITICAL THINKING EXERCISES

Note: Exercises followed by asterisks(*) have example responses listed in the Response Key *on page 253.*

Moral and Ethical Reasoning Exercises

1. In the following *Other Perspective,* three "unheard screams" are addressed. What might be considered the fourth "unheard scream"?*

OTHER PERSPECTIVES

UNHEARD SCREAMS

In "Unheard Screams," Jacqui Scipio-Bannerman, RNC—a manager at a Women and Children's Health Clinic—tries to persuade an HIV-positive, pregnant teenager to agree to highly active antiviral therapy (HAART).[18] After taking a deep breath to calm her own emotions, Jacqui said, "I can't tell you what to do. I can only support your decision. But I can tell you that infants have a much worse time dealing with HIV than adults. Whatever difficulties you have with the virus or the medication, multiply them and think about your baby having them. There are no guarantees with or without the medication. But you must be prepared to deal with the consequences of whatever choice you make." Jacqui and the doctor waited for a response. There was none. The young patient snatched the prescriptions and left the room. Jacqui felt that in that quiet room, there were silent screams. The patient was screaming her fear. The nurse was screaming her anger. The infectious disease physician was screaming his frustration. As loud as their screams were, in that little room you couldn't hear a sound.

2. What would you do if you were "Me" in the following scenario*:

Scenario
WHAT WOULD YOU DO?

My father was admitted to an intensive care unit and wasn't expected to live. I was approached by a physician, who asked, "Do you want us to resuscitate him if he arrests again?" Since my father never wanted to talk about these things, I didn't know what he'd want. I also didn't feel it was my place to answer. I called my mother and asked her the question. Here's how the conversation went:

Me: "Mom, they want to know if they should resuscitate Dad if he arrests again."

Mom: "You don't know what you're asking me."

Me: "Yes, I do. I know it's hard, but you're supposed to speak in *his* voice. Not what *you* want—what you think *he* wants."

Mom: "That's the problem. All my life when I've tried to guess his decisions, he's always done just the opposite. Even when I've said to myself, 'I think he'll do (whatever) only because it's the opposite of what I think he'd do,' I've still been wrong."

3. Which of the seven moral and ethical principles (autonomy, beneficence, justice, fidelity, veracity, confidentiality, accountability) apply to the following statement? More than one may apply.*

    By choosing to be a nurse, you must see that your patients receive competent care.

4. Get in touch with end-of-life issues. In a journal or in a group, discuss your thoughts on the following article: Penny, J. End of life care: When twilight draws near. Retrieved March 27, 2007 from www.onlinece.net/courses.asp?c ourse5237&action5view.

5. Decide where you stand in relation to achieving the following learning outcomes from page 117.

    a. Develop or adopt a personal code of conduct based on your personal values and content in this chapter.

    b. Compare and contrast the terms *moral reasoning* and *ethical reasoning*.*

    c. Make prudent decisions based on ethical principles, codes, and practice standards. To evaluate your ability to achieve this outcome, apply the *10 Key Questions* on the inside back cover to the following scenario.

Scenario
**WHAT
WOULD
YOU DO?**

The LaRusas have cared for their 40-year-old daughter, Marilou, at home for 20 years, since she became totally comatose after a car accident. All diagnostic studies indicate that Marilou will never regain consciousness. The LaRusas are almost 80 years old. Because they are concerned that they won't be able to care for her, they are considering stopping tube feedings and allowing her to die. Because the family has relied heavily on your decisions for the past 5 years, they ask you what to do. How can you best help the LaRusas make this decision?

Evidence-Based Practice Exercises

1. Find a research article on a topic you find interesting. Then do the following:
   a. Summarize in your own words what the researchers studied, what they found, how it might be used in practice, and what questions are raised by the summary.
   b. Determine where you can find out more about the research topic.
   c. Decide whether you can safely apply the findings to practice, or whether you need expert advice.
   d. List some questions that reading the article raises.
2. Together with a partner or group, discuss the self-paced tutorial and refresher for research for beginners at http://library.nyu.edu/research/health/tutorial/beginners.htm.
3. Explain why it's important to do QI studies from the following perspectives, and then give an example for each type of study:
   a. Outcomes evaluation (focuses on results)
   b. Process evaluation (focuses on how care was given)
   c. Structure evaluation (focuses on setting)
4. Learn more about transforming knowledge to evidence-based practice. With a partner or in a group, go to www.acestar.uthscsa.edu/Learn_model.htm and discuss the eight underlying principles of knowledge transformation, and the various phases of the ACE Star Model shown on page 125.
5. With a partner, or in a group, apply the 10 critical thinking questions on the inside back cover to nursing research and evidence-based practice.
6. Compare where you stand in relation to being able to achieve the following learning out comes from page 117.
   a. Explain the relationship between nursing research and evidence-based practice (EBP).*
   b. Describe your responsibilities in relation to nursing research, EBP, surveillance, and QI.*
   c. Explain why it's important to choose refereed (peer-reviewed) journals when looking for research articles.*

Teaching Others: Promoting Independence

Your role as a teacher—helping patients, families, and peers to acquire the knowledge and skills they need to be independent—can be one of the most rewarding, time-saving, and cost-effective things you do. Patients are discharged "quicker and sicker" than they were in the past, and many are managing complex problems independently at home—they need competent, knowledgeable teachers.

Whether you're dealing with patients, students, or peers, being an effective teacher requires working closely together with the learners to identify (1) what must be learned, (2) how they want to learn it, and (3) what resources can best be used to facilitate learning. The following steps can help you think critically about how to teach others.

10 Steps for Teaching Others

1. Determine the desired outcome(s) together with the learner. What exactly must the person be able to do when you complete your teaching? *Example:* The person will be able to regulate insulin dosage based on blood glucose readings.

2. Find out what the person already knows and then decide (1) what exactly the person must learn to achieve the desired outcome and (2) how much time you have before the person must know it.
   - Determine readiness to learn: Ask what the biggest concerns are, and listen carefully.
   - Determine preferred learning styles (e.g., doing, observing, listening, or reading on page 58) and use this information to plan teaching. *Example:* If you're teaching injection technique to *doers*, have them start by doing something, like handling a syringe. If they'd rather read, start by giving them a pamphlet.
   - Identify barriers to learning (e.g., consider language, reading skills, developmental problems, or problems with motivation).
   - Encourage people to ask questions, get involved, and let you know how they'd like to learn. *Example:* "Let me know if you have a better way of learning this. Not everyone learns the same way."

3. Reduce anxiety by offering support. *Example:* "Everyone is nervous when first learning to change dressings, but once you've done it a couple of times, it will be much easier."

4. Minimize distractions, and teach at appropriate times. Pick a quiet room, and choose times when the learners are likely to be comfortable and rested.

5. Use pictures, diagrams, and illustrations. These visual aids enhance comprehension and are better remembered.

6. Create mental images by using analogies and metaphors. *Example:* "Insulin is like a key that opens the cell's door to allow sugar to enter. If you don't have the key (insulin), the sugar can't get into the cell. The cell starves, and sugar accumulates in the blood, damaging kidneys and vessels."

7. Encourage people to remember by using whatever words best trigger their mind. *Example:* Someone may say, "I need to have three things: the soaking-dressing stuff, the scrubbing stuff, and the after-dressing stuff."

8. Keep it simple. The explain-it-to-me-as-if-I-were-a-10-year-old approach works especially well for complex situations. If you can't make it simple, you're not ready to teach it.

9. Tune into your learners' responses and change the pace, techniques, or content if needed. If they don't remember important content, take time to review it; if they don't seem to understand what you're saying, write it down or draw a picture.

10. Summarize key points, and don't leave learners empty-handed. Even the best learners may have trouble remembering what they just learned. Give them the important points in print or on videotape so that they can refresh their memory later.

CRITICAL MOMENTS

TEACHING "WHY" PROMOTES INDEPENDENCE

Knowing *why* something must be done empowers people to problem solve independently. Always explain the principles and rationales for treatments. If they know the reasons behind the treatments, they'll be able to make decisions about what to do when things go wrong.

Teaching Yourself: Grab the Spoon

I used to love to be spoon-fed information. I didn't know how to teach myself, and I wanted teachers to do it. Then I learned how to teach myself. I realized that often teachers were trying to "feed me" more than I could learn at one time. Sometimes they "fed me" in a different order than I wanted, and sometimes it felt like I got "food" all over my face but not in my brain. Now I know that I can teach myself better than anyone else can—I grab the spoon and feed myself.

This section helps you learn how to grab the spoon and feed yourself. When you know how to teach yourself, you save time and feel more intelligent and confident. You learn in ways that help you understand deeply. Therefore, you *remember* what you learn.

When you encounter something new, take charge and reason your way through the learning experience. Apply the strategies in this section and be confident in your ability to learn. Don't be afraid to ask questions. Remember, you are your own best teacher

Memorizing Effectively

Critical thinking takes more than memorizing facts—you must know how to *apply* information in context of various situations. Still, learning how to memorize effectively does enhance your ability to think critically: You must be able to *recall facts* to progress to *higher levels* of thinking, such as knowing *how to apply and analyze information*. For example, if you aren't able to recall what *normal* health assessment findings are, you won't be able to analyze your patient's data to decide whether there are any *abnormal* findings. Because nursing requires a lot of memorization, especially in the beginning, use the following strategies to memorize and learn efficiently.

Learning and Memorization Strategies

1. **Remember the "use it or lose it" rule.** If you haven't been using information, refresh your memory by using it again. An example of "use it or lose it" is when you forget your multiplication tables because you depend on calculators without doing the math on your own now and then.
2. **Work to *understand* information before you try to memorize it.** Once you make sense of the information, you can identify the most important things to remember.
3. **Don't try to memorize *everything*.** Separate the most important things from all the other information. Looking at the most important things, lifted out, removes clutter and helps you avoid the problem of TMI (too much information).
4. **Look for *relationships* between the facts, and group related facts together.** Your brain remembers *groups of information* better than *isolated facts*. This is like putting information in folders, rather than cluttering your desktop with individual documents. Looking for relationships between and among the facts also helps you *remember* because you are *using* the information. Mind mapping (concept mapping) is great for helping you see relationships (see pages 263-265).
5. **Create a memory hook—put the information into context.** For example, suppose you're studying *pneumonia* in class, and you cared for "Fred" who had pneumonia when you were doing your clinical experience. Visualize "Fred" and how he compared with the textbook picture ("Fred" becomes your memory hook).

    If you don't have a real situation to connect with, play around with the information until something comes to mind that helps you remember (e.g., a rhyme, a picture, a story). For example:

    - **Use a mnemonic** (a memory jog that makes an association between something that's easy to remember and something that's hard to remember). *Example:* TACIT helps you remember what to assess for medications (Therapeutic effect, Allergic or Adverse reactions, Contraindications, Interactions, Toxicity/overdose).

- **Create an acrostic** (a catchy phrase that helps you remember the first letters of the information you're trying to remember). *Example: Maggie chewed nuts every place she went* gives the first letters of things you must assess in neurovascular assessment: movement, color, numbness, edema, pulses, sensation, and warmth.

6. **Use your preferred learning style and as many senses as possible.** *Examples:* (1) Say words as you write and read them. (2) Sing what you're trying to remember to the tune of a favorite song. (3) Light a scented candle. (4) Play your favorite music.

7. **Organize and reorganize information.** This helps you see different patterns, and you remember because you're *using* the information.

8. **Review the information briefly before going to sleep.** Studies show that even if you're a "morning person," information moves into long-term memory better if reviewed late in the day, immediately before going to bed.

9. **Quiz yourself *without* your notes.** Just because you can *recognize* information in your notes, it doesn't mean you'll be able to *recall* it without your notes.

10. **Know yourself and use self-discipline.** Identify the circumstances that help you retain information and plan your schedule to include those circumstances. If you study better in the morning, go to bed early enough that you can get up early and feel rested. If you're easily distracted or sidetracked, turn off your cell phone and e-mail. Go to the library or put a *Don't Disturb* sign on your door.

11. **Seek out mentors and role models**—teachers, other nurses, friends, and peers. They help you clarify your thoughts and set goals better than any textbook.

CRITICAL MOMENTS

TEACHING OTHERS HELPS YOU LEARN
When you want to learn something, offer to teach it to someone else. You learn and recall best what you teach someone *else.*

Test Taking: Improving Grades and Passing the First Time

Test taking can be frustrating and anxiety-producing. We all have been in the position of knowing something well, yet struggling on the test. Many complex, creative critical thinkers struggle with trying to "match" right answers on a test. Lots of us can reason well in real situations but struggle with test taking. As a friend once said to me, "I need to be in real situations to think well." This section helps you use critical thinking to identify the best way to prepare for—and take—tests. Using the strategies in this section can help you reduce test anxiety, improve your confidence and grades, and pass tests on the first try.

Strategies for Successful Test Taking

Staying up on course work and studying each week—rather than cramming at the end of courses—is a key for doing well on exams. But it isn't the *only* key. Good test-taking skills are equally as important. This section gives general strategies to use when taking any test, followed by specific strategies for taking NCLEX and other standard tests.

Preparing For Tests

- **Know yourself.** Identify your usual test-taking behaviors (e.g., do you get overly anxious? Do you tend to run out of time? Are you better at one type of test than another?). Seek help for areas you'd like to change.
- **Know the test plan.** Find out what types of questions are going to be asked and what information is the most important to study. If the teacher doesn't share this information, review course objectives, text objectives, and summaries—often these will help you decide what's most important.
- **Find out how long you have to take the test,** what resources you're allowed to bring, and whether you get penalized for guessing.
- **Prepare with an attitude of, "I can do this—I just have to figure out how."** You *are* capable. Sometimes you need to remind yourself of this to acquire the positive attitude that's so important.
- **Get organized and budget your time.** Decide what you need to study, what your resources are (for example, notes, books, tutors, peers), and when and how you'll prepare for the test.
- **Join a study group**—be sure the group stays on task and on time.
- **Know the parts of a question, how to read questions, and how to make educated guesses** (See Boxes 4-3 and 4-4 on pages 139 and 140).
- **Practice taking the test under the same conditions you will experience when you actually take it.** For example, if it's a computerized test, practice on the computer.

Taking Tests

- **Arrive early for warm-up.** Give yourself time to calm down, get focused, and scan your review materials. Reviewing practice questions is also a good way to get your brain in test-taking gear.
- **Pay attention to verbal and written instructions.** Jot down notes to be sure you remember the instructions.
- **If allowed, skim the whole test and plan your approach.** For example, begin by answering the types of questions you *like* before tackling types you *don't like* (you may like matching questions better than essay). *Completing what you like and know first* reduces anxiety and gets your brain in the test-taking mode before you tackle more difficult questions.
- **Watch your time, and note how the questions are weighted.** If a question is worth 50% of your grade, you might want to save 50% of your time to work on that question.

BOX 4-3	TEST QUESTION COMPONENTS

1. **The background statement(s):** The statements or phrases that tell you the *context* in which you're expected to answer the question (e.g., the words in italics in the following example):
   Example test question: You're caring for *someone who has severe asthma, is wheezing loudly, is confused, and can't sleep.* You check the orders and note that a sedative can be given for sleeplessness. Knowing the possible effects of giving a sedative to an asthmatic, <u>*what would you do?*</u>
   a. Give the sedative to help the patient relax.
   b. Withhold the sedative, because it aggravates asthma.
   c. Withhold the sedative, and monitor the patient closely.
   d. Give the sedative, but monitor the patient carefully.
2. **The stem:** A phrase that asks or states the intent of the question (e.g., the underlined words above)
3. **Key concepts:** The most important concepts addressed in the background statement(s). In the example above, the key concepts are "severe asthma," "wheezing loudly," and "effects of giving a sedative to an asthmatic."
4. **Key word(s):** The words that specify what's being asked and what's happening. In the example above, the key words are "severe," "loudly," and "confused." These words specify that the asthma problem is severe. "Would you do" specifies that you're being asked for an appropriate action to take.
5. **The options (choices):** These include one correct answer (called the keyed response) and three to five distracters (incorrect answers). In the example above, (c) is the keyed response, and the rest are distracters.

- **Focus on what you know.**
  1. If allowed, skip difficult questions and come back to them later. Mark the easy questions and do them first.
  2. For essay tests and short-answer questions: (1) Jot down key points you need to address before writing your essay. When you finish, check your essay to be sure you hit all the major points. (2) If you have time at the end, come back to these questions and ask yourself, *What else can I say?* or *What did I miss?*
- **If you don't understand a question, ask for clarification.** If **you're** not allowed to ask questions during the test, write something like, "I wasn't sure what you meant so I'm answering the question assuming you meant...." If allowed, write this on your answer sheet.
- **When in doubt, don't change answers.** Your first response is more likely to be correct.
- **For case history questions, read the questions about the case history *first.*** Then read the histories, looking for the answers.
- **If you're stuck on a question,** try sketching a picture, map, or diagram to help you conceptualize the answer.

BOX 4-4	GUIDELINES FOR MAKING EDUCATED GUESSES

Definition of an educated guess: *Applying test-taking strategies to choose a right answer when you're unsure from content alone (when none of the options seem to jump out at you)*

1. Be sure you understand the test directions.
2. Find out whether you're penalized for guessing.
3. Read the question *twice*, asking yourself the following:
    *   **What** does the stem ask (see Test Question Components, Box 4-3, page 139)
    *   **Who** is the client? (age, sex, role, etc.)
    *   **What** is the problem? (diagnosis, signs, symptoms, behavior, etc.)
    *   **What rationale** is offered in the question? (e.g., to prevent respiratory complications… Because the cast is damp…)
    *   **What time frame** is being addressed? (e.g., immediately before surgery, on the day of admission, or when?)
4. Study all the answers.
    *   Eliminate answers you know are outright wrong.
    *   Look for answers that are wrong based on the directions.
    *   Look for clues in the questions or answers that might help you narrow it down further to the most likely best answer (see strategies 5 and 6 below).
5. Use the following rules together with your knowledge to make educated guesses:
    *   **Initial** = **Assessment**. The word *initial* used in a question usually requires an assessment answer. (What would you assess?)
    *   **Essential** = **Safety**. The word *essential* used in a question usually requires a safety answer. (What's required for safety?) Remember: "Keep them breathing, keep them safe."
    *   **Opposites Attract Right Answers.** If you have two answers that are opposite to one another, the *right* answer is usually *one* of the two opposites.
        Example: The correct answer below is likely to be (a) or (b) because they're *opposites*.
        a. Turn the client on to the right side.   c. Encourage fluids.
        b. Turn the client on to the left side.   d. Ambulate the client.
    *   **Odd Man Wins.** The option that's most different in length, style, or content is usually the right answer. The right answer is often the longest one or the shortest one. *Example:* The correct answer below is likely to be (b) because it's the "odd man."
        a. Decreased temperature   c. Decreased respirations
        b. Rapid pulse   d. Decreased blood pressure
    *   **Same Answer** = **Neither One**. If two responses say the same thing in different words, they can't both be right, so neither one is right. *Example:* Tachycardia and rapid heartbeat as two answer options
    *   **Repeated Words Means Right**. If the answer contains the same word (or a synonym) that appears in the question, it's more likely to be a correct response. *Example:* The word *hypotension* in question, the word *hypotension* or *shock* in answer.
    *   **Absolutely Not.** Answers that use "absolutes" aren't usually the right response. *Example:* always, never, all, none.
    *   **Generally So.** Answers that use qualifiers that make the response more "generally so" tend to signify right answers. *Examples:* usually, frequently, often.
6. When answering questions about setting priorities, remember Maslow's Hierarchy of Needs (Box 5-3, page 182).

Adapted from Alfaro-LeFevre, R. Workshop handouts. Strategies developed with the help of Judith Miller (http://judymillernclexreview.com) and Deanne Blach (www.DeanneBlach.com).

After the Test

- **If you do poorly, don't think it's the end of the world.** Even the best minds have failed tests (Einstein flunked algebra; Edison was considered unteachable). Instead, *do* something. Explain your difficulty to your instructor; ask for suggestions on how to prepare better or whether you can do extra credit work.
- **If there's a test review, be sure to go—you'll *learn*.** Too many students think that this is an opportunity to skip class, since "nothing much will be happening."

Strategies for NCLEX and Other Standard Tests*

The following summarizes important points on NCLEX and gives strategies for taking standard tests such as certification exams.

Fast Facts on NCLEX

- Based on surveys of skills that new graduates must have (surveys are done every 3 years)
- Taken on computer; takes up to 6 hours. As soon as you answer enough questions to predict that you will pass or fail, the computer shuts down. You answer a minimum of 75 questions, 15 of these are being tested for reliability. The maximum number of questions is 265.
- Questions require analysis and application. If you answer easy questions correctly, you move on to higher level questions. You can't go back and change answers. Don't skip questions—try your best on each one. Pace yourself at about 1 minute per question.
- Types of questions:
  1. The majority are multiple-choice questions that require selection of one answer.
  2. There are a few "alternate item questions": these require selecting one or more responses, filling in the blank (including calculation and prioritizing questions), or clicking and dragging the mouse to select a "hot spot."
  3. All items may include charts, tables, or graphs.
- Integrates four processes throughout:
  1. Nursing process
  2. Teaching and learning
  3. Caring
  4. Communication and documentation
- Addresses the following needs:
  1. Safe, effective care, including care management (21%-33% of the test)
  2. Safety and infection control (8%-14% of the test)

---

*Adapted from Alfaro-LeFevre, R. Workshop handouts. Strategies developed with the help of Judith Miller (http://judymillernclexreview.com) and Deanne Blach (www.DeanneBlach.com).

  3. Health promotion and maintenance (6%-12% of the test)
  4. Psychosocial integrity (6%-12% of the test)
  5. Physiologic integrity (around 50% of the test)
  6. Basic care and comfort (6%-12% of the test)
  7. Pharmacology and intravenous (IV) therapy (13%-19% of the test)
  8. Risk reduction (13%-19% of the test)
  9. Physiologic adaptation (11%-17% of the test)
- Stresses assessment and monitoring (safe, effective care)
  1. Preprocedure, intraprocedure, and postprocedure assessment
  2. Pre–drug administration, intra–drug administration, and post–drug administration assessment
  3. Delegation (what should you delegate, to whom, and when?)
  4. Prioritization (what should you do first?)
- Includes questions on all major specialties, as well as advance directives, injury prevention, family systems, cultural diversity, legal rights and responsibilities, error prevention, bioterrorism, disaster response, human sexuality, and mental health.

Preparing for NCLEX

- Get review books early, and use them as you progress through your program. This helps you be familiar with the types of questions you will have to answer and also helps you learn.
- Complete at least 2000 computerized practice questions, since this will significantly increase your chances of passing the first time. Pages 279-286 give example practice questions you can try.
- To increase learning and retention, when you get a question wrong, look up the information immediately so that you understand *why* you chose the incorrect response.
- Be sure you reviewed the general strategies for test taking listed earlier in this section.
- For Internet resources for studying and test taking, see http://evolve.elsevier.com/Alfaro-LeFevre/CT.

CRITICAL THINKING EXERCISES

Note: Exercises followed by asterisks (*) have example responses listed in the Response Key *on page 254.*

Teaching Others, Teaching Ourselves, Test Taking

1. Giving examples from your life experience, explain how the two following *Other Perspectives* relate to you.

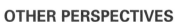

OTHER PERSPECTIVES

HOW LITERATE ARE YOU?
"The illiterate of the twenty-first century will not be those who cannot read and write, but those who cannot learn, unlearn, and relearn."—*Alvin Toffler, author of* Future Shock[19]

FIGURING THINGS OUT FOR YOURSELF: THE BEST WAY TO LEARN
Figuring things out for yourself goes something like this: "Let's see, how can I understand this? Is it to be understood on the model of this experience or that? Shall I think of it in this way or that? Let me see. Ah, I think I see. It's just so…but, no, not exactly. Let me try again. Perhaps I can understand it from this point of view…OK, now I think I'm getting it."[20]—*Author Richard Paul*

2. Explain why knowing how to teach others efficiently is essential to meeting nursing outcomes.*
3. Describe five strategies that can help you memorize effectively.*
4. Using page 58 as a guide, compare and contrast how you best learn with how learners may learn who have different learning preferences than yours.
5. With a partner, or in a group, apply the 10 critical thinking questions on the inside back cover to teaching yourself, teaching others, and test taking.
6. If you have to take NCLEX, complete the practice questions on pages 279-286.
7. Decide where you stand in relation to achieving the following learning outcomes from page 117:
   a. Use critical thinking to create individualized teaching plans.
   b. Address the roles of memorizing and reasoning in teaching ourselves.
   c. Describe at least five strategies that can help you improve your test scores and ability to pass NCLEX on the first try.

KEY POINTS / SUMMARY

- Seven principles guide ethical reasoning: autonomy, beneficence, justice, fidelity, veracity, confidentiality, and accountability.
- Practice standards, ethics codes, and bills of rights also guide ethical conduct. The following are common values addressed in ethical codes and standards: maintaining client confidentiality; acting as client advocate; delivering care in a nonjudgmental and nondiscriminatory way; being sensitive to diversity and culture; promoting autonomy, dignity, and rights; and seeking resources for solving ethical dilemmas.
- Page 122 gives steps for moral and ethical reasoning. Advance directives help us make decisions about cardiac resuscitation and other end-of-life treatments.
- EBP requires integrating (1) the best research evidence, (2) clinical expertise, and (3) patient preferences into clinical practice.
- Page 127 addresses five main responsibilities of nurses related to nursing research, surveillance, QI, and EBP.
- ACE Star Model of Knowledge Transformation (page 125) provides a framework for transforming knowledge to EBP.
- ANA standards of performance stress that nurses must apply research to practice. Morally, ethically, and professionally, we must continue to question current practices and develop new knowledge.
- Pages 127-128 answer "frequently asked questions" about staff nurses' role as it relates to research and EBP.
- QI studies examine health care from three different perspectives: (1) outcomes (evaluates results); (2) process (evaluates on how care was given), (3) structure.
- To be an effective teacher, work closely together with learners to identify (1) what must be learned, (2) how they want to learn it, and (3) what resources can best be used to facilitate learning.
- Today's workplace requires you to have excellent independent learning skills.
- Improving test performance and passing the first time requires that you know yourself, the test format, test-taking skills, and how to make educated guesses.
- Learning how to memorize effectively enhances your ability to think critically: You must be able to *recall facts* to progress to *higher levels* of thinking, such as knowing *how to apply and analyze information*.
- Pages 138-142 give strategies for successful test taking.

REFERENCES

1. American Nurses Association. (2001). *Code of ethics for nurses with interpretive statements.* Washington DC: Author.

2. Garity, J. (2005, July 26). Ethics column: "Relationship of the ANA Code of Ethics to nurses' collaborative efforts." *Online Journal of Issues in Nursing.* Retrieved March 24, 2007 from http://nursingworld.org/ojin/ethicol/ethics_16.htm.

3. Taylor, C., Lillis, C., Lamone, P. (2008). *Fundamentals of nursing: The art and science of nursing care* (6th ed.). Philadelphia: Lippincott Williams & Wilkins.

4. Jacobson, L. (January 2007). e-Mail communication.

5. Sackett, D., Straus, S., Richardson, W., Rosenberg, W., & Haynes, R. (2000). *Evidence-based medicine: How to practice and teach EBM.* Edinburgh, Scotland: Churchill, Livingstone.

6. Pravikoff, D., Annelle, B., Tanner, A., Pierce, S. T. (2005). Readiness of U.S. nurses for evidence-based practice. *American Journal of Nursing, 105*(9), 40-51.

7. Watkinson, A. (2006). Using summaries to make research more accessible. *Author Editor Newsletter.* Retrieved March 21, 2007 from http://www.nurseauthoreditr.como/article.asp?id=44.

8. Oermann, M., Floyd, J., Galvin, E., & Roop, J. (2006). Brief reports for disseminating systematic reviews to nurses. *Clinical Nurse Specialist, 20*(5), 233-238.

9. American Association of Critical Care Nurses. Practice alert: Oral care in the critically ill. *AACN News 23*(8). Retrieved April 5, 2007, from www.aacn.org/AACN/aacnnews.nsf/GetArticle/ArticleThree238#Practice%20Alert%3A%20Oral%20Care%20in%20the.

10. Horn, S., Buerhaus, P., Bergstrom, N., & Smout, R. (2005). RN Staffing time and outcomes of long-stay nursing home residents: Pressure ulcers and other adverse outcomes are less likely as RNs spend more time on direct patient care. *American Journal of Nursing, 105*(11), 58-70.

11. Kalisch, B. (2006). Missed nursing care: A qualitative study. *Journal of Nursing Care Quality, 21*(4), 306-313. Retrieved April 2, 2007, from www.nursingcenter.com/prodev/ce_article.asp?tid=671279.

12. Aiken, L., Clarke, S., Sloane, D., Sochalski, J., & Silber, J. (2002). Hospital nurse staffing and patient mortality, nurse burnout, and job dissatisfaction. *JAMA, 288*(16), 1987-1993.

13. Rogers, P., & Bocchino, N. (1999). Is it possible? *American Journal of Nursing, 99*(10), 27-34.

14. Joint Commission releases revised restraints standards for behavioral healthcare. *Medscape Medical News.* Retrieved April 5, 2007, from http://doctor.medscape.com/viewarticle/411832.

15. Burns, N., and Groves, S. (2007). *The practice of nursing research: Conduct, critique, and utilization* (6th ed.). Philadelphia: WB Saunders.

16.   American Association of Critical Care Nurses. (2007). AACN standards for establishing and sustaining healthy workplace environments. Retrieved August 10, 2007, from   www.aacn.org/aacn/pubpolcy.nsf/Files/HWEStandards/$file/HWEStandards. pdf.

17.   Riley, M. (November, 2006). e-Mail communication.

18.   Scipio-Bannerman, J. (2007) Unheard screams. Retrieved March 20, 2007, from http:// community.nursingspectrum.com/MagazineArticles/article.cfm? AID=21826.

19.   Toffler, A. (2000). In S. Thorpe *How to think like Einstein* (p. 26). Naperville, IL: Sourcebooks.

20.   Paul, R. (1993). *Critical thinking: How to prepare students for a rapidly changing world.* Santa Rosa, CA: Foundation for Critical Thinking.

Practicing Clinical Judgment Skills: Up Close and Clinical

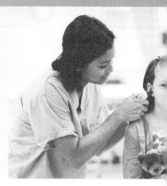

This chapter at a glance...

1. Identifying Assumptions (page 152)
2. Assessing Systematically and Comprehensively (page 155)
3. Checking Accuracy and Reliability (Validating Data) (page 159)
4. Distinguishing Normal from Abnormal and Identifying Signs and Symptoms (page 160)
5. Making Inferences (Drawing Valid Conclusions) (page 162)
6. Clustering Related Cues (Data) (page 163)
7. Distinguishing Relevant from Irrelevant (page 165)
8. Recognizing Inconsistencies (page 167)
9. Identifying Patterns (page 169)
10. Identifying Missing Information (page 170)
11. Promoting Health by Identifying and Managing Risk Factors* (page 171)
12. Diagnosing Actual and Potential Problems (page 173)
13. Setting Priorities (page 180)
14. Determining Client-Centered (Patient-Centered) Outcomes (page 184)
15. Determining Individualized Interventions (page 188)
16. Evaluating and Correcting Thinking (Self-Regulating) (page 192)
17. Determining a Comprehensive Plan/Evaluating and Updating the Plan (page 194)

---

*This skill deals with identifying risk factors in healthy people. The next skill, Diagnosing Actual and Potential Problems, deals with risk factors in the context of people with existing health problems.

Decide where you stand in relation to each of the following learning outcomes:

Learning Outcomes

After completing this chapter, you should be able to:

1. Explain why each skill in this section promotes clinical judgment.
2. Explain how to accomplish each skill in this section.
3. Describe your thinking in various situations (e.g., clearly express how you came to a conclusion or made a decision).
4. Develop a comprehensive, patient-centered plan of care.

Chapter Overview

This chapter helps you practice clinical reasoning skills in nursing situations that are based on real experiences (the names and some facts have been changed to give anonymity). Organized in logical progression according to how the skills might be used in the nursing process, each skill is presented in the following format: (1) name of the skill, (2) definition of the skill, (3) why the skill promotes clinical judgment, (4) how to accomplish the skill, and (5) practice exercises.

Clinical Judgment (Clinical Reasoning) Skills: Dynamic and Interrelated

The skills in this section are listed as *separate skills*. In real life, these skills are dynamic and interrelated. Some skills depend on—and facilitate—each other. For instance, you may *recognize inconsistencies (Skill 8 in this section)* in how someone responds to your care. This should trigger you to wonder, Have I *identified assumptions (Skill 1)?*

You think in more dynamic ways than I can describe in a book—your mind does more than one thing at a time. Think about what goes on in your head when you drive a car. You navigate the roads, adjusting to changing conditions. At the same time, you may think about what needs to be done later in the day, and even follow a radio report. It's the same with clinical reasoning skills. You often adjust your thinking on a minute-to-minute basis, considering more than one thing at a time.

As you gain experience, you'll use these skills in very dynamic ways. As a beginner, you're likely to do the first skill, *Assessing Systematically and Comprehensively*, in a methodical, step-by-step way. Later, when you have more knowledge and experience, you'll learn to *prioritize your assessment* depending on the patient's situation (addressed in *Skill 13*).

Why Practice These Skills Separately?

Think about this analogy: Tennis players practice interrelated *tennis skills* (foot placement, ball placement, swing, etc) separately to analyze and improve their *overall* game. This section helps you practice interrelated *intellectual skills* separately to help you analyze and improve your *overall ability* to reason in clinical situations. To keep the length of this chapter manageable, this chapter focuses mainly on *reasoning in the context of problems*. However, remember that critical thinking in nursing also requires you to constantly look for areas that are satisfactory, but could be improved.

How to Get the Most out of This Section

1. To get the most out of these exercises, don't try to do too many at once. Some of these exercises, as in real life, are time-consuming. The purpose of the exercises isn't to do them as quickly as possible. Rather, take your time and get in touch with your thinking. If possible, get at least one other person to complete the exercises with you. You learn more by discussing the skills with others.
2. Your brain is a tricky thing—describing what goes on in someone's head to complete each skill is difficult. If you have trouble with a section, read on and come back to it later. Explanations and practice exercises in later sections are likely to help you.
3. If you encounter diseases or drugs you don't know, look them up. This helps you build your own mental storehouse of problem-specific facts, because you apply the information to the exercise. You remember best information that you *use*.
4. Before starting this section, be sure you have a good understanding of the following terms—listed in order of how you can best learn them (you need to know the first term to understand the second term, and so on).

Required Vocabulary

Definitive diagnosis: The most specific, most correct diagnosis. For example, someone is admitted with an initial diagnosis of respiratory distress. Then, after studies are completed, the definitive diagnosis is congestive heart failure. To identify the best treatment, you must determine the most specific diagnosis.

Causative factor: Something known to create or contribute to a problem. For example, dizziness is known to cause falls.

Risk factor: Something known to cause, or be associated with, a specific problem. For example, smoking is a risk factor for cancer; having a family history of breast cancer is a risk factor for breast cancer.

Related factor: Used interchangeably with *risk factor*.

Potential problem or risk diagnosis: A problem or diagnosis that may occur because of certain risk factors present. For example, someone who's on prolonged bed rest has a potential or risk for *impaired skin integrity*. Often used interchangeably with *high-risk problem*.

Data: Pieces of information about health status. For example, vital signs.

Objective data: Information that you can clearly observe or measure. For example, a pulse of 140 beats per minute. To remember this term, remember this:

O-O: **O**bjective data are clearly **O**bservable

Subjective data: Information the patient states or communicates. These are the patient's perceptions. For example, "My heart feels like it's racing." To remember this term, remember this:

S-S: **S**ubjective data are **S**tated (or written or communicated in sign language).

Signs and symptoms: Abnormal data that prompt you to suspect a health problem. Signs are objective data. Symptoms are subjective data. For example, fever is a sign of infection; chest pain is a symptom of heart disease.

Cues: Data that trigger you to think about a certain aspect of someone's health. Often used interchangeably with signs and symptoms.

Continued

Defining characteristics: Signs and symptoms usually present with a diagnosis or problem.
Baseline data: Information collected before treatment begins.
Database assessment: Comprehensive data collection performed to gain complete information about all aspects of health status (e.g., respiratory status, neurologic status, circulatory status).
Focus assessment: Data collection that aims to gain specific (focused) information about only one aspect of health status (e.g., neurologic status).
Infer: To suspect something or to attach meaning to a cue. For example, if an infant doesn't stop crying, no matter what's done for him, you might infer that *he's in pain.*
Inference: Something we suspect to be true, based on a logical conclusion. For example, the italicized words in the preceding definition.

1. IDENTIFYING ASSUMPTIONS

Definition
Recognizing information taken for granted or presented as fact without evidence (e.g., you might assume a woman on a maternity unit has just had a baby)

Why This Skill Promotes Clinical Judgment
Clinical reasoning requires that you make judgments based on the best available evidence. This means double-checking your thinking to overcome your brain's natural tendency to grasp things at an intuitive (gut) level. By identifying assumptions, you begin to apply logic to the situation and avoid jumping to conclusions and making errors in judgment.

Guidelines: How to Identify Assumptions
The best way to identify assumptions is to *look* for them by asking questions like, What's being taken for granted here? and How do I know that I've got the facts right? *Recognizing inconsistencies, checking accuracy and reliability, identifying patterns,* and *recognizing missing information*—skills you'll practice later also help you identify assumptions.

> **RULE**
>
> Identifying assumptions requires doing a comprehensive, focused assessment. This means getting information from patient records, other caregivers, significant others, and applicable literature (e.g., information from a drug manual about medications being taken). But **always consider *your direct assessment of the patient* to be the primary source of information.**

OTHER PERSPECTIVES

AVOIDING MAKING ASSUMPTIONS

"Heightened awareness often precedes a change in behavior. For example, once you know you tend to make assumptions, you soon begin to double-check your thinking."[1]—*Carol Matz, RN, MSN*

AVOIDING ASSUMPTIONS BASED ON CULTURE

"Giving culturally competent care means being careful to avoid making assumptions about patients' beliefs based on cultural, ethnic, or religious background, alone. For example, nurses ask me if all Hispanic patients believe in the evil eye ('el mal de ojo'). The answer is, "No." Each patient—regardless of culture—is an individual, with varying levels of education, experience, and assimilation into mainstream America. Learning the common beliefs, traditions, and health practices of other cultures is important. But, to truly give culturally competent care—to help patients feel respected and supported within their own beliefs—we must *assess with an open mind* and a true desire to understand each *individual's* perspective about what's influencing that individual's health."[2]
—*Darlene N. Silver, MSN, RN, IBCLC*

Practice Exercises: Identifying Assumptions

Note: Example responses are on page 254.

1. Explain why the following statement is an assumption: We need to teach this patient how to stick to a low-salt diet because he eats whatever he wants even though his doctor told him not to eat salt.
2. What could happen if you planned nursing care based on the preceding assumption?
3. Read the following scenarios, and then answer the questions that follow them.

Scenario One

Anita plans to teach Jeff about diabetes today. She's well prepared and decides she'll create a positive attitude for Jeff by telling him about all the advances in diabetic care. She doesn't have much time, so she introduces herself and starts telling him how much easier it is to manage diabetes than it used to be. She goes on to explain how easy it is to learn the required diet, monitor blood sugar, and take insulin. Jeff listens to all Anita has to say, asks a few questions, and then leaves with his wife. As they drive off, he says to his wife in a discouraged tone, "She sure is a know-it-all, isn't she?"

a. Based on the information provided, what assumption does it seem Anita made about creating a positive attitude?

b. What key thing did Anita forget to do that might have helped her avoid making this assumption?

c. Why do you think Jeff said Anita is a know-it-all?

Scenario Two

Four-year-old Bobby is in the emergency department with his mother. He fell off his bike and had an initial period of unconsciousness lasting about a minute. He's been examined, has no skull fracture, and is now awake and alert and ready to go home with his mother. The nurse gives his mother a computer printout of instructions for checking Bobby's neurologic status and says, "Let me know if you have questions."

a. What assumption does it seem the nurse has made?

b. What might happen if the nurse's assumption is incorrect?

Scenario Three

A friend told me this story: I was working evenings in the emergency department of a seaside hospital. We admitted a 54-year-old man, whom I'll call Mr. Schmidt. He told me, "I just got here for vacation, and I'm not feeling so great. I had pneumonia at home, got treated, and thought I was better. Now my breathing feels lousy again." A check of his vital signs while he was sitting quietly revealed the following: T 99° P 138 R 36 BP 168/80. As I helped him to the stretcher, he became significantly more short of breath. I checked his lung sounds and heard a lot of congestion. I notified the physician and voiced my concern that Mr. Schmidt seemed quite ill. The doctor examined him and ordered an ECG and chest x-ray study. During this time we got very busy. I was helping another patient when the physician came to me and said, "I want you to give Mr. Schmidt 80 mg of furosemide (a diuretic) IV now and discharge him. "I looked at him skeptically and said, "Discharge him?" He said, "Yes. I'm sure the diuretic will help him get rid of this fluid." Tactfully, I asked, "Can we give him some time to see how he responds?"

The physician responded: "No. This place is wild. I'm sending him home. He's going to a private physician in the morning. He'll be fine once he gets rid of some fluid. Discharge him with instructions to call if he doesn't feel better." Reluctantly, I went to give Mr. Schmidt the furosemide. I still had trouble with the idea of sending this man home before knowing his response to the IV diuretic. Then I decided to use my own clout as a nurse: I had established a rapport with the Schmidts, and they trusted me. Before I gave the drug, I said, "I realize the doctor has discharged you, but I'd be interested to see if there's any change in blood pressure after you get rid of some fluid. How would you feel about sitting in the waiting room, and I'll check your blood pressure in an hour?" Both the Schmidts thought this was a good idea and went off to the waiting room. Only 45 minutes had passed when there was a shout for help. I ran to the waiting room and found Mr. Schmidt on the floor having a grand mal seizure. He then stopped breathing.

We were able to resuscitate Mr. Schmidt, and he was admitted to the hospital, diagnosed with electrolyte imbalance and heart failure, and discharged a week later.

a. What assumption does it seem the physician made about Mr. Schmidt's response to the furosemide?

b. Why do you think the nurse was so concerned about the assumption the physician made?

c. What assumption does it seem the nurse made about how the physician would respond to her if she cautioned him about discharging Mr. Schmidt?

2. ASSESSING SYSTEMATICALLY AND COMPREHENSIVELY

Definition
Choosing an organized, systematic approach that enhances your ability to discover all the information needed to fully understand the status of a problem or a person's health

Why This Skill Promotes Clinical Judgment
Making judgments or decisions based on incomplete information is a leading cause of mistakes. Having an organized approach to assessment prevents you from forgetting something. For example, you might be interrupted while doing a physical assessment. If you use an assessment tool to guide your assessment, you know exactly where you left off and where to continue. If you consistently use the same organized approach, you form habits that help you be systematic and complete.

Guidelines: How to Assess Systematically and Comprehensively
Being *purposeful and focused* is the key to knowing how to assess systemically and comprehensively: You must decide the purpose of your assessment and choose an approach that gets the information needed to *achieve your purpose*. For example, doctors' assessments usually focus on identifying organ or body system problems. Doctors may miss key information that would be needed by nurses to determine *nursing* needs (e.g., whether the person has a risk for falls).

To avoid omission errors, most facilities develop their own standard assessment tools that nurses complete for each patient. Remember the following rule.

RULE

To ensure accurate, systematic, comprehensive assessment, use a standard tool that's designed for your particular patient situation—don't rely on memory.

Some assessment tools are designed for *data base assessment* (see pages 272-275). Others are designed for *focus* assessment (see the *Neurologic Focus Assessment Guide* on page 157). Although tools can help you develop habits that promote an organized and comprehensive approach, you must use these guides appropriately:

- Before using a tool, make the connection between what information is requested on the tool and *why* it's relevant. For example, suppose you use a neurologic focus assessment tool, and it says to collect data about how the pupils react to light. Ask *why* do I need to check the pupils and what is the significance of how pupils react to light in context of determining neurologic status?
- Collect both *subjective data* (patient's perceptions) and *objective data* (your observations).
- Remember that assessment tools don't prompt you to use all your resources. After you interview and examine your patient, ask, What other resources might provide additional information about this person's health status (e.g., medical and nursing records, significant others, other health care professionals)?
- Choose a method of assessment and use it consistently.
- Change your approach, depending on the person's health status:
  - If the person is acutely ill, assess urgent problems first (see *Skill 13, Setting Priorities*, page 180).
  - If the person has a specific complaint, assess that problem first, and then go on to complete the assessment in the same way you would if the person were healthy.
  - If the person is generally healthy, choose the method that meets your purpose and is most convenient. For example, use the head-to-toe approach, the body systems approach (Figure 3-3, page 104), or the functional health patterns approach (Box 3-9, page 103), or follow a preprinted assessment tool (page 157).
- Practice using various assessment tools and be sure you understand *why* you collect each piece of data. This will help you learn *what's relevant* to various situations.
- Keep in mind that a body systems approach to assessment helps you collect data about medical problems. Nursing frameworks, such as functional health patterns, help you collect data about human function and responses (nursing problems).
- Always assess the four major vital signs: temperature, pulse, respirations, and blood pressure. Also assess the "fifth and sixth" vital signs: pain and cough. Ask about the presence of pain or discomfort and assess closely as indicated. Ask the person to cough. Although asking the person to cough doesn't replace a thorough lung assessment, you can learn a lot from brief encounters. Say something like, "Can you cough for me, so I can hear how it sounds?" The person's ability (or inability) to comply with this request gives you a lot of information (for example, whether the person has pain with coughing, whether there's congestion, or whether the person coughs well enough to clear the airway). These brief encounters can flag patients that need more in-depth monitoring and assessment. *Note:* Some consider *pulse oximetry* to be the sixth vital sign. *Pulse oximetry*— using a probe attached to the patient's finger or ear and linked to a computerized unit—monitors the percentage of hemoglobin saturated with oxygen.

NEUROLOGIC FOCUS ASSESSMENT GUIDE

VITAL SIGNS Temp. _____ Pulse _____ Resp. _____ BP _____

(Check the boxes that apply below)

EYE OPENING
☐ Spontaneous ☐ To command ☐ To pain ☐ No response

MOTOR RESPONSE
☐ Obeys commands ☐ Localizes pain ☐ Flexion withdrawal
☐ Abnormal flexion ☐ Abnormal extension ☐ No response

BEST VERBAL RESPONSE
☐ Oriented ☐ Confused ☐ Inappropriate words
☐ Incomprehensible words ☐ No response

PUPIL REACTION
☐ Right eye: _____ Size of pupil _____ Reaction to light (brisk, sluggish)
☐ Left eye: _____ Size of pupil _____ Reaction to light (brisk, sluggish)

PURPOSEFUL LIMB MOVEMENT
Right arm
☐ Spontaneous ☐ To command ☐ Paralysis
☐ Visible muscle contraction but no movement
☐ Weak contraction; not enough to overcome gravity
☐ Moves against gravity, not to external resistance
☐ Normal range of motion; can be overcome by increased gravity
☐ Normal muscle strength

Right leg
☐ Spontaneous ☐ To command ☐ Paralysis
☐ Visible muscle contraction but no movement
☐ Weak contraction; not enough to overcome gravity
☐ Moves against gravity, not to external resistance
☐ Normal range of motion; can be overcome by increased gravity
☐ Normal muscle strength

Left arm
☐ Spontaneous ☐ To command ☐ Paralysis
☐ Visible muscle contraction but no movement
☐ Weak contraction; not enough to overcome gravity
☐ Moves against gravity, not to external resistance
☐ Normal range of motion; can be overcome by increased gravity
☐ Normal muscle strength

Left leg
☐ Spontaneous ☐ To command ☐ Paralysis
☐ Visible muscle contraction but no movement
☐ Weak contraction; not enough to overcome gravity
☐ Moves against gravity, not to external resistance
☐ Normal range of motion; can be overcome by increased gravity
☐ Normal muscle strength

Limb Sensation (prick limb with sterile needle)
Right arm:	☐ Normal	☐ Decreased	☐ Absent
Right leg:	☐ Normal	☐ Decreased	☐ Absent
Left arm:	☐ Normal	☐ Decreased	☐ Absent
Left leg:	☐ Normal	☐ Decreased	☐ Absent

Seizure Activity: Describe in nurse's notes.
Gag Reflex: ☐ Present ☐ Absent ☐ Weak

Practice Exercises: Assessing Systematically and Comprehensively

Note: Example responses are on pages 254-256.

1. Imagine that you're a school nurse and have been asked to do physical exams to screen students for possible medical problems. Identify an organized, comprehensive approach to assessing for signs and symptoms of a medical problem.
2. Suppose you make a home visit to a woman who has a newborn child and seven other children younger than 12 years old. Both the baby and the mother are healthy. Identify an organized and comprehensive approach to assessing for nursing and medical problems.
3. Read the following scenarios, and then answer the questions that follow.

Scenario One

Pearl, an 89-year-old grandmother, is admitted with a fractured ankle. She has surgery, and a cast is applied. The cast goes from her toes to the knee. Her toes are visible, and she can wiggle them freely. A small window was cut in the cast over the dorsalis pedis pulse. Routine hospital protocols state that anyone with a cast must have neurovascular checks every 2 hours. You know the following memory-jog helps you remember the things you need to check when performing a neurovascular assessment:

Maggie **C**hewed **N**uts **E**very **P**lace **S**he **W**ent, which stands for this: **M**ovement, **C**olor, **N**umbness, **E**dema, **P**ulses, **S**ensation, **W**armth

a. Using the preceding memory-jog to help you assess systematically, how would you do an assessment to determine the neurovascular status of Pearl's injured leg?
b. Why is it necessary to monitor each of the assessment parameters listed in the memory-jog to determine neurovascular status?
c. What would you do if Pearl told you her toes felt *numb and cold?*

Scenario Two

You must give Mr. Wu digoxin by mouth. You know that the memory-jog **TACIT** helps you with what you need to remember to monitor responses to medications:

Therapeutic effect (Is there a therapeutic effect?)
Allergic or **A**dverse reactions (Are there signs of allergic or adverse reactions?)
Contraindications (Are there contraindications to giving this drug?)
Interactions? (Are there possible drug interactions?)
Toxicity or overdose (Are there signs of toxicity or overdose?)

Using TACIT to focus your assessment and systematically gather information about how Mr. Wu is responding to the digoxin, answer the following questions.

a. What, specifically, would you assess to decide whether to give the digoxin?
b. Why is it important to determine all of the things listed in the mnemonic TACIT?

Scenario Three

You just admitted Gerome, who fell off his bike, hit his head, and had a short period of unconsciousness. He is now awake and alert but is admitted for 24 hours of neurologic monitoring. The physician orders neurologic assessments every hour.

Using the *Neurologic Focus Assessment Guide* on page 157, respond to the following questions:

a. How would you assess Gerome to determine the status of each of the neurologic assessment parameters addressed in the guide?
b. Why is each piece of data on the focus assessment guide relevant to determining neurologic status?
c. What would you do if, on admission, Gerome demonstrates normal neurologic assessment findings but 2 hours later demonstrates extreme drowsiness (that is, he awakens only if you shake him and call his name)?
d. What would you do if one pupil started to become more sluggish in its response to light than the other?
e. What would you do if you noted a general pattern of the pulse getting slower than baseline pulse?

3. CHECKING ACCURACY AND RELIABILITY (VALIDATING DATA)

Definition

Collecting more data to verify whether information you gathered is correct

Why This Skill Promotes Clinical Judgment

Clinical judgments must be based on evidence. Verifying that your information is accurate, factual, and complete helps you avoid making decisions based on incorrect or incomplete data. Checking accuracy and reliability also promotes *comprehensive data collection* because you gather more data to double-check your information.

Guidelines: How to Check Accuracy and Reliability

1. Review the data you gathered and ask questions like these:
    - Do the objective data (what you observed) support the subjective data (what the patient stated)?
    - How do I know this information is reliable?
    - Does this information make sense in the context of this situation?
    - How does this information compare with similar data collected in a different way or at another time (e.g., how does an oral temperature compare with a rectal temperature)?
2. Focus your assessment to gain more information about whether your information is correct. For example, an elderly person may have told you that she

took her medicine. To verify this, interview significant others or caregivers, check pill containers to see if pills are gone, and ask whether there is any record kept when pills are taken. Remember the following rule.

RULE

More than one source, more likely of course. The more information you have coming from different sources, indicating the same thing, the more likely it is that your information is valid and reliable. For example, verify *what your patient says* by *checking with family members and patient records.*

Practice Exercises: Checking Accuracy and Reliability (Validating Data)

Note: Example responses are on page 257.

For each of the following, determine how to validate whether the information is accurate and reliable:

1. The off-going nurse tells you that Mrs. Molina is depressed and angry about being in the hospital.
2. Mr. Nola tells you he thinks his blood sugar was 104 when he tested it an hour ago.
3. You take a blood pressure from the left arm and find it to be abnormally high.
4. A team member tells you that Mr. McGwire needs teaching about diabetic foot care because this is his third admission for foot ulcers.

4. DISTINGUISHING NORMAL FROM ABNORMAL AND IDENTIFYING SIGNS AND SYMPTOMS

Definition

Analyzing patient data and deciding what's within normal range and what's outside the usual range for normalcy; then deciding when abnormal data may be signs or symptoms of a specific problem

Example: If a 62-year-old man who takes no medications has a pulse of 42 beats per minute, you know that this is *abnormal*. It may be a *sign* of a heart problem because a normal pulse rate rarely drops below 55 to 60 beats per minute in someone this age who takes no medications (some cardiac medications lower the heart rate).

Why This Skill Promotes Clinical Judgment

Recognizing abnormal data and signs and symptoms is the first step to problem identification: Signs and symptoms are like red flags that prompt you to suspect a problem. If you miss these red flags, you miss recognizing problems and opportunities for early intervention.

Guidelines: How to Distinguish Normal from Abnormal and Identify Signs and Symptoms

Identifying signs and symptoms requires you to apply knowledge of what are considered normal findings. If your patient's findings are *outside the normal range*, then you have identified a *possible sign or symptom*. You must use all your senses (sight, hearing, touch, and smell) to gain all the relevant information you need (e.g., if you see cloudy urine, smell it to check its odor).

Ask the following questions:

1. **How does my patient's information compare with accepted standards for normal for someone of this age, culture, disease process, and lifestyle?** If the patient's information isn't within normal accepted standards, this is a possible sign or symptom of a problem.

2. **Is my patient taking any medications that change normal function?** For example, someone may be taking a heart medication that lowers heart rate; in this case an abnormally low heart rate is actually normal. Check action and side effects of all medications.

3. **How does my patient's current information compare with the previously collected data?** This question is especially helpful in situations where the patient has chronic signs and symptoms and you need to decide whether the signs and symptoms are getting *worse*. For example, an asthmatic may always be slightly wheezy. However, if this same person is now wheezier than before, this increased wheeziness is a sign of *increasing problems*.

Practice Exercises: Distinguishing Normal from Abnormal and Identifying Signs and Symptoms

Note: Example responses are on page 257.

1. Place an S next to the data below that are signs or symptoms of a possible problem or signs or symptoms of a problem that's getting worse. Place an O if it's neither a sign nor a symptom. Place a question mark if you need more information to decide.

   a. ___ Temperature of 99.68° F
   b. ___ Bilateral pulmonary rales
   c. ___ Someone tells you she rarely sleeps more than 3 hours at a time
   d. ___ Someone's nasogastric drainage has turned from brown to red
   e. ___ Someone's abdominal incision is slightly red around the sutures
   f. ___ A 2-year-old is inconsolable when his mother leaves the room
   g. ___ Someone with no health problems has developed ankle edema

> h. ___ Someone tells you he bathes every other week
> i. ___ Someone on kidney dialysis never urinates
> j. ___ Pulse of 54 per minute

2. For each question mark you placed above, explain what else you want to know before you decide whether the information is abnormal (and therefore a sign or a symptom).

5. MAKING INFERENCES (DRAWING VALID CONCLUSIONS)

Definition
Making deductions or forming opinions that follow logically by interpreting patient cues (subjective and objective data)

To clarify, study the following examples.

Cue	Corresponding Inference
Frowning	Seems worried
White blood cell count = 14,000	Probable infection
Deaf	Probable communication problems

Why This Skill Promotes Clinical Judgment
Your ability to interpret data and draw valid conclusions (make inferences) is essential to determining health status. If you draw incorrect conclusions, your judgment will be flawed.

Making correct inferences helps you focus your assessment to look for additional relevant information. For example, if you infer that an elevated white blood cell count may indicate an infection, you know to look for signs and symptoms of infection.

Guidelines: How to Make Inferences (Draw Valid Conclusions)
Making correct inferences requires knowledge of common health problems, knowledge of human behavior, knowledge of cultural and spiritual influences, and knowledge of the patient as a person. For example, to make the inference of *probable infection*, you need to know the signs and symptoms of infection. To make the inference that someone's lack of eye contact indicates that he's not trustful, you must know how eye contact is used in his particular culture (in some cultures, direct eye contact may be disrespectful).

To avoid jumping to conclusions, begin your statements about inferences by saying, *I suspect this information indicates....* Using this phrase reinforces that you to need to collect more data to decide if your suspicions are correct. Once you have enough evidence to support your inference, you can know that you are probably correct. Also remember that critical thinking requires you to think about *alternate conclusions and ideas*. If you make an inference, try to think of some other things that you could also reasonably infer. For example, you may infer that a patient is angry with you because she is shouting and irritable. Ask yourself, *Could she really be mad about something else?*

More than one cue, more likely it's true—more than one source, more likely of course. Avoid making inferences based on only one cue (the more facts and sources you have to support your inference, the more likely it is that your inference is correct). Once you make an inference, verify whether it's correct by gathering more information and looking for additional cues.

CRITICAL MOMENTS

WHEN DRAWING CONCLUSIONS ABOUT SIGNS AND SYMPTOMS: REMEMBER M & M
Always ask, *Could these signs and symptoms be related to medical or medication problems that are undiagnosed?*

Practice Exercises: Making Inferences (Drawing Valid Conclusions)

Note: Example responses are on page 258.

Make an inference about each of the following data (begin your inference by writing, *I suspect this information indicates…*).

1. Temperature of 102.8° F for 3 days
2. A mother tells you she can't afford prenatal care
3. A diabetic is 100 pounds overweight and says his blood sugar is always out of control, even though he watches his food intake and takes his insulin regularly
4. A 5-year-old child whose mother told you he broke his leg falling down the stairs keeps looking at his mother before answering any of your questions
5. A usually active, alert grandmother has unkempt appearance and seems a bit confused

6. CLUSTERING RELATED CUES (DATA)

Definition

Grouping data together in a way that it helps you see relationships among the data

Example: Suppose you grouped the following cues together: 2 years old; temperature 100.8° F; pulse 150 per minute; rash all over trunk; recent measles exposure; never had measles; screaming that he wants his mother. If you consider the relationship among this data, you should suspect that the child's rapid pulse is related to his screaming and elevated temperature rather than a sign of cardiac problems. If you consider *all of the data*, you'll probably suspect that these symptoms indicate the child may have measles.

Why This Skill Promotes Clinical Judgment

Grouping information applies the scientific principle of classifying information to enhance ability to see relationships between and among data. It helps you get a beginning picture of patterns of health or illness. A good way to remember the importance of clustering related data is what I call "the puzzle analogy." When you put together a puzzle, you begin by putting all the edges of the picture in one pile, all the pieces of a certain color in another pile, and so on. Putting the pieces in piles helps you begin to see patterns. The same principle applies to health assessment data, but in health care, you cluster *signs and symptoms*.

Guidelines: How to Cluster Related Cues (Data)

1. How you cluster data depends on your purpose:
   - If you're trying to determine the status of medical problems or physiologic responses, cluster the data according to body systems (see Figure 3-3, page 104).
   - If you're trying to determine the status of nursing problems, cluster the data according to a nursing framework (for example, see Box 3-9, page 103).
2. Mind mapping, or concept mapping (pages 263-265), is especially helpful for identifying relationships. Mapping relationships between and among patient cues helps you visualize factors that contribute to one another.

Practice Exercises: Clustering Related Cues (Data)

Note: Example responses are on page 258.

Read the following scenarios, and then answer the questions that follow.

Scenario One

The 16-year-old baby-sitter next door calls and tells you that Jack, the 8-year-old she's watching, was stung by a bee on the ear an hour ago. She tells you the ear is swollen and asks you to come and check him. You go over and examine the child. He asks you if he might die "like the kid on TV did." The baby-sitter tells you she's afraid because she doesn't know where the mother is. You check the ear and find it red, swollen, and free of the stinger. When asked, Jack tells you he was stung before but that wasn't as scary. Jack has no rash and no wheezing. He asks if he could have a Popsicle and watch TV. His pulse and respirations are normal.

Cluster the information that will help you determine the following:
a.   Jack's physical health status
b.   Jack's human responses
c.   The baby-sitter's learning needs

Scenario Two

It's 11 am and you just admitted Mr. Nelson, a 41-year-old businessman who has acute abdominal pain. He's never been in the hospital and tells you he hates everything about hospitals. He's been vomiting for 2 days and is unable to keep any food down. His abdomen is distended, and he has no bowel sounds. He is scheduled to go to the operating room at 2 pm for emergency exploratory surgery. He tells you he's worried because his brother died in the hospital after a car accident. Suddenly he doubles over and says, "This is really getting worse!" You take his vital signs, and they are as follows: T 101° P 132 R 32 BP 140/80. These signs are the same as those taken an hour ago, except that before, his pulse was 104.

Cluster the information that will help you determine the following:
a.   Mr. Nelson's physical status
b.   Mr. Nelson's human responses

7. DISTINGUISHING RELEVANT FROM IRRELEVANT

Definition
Deciding what information is pertinent to understanding the situations at hand and what information is immaterial

Why This Skill Promotes Clinical Judgment
When faced with a lot of information, narrowing it down to only the *pertinent facts* prevents your brain from being cluttered with unnecessary facts. *Deciding what's relevant* is also an example of one of the principles of the scientific method: classifying or categorizing information into groups of related (relevant) information.

Guidelines: How to Distinguish Relevant from Irrelevant
This skill is closely related to *Skill 6, Clustering Related Cues.* Here, however, we're looking at this skill a little differently. In *clustering related cues,* you simply put related information together (for example, you put all the respiratory data in one place, all the nutritional data in another, and so on). In this skill, you *analyze* the data you put together and decide what information is related to a specific health concern. For example, if you suspect constipation, and you note that the person has a sedentary life, poor roughage intake, and takes iron supplements, it's likely that this information is relevant to the constipation.

Distin*guishing relevant from irrelevant* is especially difficult for novices because being able to do **this** depends on having *problem-specific knowledge and experience.* **If you're a novice, you'll find that this skill will get easier as you gain more clinical experience.**

Here are some strategies that can help you determine what's relevant, even with limited knowledge:
1. List the abnormal data you collected.
2. Then ask yourself, *Could there be any connection between this (abnormal data) and that (abnormal data)?*
3. As appropriate, ask the person or significant others, *Do you think there's any relationship between this (abnormal data) and that (abnormal data)?*

Practice Exercises: Distinguishing Relevant from Irrelevant
Note: Example responses are on page 258.

Consider the following scenarios, then answer the questions that follow them.

Scenario One
You work in community health and make a visit to Mrs. Blondell, who is 80 years old and had a cerebrovascular accident (CVA) a month ago. Today you notice she seems to be increasingly confused: She knows where she is, but forgets what day it is and doesn't seem to remember her daily routine. You know that confusion in the elderly can be caused by any of the following: medications, infection, decreased oxygen to the brain, electrolyte imbalance, and brain pathology. You assess Mrs. Blondell and gather the data listed below.

Consider the following data, and decide its possible relevance to the problem of confusion. Put an *R* in front of the things that are relevant.
a. _____ Recently started taking buspirone hydrochloride for anxiety
b. _____ Temperature: 100.8° F. orally
c. _____ History of a myocardial infarction 5 years ago
d. _____ Seems dehydrated
e. _____ Has no allergies
f. _____ Regular diet

Scenario Two
You assess Mrs. Clark, a 32-year-old diabetic who is in for a routine visit. When you ask how the new diet is going, she breaks down into tears, saying, "I'm never going to be able to do this!"

Consider the following data and decide its possible relevance to her problem with sticking to the diabetic diet. Put an *R* in front of the things that are relevant.
a. ____ Diagnosed with diabetes 2 months ago
b. ____ Vital signs within normal limits

c.   ___ Complains of constipation
d.   ___ Married with three school-age children
e.   ___ Loves to cook
f.   ___ Has always been 50 pounds overweight
g.   ___ Allergic to aspirin

8. RECOGNIZING INCONSISTENCIES

Definition
Realizing when data contradict each other
     For example, suppose you're caring for Fred after chest surgery and he tells you that he has no pain. However, he moves very little and barely breathes when you ask him to take a deep breath. The way this person is moving is *inconsistent* with his statements of being pain-free.

Why This Skill Promotes Clinical Judgment
Recognizing inconsistencies prompts you to investigate issues more closely. It sends up a red flag that tells you to probe more deeply to get to the facts. It also helps you focus your assessment to clarify the issues. For example, with Fred in the preceding section, you might say, "It seems to me that you aren't moving very well.... I suspect you have more pain than you admit. I want you to be comfortable, so that you move well and are able to take deep breaths to clear your lungs. Are you sure there isn't a particular spot that's bothering you?"

Guidelines: How to Recognize Inconsistencies
One way to recognize inconsistencies is to compare what the patient states (subjective data) with what you observe (objective data). If what the *person states* isn't supported by what *you observe*, you have inconsistent information and need to investigate further.
     Recognizing inconsistencies requires problem-specific knowledge. For example, suppose you have the following data:
Subjective Data: Patient states, "I must have strained my back lifting my child. My right side is killing me."
Objective Data: Fever of 102.4° F; cloudy, foul-smelling urine.
     If you know how back injuries usually present, you know that the subjective and objective are *inconsistent* with a back injury and *more consistent* with a urinary tract infection.

To Recognize Inconsistencies with Limited Knowledge:

1. Determine the signs and symptoms of the problem you suspect by looking up the problem in a reference. For example, if you suspect pneumonia, look up the signs and symptoms of pneumonia.

2. Compare the information in the reference with your patient's data. If your patient's signs and symptoms are *different* from those listed in the reference, you have *inconsistencies* and must investigate further. Assess the person more closely, and consider other problems that the signs and symptoms might represent. For example, are the signs and symptoms more consistent with a cold or flu than pneumonia?

Practice Exercises: Recognizing Inconsistencies

Note: Example responses are on page 258.

Read the following scenarios; then answer the questions that follow them.

Scenario One

You interview Cathy in the prenatal clinic 2 weeks before delivery. You ask her how she feels about the baby coming. She tells you she's happy that she gets to see the baby in only 2 weeks. When you ask her if she has any questions about the delivery, she tells you she's been going to birthing classes with her boyfriend and feels like she knows what to expect.

You review her records and notice that her first clinic visit was 2 weeks ago, when she came with her mother.

a. Identify inconsistencies in the preceding scenario.
b. Explain what you might do to clarify the inconsistencies you identified.

Scenario Two

You're in the grocery store and a woman who appears to be about 20 years old comes up to you and says, "Please help me! I can't breathe, and my heart is racing. I think I'm having a heart attack!" You help her sit down, then take her pulse, and find it to be 100 per minute, regular, and strong. Her respirations are 36 per minute. She tells you she has no pain but asks the store manager to call an ambulance. As you wait for the ambulance, she tells you this has happened to her several times before and that she has had an electrocardiogram, which showed normal cardiac function. Then she says, "But I know I'm having a heart attack! I'm so scared!"

How consistent are this woman's signs, symptoms, and risk factors with those of a cardiac problem?

9. IDENTIFYING PATTERNS

Definition
Putting together pieces of information and deciding what they indicate about overall health status

For example, you cluster together cues of chronic productive cough, wheezing, and exercise intolerance and decide that they indicate a pattern of respiratory problems. Keep in mind that *identifying patterns* means looking at signs and symptoms *over a period of time*, not just as single incidences. You may have had a headache last week, but this doesn't indicate a pattern you need to worry about.

Why This Skill Promotes Clinical Judgment
Identifying patterns helps you (1) get a beginning picture of problems, and (2) recognize gaps in data collection. Once you recognize gaps in data collection, you can decide how to focus your assessment to gain that missing information. Using the puzzle analogy, when you put some pieces together, you start to see what the end picture will be. You also find it easier to finish the puzzle after you see patterns start to form.

Here's an example of how *identifying patterns* helps you discover missing pieces of information. Suppose you clustered together the following data:

- No bowel movement in 3 days
- Abdominal fullness
- States he's been "constipated off and on for the past month"

You may decide that these cues represent a pattern of *altered bowel elimination*. Having recognized this pattern, you know to focus your assessment to gain more information and decide exactly what the problem with bowel elimination is. For example, you ask, "What does *off and on* mean?" The person responds, "I get so constipated I have to take laxatives, and then I get diarrhea." This added information is likely to make you suspect that the bowel elimination problem is being caused in part by laxative abuse. You then explore his knowledge of dietary concerns and the problems caused by laxatives. You also need to ask when the person had a physical exam by a doctor and whether this bowel problem was evaluated. (Remember that changes in bowel elimination may be a sign of cancer.)

Guidelines: How to Identify Patterns
To identify patterns:
1. Analyze the cues you put together and decide which of the following patterns they represent:
   - No signs and symptoms present = **Normal Pattern**
   - Risk factors present = **Risk for Abnormal Pattern**
   - Signs and symptoms present = **Abnormal Pattern**

2. After you get a beginning idea of the patterns, look for gaps in data collection by asking, *What other information might clarify my understanding of this pattern?*

Practice Exercises: Identifying Patterns

Note: Example responses are on page 259.

Matching: Decide which numbers best match the phrases in the letters that follow:

1. Potential (risk) for impaired bowel elimination pattern
2. Potential (risk) for ineffective sexual-reproductive pattern
3. Probably normal sleep-rest pattern
4. Impaired respiratory function pattern
5. Probably normal coping pattern

a. Bilateral rales; respirations increased to 34 per minute; coughing up thick, white mucus

b. States, "I can cope with my illness, so long as I have help from my husband." Manages daily self-care; has husband cook all meals; passes the time by knitting blankets for the homeless

c. Eats little roughage; just started taking codeine every 4 hours; drinks about three glasses of water daily; spends most of her time in bed; normal bowel function

d. Works nights; sleeps 4 hours in the morning and 3 hours just before going to work at night

e. Has just been diagnosed with genital herpes; single; worried about transmitting herpes to future sex partners and future children (during delivery)

10. IDENTIFYING MISSING INFORMATION

Definition
Recognizing gaps in data collection and searching for information to fill in the gaps

Why This Skill Promotes Clinical Judgment
Recognizing gaps in information and filling in those gaps prevents you from making one of the most common clinical reasoning errors: making judgments based on incomplete information. It also helps you gain a deep understanding of the situations at hand.

Guidelines: How to Identify Missing Information
1. Don't try to do it all in your head—reflect *on the recorded data* and ask, *What's missing here?*

2.   If you're not sure if you really need more information, ask questions like, *What difference will it make?* or *How will knowing this information change the approach to treatment?* If the information won't change your approach, then you may not need to take the time to gather it.

3.   Other strategies for recognizing missing information include accomplishing all of the following clinical judgment skills from this section: *identifying assumptions; checking accuracy and reliability of data; clustering related cues; recognizing inconsistencies; identifying patterns;* and *evaluating and correcting thinking*

Practice Exercises: Identifying Missing Information

Note: Example responses are on page 259.

Go back to the practice exercises for the previous skill, *identifying patterns.* For each pattern represented by the information listed in *a* to *e*, decide what information might be missing that could add to your understanding of the pattern.

11. PROMOTING HEALTH BY IDENTIFYING AND MANAGING RISK FACTORS

Note: This skill deals with *identifying risk factors* in <u>healthy</u> people. The next skill, *diagnosing actual and potential problems* deals with identifying risk factors in the context of people with <u>existing health problems</u>.

Definition

Preventing health problems by early detection and treatment of factors that cause—or put someone at risk for—decreased well-being

Why This Skill Promotes Clinical Judgment

Critical thinking is proactive. You don't wait for problems to appear to put a plan into action. By identifying risk factors, you apply the proactive *predict, prevent, manage, promote (PPMP)* approach, rather than the reactive *diagnose and treat (DT)* approach (see pages 74-77).

Guidelines: How to Identify and Manage Risk Factors

1.   Assess people's awareness of—and motivation for—identifying and managing risk factors. For example, do they know what's required for adequate nutrition, rest, exercise, and spiritual and psychologic well-being? Are they willing to do what's needed to reduce risks? *Not knowing about risk factors* and *not wanting do something about them* are risk factors in themselves.

2.   Keep growth and development in mind. **Examples:**

- A woman who is pregnant or planning on becoming pregnant must consider risk factors for both herself and the fetus when taking medications. She should know that inadequate intake of folic acid increases risk of spontaneous abortion and other problems such as spina bifida in the infant.
- After menopause, women should be aware that they should be screened for decreased bone density.

3. Look for risk factors that are known to put people at risk for a variety of common problems. **Examples:** Obesity, poor diet, high cholesterol, tobacco use, immobility, sedentary life, stressful life, poor sleeping habits, allergies, chronic illness, extremes of age (very young or old), low socioeconomic status, illiteracy, sun exposure, and excessive use of medications, alcohol, or illicit drugs.

4. Also assess for the following:
    - Genetic, cultural, or biologic factors (e.g., race, family history, and personal history predisposing one to health problems)
    - Behavioral factors (e.g., problems with anger management, attention-deficit disorders)
    - Psychosocial and/or economic factors (e.g., lack of significant others, poverty)
    - Environmental factors (e.g., air quality)
    - Age-related factors (e.g., women after menopause are at risk for osteoporosis; infants are at risk for ear infection)
    - Sexual-pattern factors (e.g., whether one is sexually active and with whom)
    - Safety-related factors (e.g., whether seat belts are worn, whether the home environment is safe for children)
    - Disease-related factors (e.g., someone with chronic lung disease is at risk for pneumonia; someone with diabetes is at risk for skin problems)
    - Treatment-related factors (e.g., complicated medication or treatment regimen)

5. Teach the importance of managing risk factors to prevent costly, debilitating illnesses in the future.

6. **For more strategies on risk management:** Go to the Web page of Harvard Center For Risk Analysis (www.hcra.harvard.edu), which is dedicated to promoting reasoned public responses to health, safety, and environmental hazards. It also gives statistics and approaches for problems like stroke, heart disease, suicide, cancer, and drowning and other accidents. The Centers for Disease Control and Prevention Web page (www.cdc.gov) has a wealth of information on disease and disability prevention. Also, look up "risk factors" in the index of up-to-date textbooks. Usually you can find excellent tables on common diseases and risk factors that present information in an easy-to-understand format.

Practice Exercises: Promoting Health by Identifying and Managing Risk Factors

Note: Example responses are on page 259.

1. You assess a 25-year-old man and determine that he is healthy. What questions might you ask to identify risk factors for possible problems?
2. You assess a 72-year-old woman and find that she is healthy, but she says "I tend to be a little clumsy—I lose my balance." Why should you be concerned about this?
3. You're at a barbecue talking casually with the 50-year-old husband of one of your friends. He says, "I guess I'm getting to the age where I should be doing more to look after myself. How can I find out my risk factors?" How do you respond?

12. DIAGNOSING ACTUAL AND POTENTIAL PROBLEMS

Note: This skill deals with *identifying risk factors* in the context of people with existing health problems. *Skill 11* deals with risk factors in the context of healthy people.

Definition

Labeling the actual and potential problems in the most accurate way possible, based on evidence from the health assessment

This skill includes (1) choosing the name that *best* describes the problem (the definitive diagnosis), (2) determining the cause(s) or related factors of the problems, and (3) providing the evidence that leads you to believe the diagnosis is present.

Why This Skill Promotes Clinical Judgment

This skill is important for several reasons:

1. Making *definitive diagnoses* (the most specific, correct diagnoses) is key to being able to determine the *specific actions* designed to prevent, manage, or resolve them. If you miss problems, are too vague about the problems, or name them incorrectly, you have made a diagnostic error that may cause you to:
   - Initiate actions that *aggravate* the problems or *waste time.*
   - Omit essential actions required to prevent and manage the problems.
   - Allow problems to go untreated.
   - Influence others to make the same mistake you did.

RULE

> Making the *definitive diagnosis*—the most specific appropriate diagnosis —is the key to appropriate specific treatment. If you have limited time with the patient and you suspect a problem, but are unable to make a *definitive diagnosis,* rather than jumping to conclusions, it's prudent to say something like this: "We don't have enough information with the limited time we've had, but there seems to be some sort of issue with [fill in the blank] or….there seems to be a pattern of [fill in the blank]."

2. You don't fully understand the problem(s)—or know what to do about them—until you clearly identify what's *causing or contributing* to them.
3. *Predicting potential problems* helps you:
   - Know what signs and symptoms to look for when monitoring the patient.
   - Anticipate what could happen if things get worse (therefore allowing you to plan ahead to be prepared)
4. *Providing the supporting evidence* that led you to the diagnosis helps others understand the problem better. For example, compare the two following problem statements, and decide which one gives a better picture of the problem.
   - Potential for violence
   - Potential for violence related to history of violence as evidence by denial of anger management problems and refusal to attend anger management programs.

The above gives a summary statement for diagnosis. Alternatively, use a diagram or map as noted in Figure 5-1.

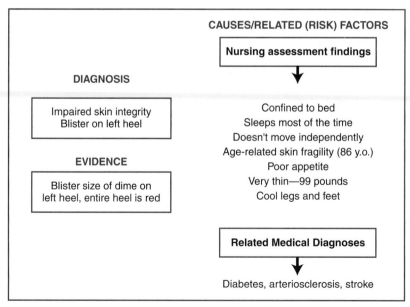

Figure 5-1 Using diagrams and maps to illustrate diagnosis.

Guidelines: How to Diagnose Actual and Potential Problems

The ability to identify and predict problems depends on your clinical knowledge and expertise, and your knowledge of the patient *as a person*. As addressed in Chapter 3, experts can usually identify problems more quickly than novices because they've "seen it all before." They have better hunches about what the problems might be, and they move through problem identification in rapid, dynamic ways.

If your knowledge and expertise are limited, you are at risk of making any one of the following diagnostic errors:

- Choosing a diagnosis without considering whether the data may represent a *different problem altogether* (e.g., assuming indigestion signifies gastric reflux instead of possible coronary problems)
- Not considering all the relevant data because of a narrow focus (e.g., not looking for other coronary symptoms because you decide that the person has indigestion)
- Failing to recognize personal biases or assumptions (e.g., thinking that someone isn't very smart because she doesn't speak your language)
- Making a diagnosis that's too general (e.g., using *pain* instead of *acute pain* or *chronic pain*).
- Overanalyzing ("analysis paralysis") and delaying taking action

Identifying Actual Problems

1. Verify that your information is correct and complete. If you're not sure what to do next, make *patient safety number one*: Report signs and symptoms to a more qualified nurse before going on to complete problem identification.
2. Avoid drawing conclusions or identifying problems based on only *one cue* or one source ("More than one cue, more likely it's true. More than one source, more likely of course").
3. Cluster abnormal data (signs and symptoms): Cluster according to body systems to identify medical problems and according to a nursing framework to identify nursing problems. Looking at data from *both* medical and nursing perspectives help you see *different* problems.
4. Consider the signs and symptoms and ask yourself what information you could have missed.
5. Create a list of problems that may be suggested by the signs and symptoms. Box 5-1 on the next page gives a helpful checklist to consider possible problems.
6. After you complete your list of suspected problems, compare your patient's signs and symptoms with the signs and symptoms or defining characteristics of the problems you suspect. Some call this phase "testing hunches (hypotheses)."
7. Name the problems by using the term that most closely matches your patient's signs and symptoms. **Example:** If your patient's signs and symptoms match the signs and symptoms of *anxiety*, better than *fear*, label the problem *anxiety*.
8. Determine what's causing or contributing to the problems.

BOX 5-1	CHECKLIST FOR IDENTIFYING ACTUAL AND POTENTIAL PROBLEMS

1. List current medications (include over-the-counter and herbal drugs). Ask yourself whether any of the patient's problems could be related to any of the medications (remember **SODA**).
    Side effect?
    Overdose?
    Drug interaction?
    Allergy or **A**dverse reaction?
2. List current and past allergies, diseases, surgeries, or trauma.
3. Consider whether any of the patient's current problems are related to Questions 1 or 2 above.
4. Complete the following checklist: (Circle those that apply)

Is there a problem with breathing?	Yes	No	AR[1]	Pos[2]
Is there a problem with circulation?	Yes	No	AR	Pos
Is there a problem with comfort?	Yes	No	AR	Pos
Is there a problem with nutrition?	Yes	No	AR	Pos
Is there a problem with urinary or bowel elimination?	Yes	No	AR	Pos
Is there a problem with fluid or electrolyte balance?	Yes	No	AR	Pos
Is there a problem with ability to think or perceive environment?	Yes	No	AR	Pos
Is there a problem with communication?	Yes	No	AR	Pos
Is there a problem with safety (risk for injury or falls)?	Yes	No	AR	Pos
Is there a problem with sleeping or exercising?	Yes	No	AR	Pos
Is there a risk for infection (self or transmission to others)?	Yes	No	AR	Pos
Is there a risk for impaired skin integrity?	Yes	No	AR	Pos
Is there a problem with coping or stress?	Yes	No	AR	Pos
Is there a psychologic, developmental, self-esteem problem?	Yes	No	AR	Pos
Is there a sociocultural problem?	Yes	No	AR	Pos
Is there a problem with roles, relationships, or sexuality?	Yes	No	AR	Pos
Does the person have a problem with taking medications?	Yes	No	AR	Pos
Does the patient require teaching?	Yes	No	AR	Pos
Is there a problem with health maintenance at home?	Yes	No	AR	Pos
Is this admission going to cause difficulties at home?	Yes	No	AR	Pos
Is there a problem with personal or religious beliefs?	Yes	No	AR	Pos
Is there a problem with coping or managing stress?	Yes	No	AR	Pos
Could this person be pregnant?	Yes	No	AR	Pos

[1]AR = At risk for problem (no signs and symptoms present, but risk factors are evident).
[2]Pos = Possible problem (insufficient data, but you suspect a problem).

RULE

Diagnosis is *incomplete* until you identify not only the problems, but also the *underlying causes and risk factors* of the problems. You can't adequately prevent or treat the problems unless you understand both problems *and* what's causing or contributing to them. (See *Skill 15, Determining Specific Interventions,* on page 188.)

- Always ask yourself whether it's possible that medications, allergies, or untreated (or inadequately treated) medical problems are causing the problems. If so, follow procedures to activate the chain of command to notify the professional most qualified to manage the problem.
- Ask the person and significant others if they can identify factors that are contributing to the problems.
- Consider whether there are factors related to age, disease process, medications, or life changes that could be contributing to the problems.

9. As appropriate, use the following strategies:
- Draw a map to clarify relationships between problems and signs, symptoms, or risk factors.
- Use the worksheet on the next page to systematically consider possible causative factors.

10. If a summary diagnostic statement is required:
- Use the memory-jog PRE (problem, related or risk factors, evidence) to describe the following:
  Problem
  Related factors (cause, risk factors)
  Evidence that led you to conclude the problem exists
- Use "related to" to link the problem and its cause. **Example:** *Acute pain related to left rib fracture as evidenced by statements of extreme tenderness in the left rib cage area*

Predicting Potential (Risk) Problems

1. Find out the patient's allergies, current and past medical and nursing problems, medications, treatments, or experiences of invasive monitoring.
2. Look up problems and complications often associated with the above. Box 3-6 on page 96 and Box 3-7 on page 97 can help you with this. **Examples:** If the person has diabetes, there is a risk for foot ulcers and poor healing. If your patient just had a myocardial infarction (MI) and has an arterial line in place, determine common potential complications of MI (e.g., congestive heart failure, arrhythmias, pericarditis, MI extension, and cardiac arrest) and of the arterial line (e.g., thrombus or emboli).
3. Look for common risk factors as addressed in *Skill 11* on page 171.
4. If a summary statement is required, use the most appropriate of the following:
- Name the potential (risk) problem by stating the problem and the risk factors, using "related to" to link the problem and risk factors. **Example:** *Risk for impaired skin integrity related to immobility and fragile skin*
- Describe the potential complication by using the letters *PC,* followed by a colon. **Example:** *PC: hemorrhage.*

SYSTEMATIC PROBLEM ANALYSIS WORKSHEET

Instructions:

1. List the focus problem, diagnosis, issue, or in box below.
2. Put a check mark in all boxes on the right that correspond to factors that contribute to the problem, diagnosis, or issue you identified.
3. Decide what factors must be managed and who will manage them.
4. Use back of page or figure of man as needed.

Actual / potential diagnosis, problem, or issue

CONTRIBUTING OR RELATED (RISK) FACTORS

1. Main reason for admission or contact?

2. Vulnerability—constitutional or age-related factors?
☐ Age _____ Weight _____ Height _____ Mental Status? _____
☐ Communication ability? ☐ Smoker? ☐ Drinker (alcohol)?
☐ Skin status? ☐ Nutrition-hydration status?
☐ Mobility or self-care problems?
☐ Bowel elimination or urine elimination problems?
☐ Immune system status? ☐ Overall health status/resilience?
☐ Other?

3. Allergy, medication, or treatment-related factors?
☐ Allergies?   ☐ Considered all meds (Rx, OTC, herbal)?
☐ Treatments?

4. Co-existing medical problems, injuries, or pathophysiology?
☐ Neuro?   ☐ Resp? ☐ Cardiac-circulatory?   ☐ GI? ☐ GU?
☐ Diabetes? ☐ Hypertension?   ☐ Depression?   ☐ Other?

5. Environmental factors? Patient identified factors?
☐ Current environment (include work)?   ☐ Role-related?
☐ Other factors?

6. Comfort factors? Mobility problems? Self-care problems?
☐ Pain level? ☐ Pain management? ☐ Self-mobile? ☐ Other?

7. Socioeconomic, spiritual, cultural factors?
☐ Family issues? ☐ Coping problems? ☐ Support systems limited?
☐ Other?

CRITICAL MOMENTS

TOLERATING AMBIGUITY: A GOOD THING—OR NOT
Acceptance of ambiguity is often listed as a critical thinking characteristic. Certainly there are times, as the saying goes, that there is "no black or white—only gray." But you must ask, *How much ambiguity is acceptable in this particular situation?* For example, if you were sick, would you be happy with an ambiguous diagnosis, or would you want it to be specific? Remember that clearly and specifically defining *the problem and its cause* helps you identify *specific* interventions to resolve it.

Practice Exercises: Diagnosing Actual and Potential Problems
Note: Example responses are on page 260.
1. Write a summary diagnostic statement that best describes the potential problem in the following scenario (state the problem and the related factors).

Scenario 1
You just admitted Nigel to the psychiatric unit. He is agitated but won't talk to anyone. You check previous records and note that he has a history of striking caregivers.

2. Based on the information given in the following scenario, predict the potential complications Elaine might experience.

Scenario 2
Elaine is in the recovery room after having an emergency appendectomy under general anesthesia. She's very groggy and extremely nauseated.

3. Based on the information in the following scenario, write a summary statement that best describes the problem, using the PRE format (see Point 10 on page 177).

Scenario 3
You clustered together the following data: Mrs. Pue has just been told she has terminal cancer. She refuses to take her medications. She sleeps most of the time and says she doesn't want to talk to anyone. Mrs. Pue states her situation is hopeless and she's going to die, so she'd rather not bother talking.

4. What risk factors would you look for to determine if the man in the following scenario is at high risk for respiratory problems?

Scenario 4
You're caring for a 41-year-old man who has four fractured ribs.

13. SETTING PRIORITIES

Definition

In this section, *setting priorities* is defined in three ways: (1) Differentiating between problems needing immediate attention and those requiring subsequent action, (2) deciding what problems to delegate and what problems you must manage *yourself*, and (3) deciding what problems must be addressed in the plan of care.

This skill is important for four main reasons:

1. If you don't know how to set priorities, you may cause life-threatening treatment delays. For example, if you don't know that symptoms of congestive heart failure (CHF) require immediate medical attention, the problem can progress to *pulmonary edema and death.*
2. If you give equal attention to *major* and *minor* problems, you won't be able to devote the time you need to manage the *most important* problems.
3. By deciding what you can delegate to others, you have more time for things you *must do* yourself.
4. To communicate care priorities to the health care team, all problems that *must* be managed to achieve the *overall outcomes* must be recorded in the patient record.

Guidelines: How to Set Priorities

This section addresses how to set priorities related to patient problems in the clinical setting. Page 222 in Chapter 6 *(Managing Your Time)* gives additional strategies.

1. Ask the patient to tell you the top three problems he has right *now*.

> **RULE**
>
> **Patients rarely are seen for care with an isolated problem.** Rather, they have several *interrelated* problems that contribute to one another. Determining *relationships* between the problems is key to setting priorities.

2. Apply the principles and strategies on setting priorities listed in Boxes 5-2 and 5-3 (pages 181 and 182). Note that there's more than one way to set priorities. Choose the one that makes the most sense to you in context of each patient situation.
3. Decide *what* you'll delegate and *who* you'll delegate it to (Box 5-4, page 182).
4. Determine what problems *must* be recorded in the patient record:
    -   Clarify the *overall* expected outcome(s). **Example:** Mrs. Rolan will return home and be able to manage diabetic regimen independently. (How to determine expected outcomes is addressed in the next skill *[Skill 14]* . To help you complete this section, outcomes are provided for you.)
    -   Decide *what problems must be addressed* in order to achieve the *overall outcomes*. In the case of Mrs. Rolan, she may have the following two problems:

1. Knowledge deficit: insulin administration
2. Ineffective coping related to marital problems

Only the *first* of these problems relates to the *overall* outcome, so that's the problem you must address in the plan of care.

- Assign *high priority* to recording an individualized plan of care for the following problems:
    1. Those not covered by facility standard plans, protocols, or physician's orders
    2. Those that may jeopardize the achieving of the major expected outcomes of the plan of care

---

| **BOX 5-2** | **SETTING PRIORITIES** |

Principles of Setting Priorities:

1. **Make a complete list of current medications, medical problems, allergies, and chief complaints, then refer to them frequently because they may affect how you set priorities.**
2. **Determine the *relationships* among the problems:** If problem Y causes problem Z, problem Y takes priority over problem Z. **Example:** If pain is causing immobility, *pain management* is a high priority.
3. **Setting priorities is a dynamic, changing process;** at times, the order of priority changes, depending on the seriousness and relationship of the problems. **Example:** If abnormal lab values are at life-threatening levels, they are likely to be highest priority; if your patient is having trouble breathing because of acute rib pain, managing the pain may be a higher priority than dealing with a rapid pulse (first-level priority, listed below).

Steps to Setting Priorities:

1. Assign high priority to *first-level* priority problems (immediate priorities): Remember "ABCs plus V."

    ❑ Airway problems
    ❑ Breathing problems
    ❑ Cardiac and circulation problems
    ❑ Vital sign concerns (such as high fever)

    Exception: With CPR for cardiac arrest, begin chest compressions immediately. Go online to www.americanheart.org, for the most current CPR guidelines.
2. Next, attend to *second-level* priority problems:
    ❑ Mental status change (e.g., confusion, decreased alertness)
    ❑ Untreated medical problems requiring immediate attention (e.g., a diabetic who hasn't had insulin)
    ❑ Acute pain
    ❑ Acute urinary elimination problems
    ❑ Abnormal lab values
    ❑ Risks of infection, safety, or security (for patient or for others)
3. Address *third-level* priority problems (later priorities):
    ❑ Health problems that don't fit into the above categories (e.g., problems with lack of knowledge, activity, rest, family coping)

BOX 5-3	SETTING PRIORITIES ACCORDING TO MASLOW'S HUMAN NEEDS

No. 1 priorities:	Problems with survival needs (e.g., food, fluids, oxygen, elimination, warmth, physical comfort)
No. 2 priorities:	Problems with safety and security needs (e.g., risks of injury or infection, threats to feeling secure)
No. 3 priorities:	Problems with love and belonging (e.g., family problems, separation from loved ones)
No. 4 priorities:	Problems with self-esteem needs (e.g., need for privacy, respect, independence, and positive self-image)
No. 5 priorities:	Problems with self-actualization needs (e.g., need to grow and achieve outcomes)

Summarized from Maslow, A. (1970). *Motivation in personality.* New York: Harper & Row.

BOX 5-4	DELEGATING IN THE CLINICAL SETTING*

When is It Safe to Delegate?

Delegate When...

- The patient is stable.
- The task is within the worker's job description and capabilities.
- The amount of RN time with the patient isn't significantly reduced.

Don't Delegate When...

- Complex assessment, thinking, and judgment are required.
- The outcome of the task is unpredictable.
- There's increased risk of harm (e.g., arterial puncture can cause more severe complications than venous puncture).
- Problem solving and creativity are required.

Key Points On Delegation

Delegation defined: *Transferring to a competent individual the authority to perform a selected task in a selected situation, while retaining accountability for results*

1. **Remember the "five rights of delegation."** Delegate...
   - **The right task**—one that doesn't fall under nursing's practice scope only.
   - **To the right person**—someone qualified and competent to do the job. Keep costs in mind (e.g., diet teaching by a dietician may cost more than having a nurse do diet teaching in the home).
   - **In the right situation**—see left column (When Is It Safe to Delegate?)
   - **With the right communication**—be clear and concise when describing the task, the goal, and what you want reported.
   - **With the right supervision, evaluation, and feedback**—timely evaluation of patients' responses and worker's performance is key. Let the caregiver know what he or she is doing well, and give tips for improvement.
2. **Delegate with full knowledge of...**
   - Your state practice act, and applicable standards, policies, and procedures (e.g., what you're allowed to delegate and to whom may vary from state to state and facility to facility).
   - The person's specific job description and competencies.
3. **When delegating to patients or family caregivers,** determine whether they have the required knowledge and skills.
4. **Follow up *with your direct assessment* of the patient:** You are accountable for patient outcomes. When the person you delegated knows you'll be checking results **with the patient**, she is more likely to do a good job.

> **RULE**
>
> **Set daily priorities by applying the "80/20 Rule."** Think of all the things you have to do for your patients as 100%. Then figure out the 20% that *must get done.* This is where you need to spend 80% of your time.

CRITICAL MOMENTS

REMEMBER THE CHAIN OF COMMAND, AND AVOID MALPRACTICE SUITS

Too many nurses have tunnel vision, focusing only on what they can do independently to resolve a problem. This can cause treatment delays that result in patient harm. Always ask yourself, *Could any of these signs and symptoms be due to a medication, an allergy, or a problem that requires medical management?* If the answer is yes, an immediate priority is to notify the appropriate person along the chain of command. For example, you may have to notify an instructor or supervisor before calling the doctor. Problems with nurses not initiating the chain of command early are key contributing factors to adverse patient outcomes (and malpractice suits).

Practice Exercises: Setting Priorities

Note: Example responses are on page 260.

1. If the expected outcome is *will be discharged home in 5 days and able to manage colostomy care,* which of the following problems *must* be addressed in the plan of care?
    a. Anxiety related to inability to return to work for 6 weeks
    b. Knowledge deficit: colostomy care
    c. Risk for impaired skin integrity related to colostomy drainage
2. Based on the information in the following scenario, what is your *most immediate* priority?

Scenario

Mr. Santos, a 64-year-old migrant worker, is admitted with a right calf thrombophlebitis. He is on therapy with bed rest, warm soaks, and anticoagulants. His knowledge of English is minimal. You try to teach him how to give himself anticoagulant injections. You have problems communicating, so you decide to contact social services to get a translator to attend the teaching sessions. Mr. Santos conveys to you that his leg is still painful and that he's also been getting pains in his chest.

3. Read the following scenario, and then answer questions a-c.

Scenario

You're caring for Neil, a 16-year-old football player who had surgery for a ruptured spleen 10 hours ago. He is alert, his vital signs are stable, and his abdominal dressing is clean and dry. He has incisional discomfort and hasn't been medicated for pain since surgery. He is also uncomfortable because he hasn't been able to void since surgery. He says, "I feel so lousy, I wish my mother could stay with me." When you offer to call her, he replies, "No, she's dying of cancer. I don't know what I'm going to do without her. Would you call my aunt?"

a. You identified the following nursing concerns. Using Box 5-3 on page 182 as a guide, decide how you would prioritize the needs and problems below: Place a *1* (for first priority), *2* (second priority), or *3* (third priority) in the appropriate blank.

   i. _____ Wants his aunt to come in

   ii. _____ Hasn't voided in 4 hours

   iii. _____ Has incisional pain

b. Explain why you chose the order of priorities you listed in (a).

c. The expected outcome for Neil is, *Will be discharged home after 3 days, able to change dry sterile dressings.* Neil demonstrates dressing changes the day after surgery and relates the importance of impeccable wound care. He is ambulatory and voiding well. Which of the following is *not* likely to be addressed on the care plan and why?

   i. Risk for infection related to incision

   ii. Anticipatory grieving related to loss of his mother as evidenced by statements that mother has terminal cancer and he wishes she could be with him

   iii. Deficient knowledge: dressing changes

14. DETERMINING CLIENT-CENTERED (PATIENT-CENTERED) OUTCOMES

Definition

Describing exactly what results will be observed in the patient to show the expected benefits of care at a certain point in time

Example: Twenty-four hours after endotracheal intubation for open-heart surgery, the patient will be without the tube and able to breathe independently. Before going on to complete this section, be sure you have studied pages 79-80, which describe various types of outcomes (clinical, functional, and other types) and address the role of outcomes in the context of evidence-based practice.

Why This Skill Promotes Clinical Judgment

On a daily basis, outcomes (results) are often *implied*—if you're doing something to fix a problem, you obviously expect to see *beneficial results*. However, in complex situations and when writing formal or standard plans, outcomes are stated according to *very specific rules* as noted in this section. Following the rules forces you to think things through and helps you to record a very specific outcome that guides care and facilitates evaluation of care.

Clearly described expected outcomes promote efficiency. They help you:

- Explain why the treatment plan is worthwhile.
- Keep the focus on *how the person is responding* to care, the most important measure of how well the plan is working.
- Determine priorities. You need to know *exactly what you aim to do* before you can decide what's most important and what must be done first.
- Motivate key players—knowing the benefits and time frame for outcome achievement prompts patients and caregivers to initiate actions in a timely fashion.
- Determine specific interventions designed to achieve the outcomes. As the saying goes, "If you don't know where you're going, it's hard to figure out how to get there."

Guidelines: How to Determine Client-Centered (Patient-Centered) Outcomes

Study the following principles, and then go on to the following section, which addresses how to individualize outcomes when using standard plans and critical pathways.

Principles of Client-Centered (Patient-Centered) Outcomes:

1. To describe expected outcomes, use terms that explain the *benefits* expected to be *observed in the patient* after care is given.
2. If you don't understand the difference between clinical, functional, quality of life, and other types of outcomes, or the interplay between outcomes and problems, study pages 79-81.
3. Always partner with key stakeholders to develop outcomes *together*. Be realistic, considering:
   - Physical health state, overall prognosis
   - Growth and development; psychologic/mental status
   - Spiritual, cultural, and economic needs
   - Expected length of stay
   - Available human, material, and financial resources
   - Other planned therapies for the client
4. Expected outcomes may be written from a *problem or intervention* perspective.
   - **Outcomes written for problems** describe exactly what will be observed in the patient to show that the problems are resolved (or managed). For example, what will be observed when a patient no longer has trouble feeding himself?

■ **Outcomes written for interventions** describe the *desired response* to the intervention. For example, what will be observed in the patient after you irrigate his nasogastric tube?

> **RULE**
>
> **There's a dynamic relationship between outcomes, problems, and interventions:** (1) If you aren't achieving desired results, ask, *Are we sure that we identified the problems correctly? Are we sure that we're using the correct interventions?* and *Have we included key stakeholders (e.g. patients and care providers) in decision making?* (2) To prioritize care, be sure that you have clearly determined the problems, issues, and risks that must be managed to achieve the *overall outcomes* of the plan of care (problem and risk identification is often described as being at least 50% of the work of planning care).

5. **To determine expected outcomes for problems:** Reverse the problem—describe what will be observed *in the patient* when the problem no longer exists or is managed at an acceptable level (see following diagram).

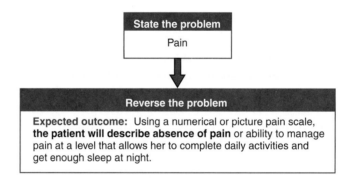

6. **To determine expected outcomes for interventions:** Describe what will be observed *in the patient* to demonstrate that the *desired response* to the intervention has been achieved (see following diagram).

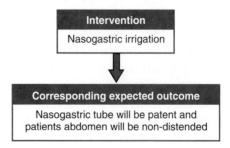

7. To ensure clarity, expected outcomes should have the following components:
   - **Subject:** Who is expected to achieve the outcome? Or, what part of the patient will be observed to demonstrate the expected benefit?
   - **Verb:** What will the person do (or what will be observed) to demonstrate outcome achievement?
   - **Condition:** Under what circumstances will the person do it?
   - **Performance Criteria:** How well will the person do it?
   - **Target Time:** By when will the person be able to do it?

   Examples: "By Friday, Jim will walk with a walker to the end of the hall." Or, "By Friday, the skin on the bottom of the heel will be intact and free from signs of irritation."

8. Use verbs for actions that are observable and measurable (actions you can clearly *see, hear, feel,* or *smell*).
   - **Use verbs like these:** explain, describe, state, list, demonstrate, show, communicate, express, walk, gain, and lose.
   - **Don't use verbs like these:** know, understand, appreciate, feel (these aren't measurable because no one can read someone else's mind to find out if they know, understand, appreciate, etc.).

9. To give a summary statement to guide evaluation, use as *evidenced by* to describe *exactly what behaviors will indicate that the outcome has been met.* **Example:** The client will demonstrate diabetes management *as evidenced by ability to state how insulin works, perform glucose monitoring, adjust insulin dose according to blood sugar level, and use sterile injection technique.*

10. In complex cases, develop both *short-* and *long-term* outcomes. Use short-term outcomes as stepping stones to long-term outcomes. **Example:** (Short-term) "After 1 week, Fred will be able to bathe and dress himself with assistance." (Long-term) "After 4 weeks, Fred will be totally independent in performing his morning care."

Practice Exercises: Determining Client-Centered (Patient-Centered) Outcomes

Note: Example responses are on page 260.

Based on the information provided, determine the most specific, client-centered outcome for each of the following:

1. Risk for impaired skin integrity related to age, obesity, and prolonged bed rest
2. Suction patient prn (as needed)
3. Powerlessness related to quadriplegia as evidenced by statements such as "I have no choices"
4. Irrigate Foley catheter every 4 hours
5. Endotracheal intubation
6. Activity intolerance related to muscle weakness secondary to prolonged bed rest as evidenced by inability to walk the length of the hall without assistance

15. DETERMINING INDIVIDUALIZED INTERVENTIONS

Definition
Identifying specific nursing actions that are tailored to the patient's needs and desires and designed to (1) prevent, manage, and eliminate problems and risk factors; (2) reduce the likelihood of undesired outcomes and increase the likelihood of desired outcomes; and (3) promote health and independence

Why This Skill Promotes Clinical Judgment
To prevent and resolve health problems, you must know how to develop safe, *individualized* interventions that are *specific to each patient's particular situation*. Keeping a focus on *individual patient needs and desires* gives the patient a sense of autonomy and helps you design a plan that's more likely to be followed. Knowing how to tailor the interventions to increase the likelihood of success and decrease the likelihood of harm is the key to efficiency and improving the quality of your patients' lives.

Guidelines: How to Determine Specific Interventions
1. Get patients and families involved in decision-making *early*. They are the ones who can help you tailor interventions in ways that are likely to succeed. Tell patients that your role is not only to take care of them, but to help them know how to take care of themselves *when you're not there*.
2. Identify interventions that aim to monitor and manage both problems and the underlying cause(s) or contributing factors, as in the box on the right.
3. Give high priority to designing interventions aimed at managing the factors *contributing* to the problems. For example, if your patient has problems coughing because of incisional pain, a high-priority intervention will be to manage the pain.
4. Use the worksheet on page 178 to systematically consider all the things that may contribute to a given problem. After you identify all the things contributing to the problems, decide what can be done to manage the contributing factors and who is responsible for managing them. For example, if your patient has a pressure ulcer and is diabetic, realize that the diabetes is a contributing factor and specify who is responsible for managing the diabetes. Sometimes there are contributing factors that you can't do anything about, but you still need to consider them. For example, you can't do anything about a risk factor of a woman being 86 years old. However, keep in mind that this woman is at risk for many potential problems and is less resilient because of her age; therefore, you should monitor her more closely and make sure to focus on prevention early.

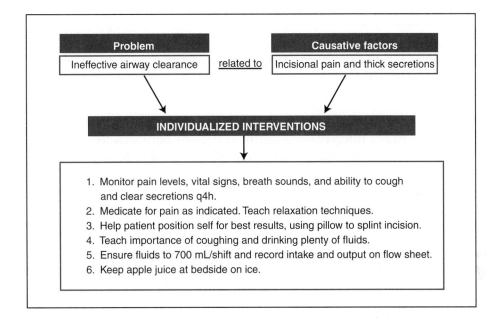

Be sure that your independent interventions are not attempting to treat a problem that needs medical management by a more qualified professional. *Example: Unrelieved pain* may indicate that there's a life-threatening problem that needs immediate medical attention; continuing to treat the pain may mask critical symptoms and put the patient at significant risk.

5. Always ask, *Are there risk factors we need to manage?* If so, identify interventions to monitor and manage the risk factors. **Example:** If the person is bed-ridden, this is a risk factor for *impaired skin integrity* and *pressure ulcers.* Monitor skin status carefully, and identify a plan for repositioning the person.

6. Identify the problems and risk factors that *must be monitored and managed* to achieve the *overall outcomes,* then ask the following:
   - How will we monitor the status of the problems and risk factors? (What will we assess? Who will assess it? How often will we assess it? How will assessments be recorded?)
   - What must be done to (1) manage or eliminate the *risk (contributing) factors?* (2) Manage or eliminate the *problems?* (3) Promote safety and reduce risk of harm? (4) Teach the person what he needs to know to be independent?

7. Consider the interventions you identified and ask the following:
   - Have I predicted how I expect this patient *in this situation* to respond to the interventions I identified?
   - Have I predicted *undesired responses* and identified ways to minimize the risk of getting them?

RULE

When predicting patient responses, consider each patient's unique situation. Identify the *desired* outcomes (the benefits of the intervention) and the *undesired* outcomes (the risks of the interventions).

- Do I know the level of evidence that supports that I will get the desired results to my interventions in this situation? For example are your interventions recommended by textbooks? By policies, procedures, standard plans? By national clinical practice guidelines?
- What can we do to increase the likelihood of getting desired results and reduce the risk of doing harm (getting undesired results) *in this specific patient's situation?*

8. Remember the PPMP (predict, prevent, manage, promote) approach:
   - Predict potential complications and be ready to manage them (Box 3-6 on page 96 and Box 3-7 on page 97 list common potential complications). Sometimes you can't do much about the *cause* of the problems, but you can prevent and manage the *symptoms and potential complications* of the problems. For instance, if someone has just had his jaws wired shut, you can't do much about it, but you must be prepared to handle the potential complication of aspiration by having suction equipment and wire cutters nearby.
   - Identify interventions that not only treat problems and risk factors, but also *promote optimum function, independence, and well-being.* **Example:** Stress the benefits of walking at least 20 minutes a day. Be sure that patients have a paper and pen to write down things they need to remember. Ask patients for things you can do to make things more convenient for them.

9. To be complete when writing nursing interventions, use the following memory-jog: *See, do, teach,* and *record.* Consider what you need to *see* (assess), what you or the patient needs to *do,* what you need to *teach,* and what you must *record.* **Example:**
   - **See:** Assess ability to walk with walker in the room before allowing the patient to go out in the hall alone.
   - **Do:** Have him walk the length of the hall three times a day.
   - **Teach:** Reinforce that research shows that walking will increase muscle strength and reduce fatigue.
   - **Record:** Record pulse and blood pressure before and after walking at least once a day.

10. Keep in mind both direct-care interventions (things you do directly for or with the patient, such as helping him get out of bed) and indirect-care interventions (things you do away from the patient, such as monitoring lab results).

Practice Exercises: Determining Individualized Interventions

Note: Example responses are on page 261.

1. Determine specific interventions for each of the following problems and corresponding outcomes.

Problem	Corresponding Expected Outcome
a. Risk for fluid volume deficit related to diarrhea and insufficient fluid intake	Will maintain adequate hydration as evidenced by drinking at least 4 quarts of clear liquids per 24-hour period
b. Anxiety related to insufficient knowledge of hospital procedures	By the end of today, will relate knowledge of hospital procedures and express ways of managing anxiety
c. Chronic pain related to arthritic joints as evidenced by statements of pain with range of motion for the past 20 years	After application of heat and assistance with range of motion, will rate pain on a scale of 0-10, and express that joint pain doesn't prohibit movement or sleep

2. Imagine you do a home visit with an 86-year-old woman who is asthmatic and is on chemotherapy for ovarian cancer. She is independent, but likes to spend much of her day reading in bed. She is 5 feet tall and weighs 93 pounds. Using the worksheet on page 178, determine all the factors she has that may contribute to a *risk for impaired skin integrity*. Then decide what, if anything, will be done to manage each contributing factor.

3. Consider the following scenario; then respond to the questions that follow.

Scenario

You make a home visit to the Supopoffs. The family is Russian and has three children, ages 5, 7, and 10. Their home is next to a forest full of deer ticks. Mrs. Supopoff is upset because she keeps finding ticks on the children, and she knows Lyme disease comes from tick bites. She's told the children not to go into the forest, but she suspects they disregard her instructions. Mrs. Supopoff is considering punishing the children when she finds a tick on them, hoping this will make them more careful.

You look up Lyme disease and learn that the best treatment is *prevention of tick bites.* You then identify the following problem and expected outcome:

Problem: Risk for infection related to tick bites.

Expected outcome: The children will have a decreased risk of tick bites and infection as evidenced by their wearing insect repellent when outside, avoiding tall grassy areas, and monitoring themselves and each other for ticks.

a. Consider the risks and benefits of the following actions:
   (1) What might happen if the children are punished when a tick is found on them?
   (2) What might happen if you reward the children for finding ticks?
b. What interventions might safely motivate the children to participate in spotting ticks and avoiding bites? Write specific interventions to achieve the expected outcome listed for this situation.

16. EVALUATING AND CORRECTING THINKING (SELF-REGULATING)

Definition
Reflecting on thinking for the purpose of improvement—for example, looking for flaws, deciding whether your thinking is focused, clear, and in enough depth—then making adjustments as needed.

Why This Skill Promotes Clinical Judgment
Developing clinical judgment skills requires you to self-regulate, which means you must constantly reflect on your thinking and ask yourself questions like, *Am I clear about what's going on here? What am I missing? How can I be more sure that my reasoning is sound? Am I holding myself to high standards? Do I know what I'll do if things go wrong?* and *What creative approaches might work here? What peers or experts can I get to dialogue with me so that I better understand the thinking that should go into a situation like this?*

RULE

To avoid judgment errors, don't settle for the first conclusion or idea you have. Reflect on thinking and consider alternative conclusions, problems, explanations, and solutions. Successful nurses aren't successful because they can come up with one right answer or explanation—they come up with many, and then choose the best one.

Guidelines: How to Evaluate and Correct Thinking (Self-Regulate)
Evaluating and correcting thinking is an ongoing process. Because the nursing process is a major tool for critical thinking, the following box gives example questions you should be asking at various phases of the nursing process.

REFLECTING ON VARIOUS PHASES OF THE NURSING PROCESS

Assessment
- Were the patient and the key stakeholders involved in the process as much as possible?
- How well do I understand my patient's perceptions?
- What assumptions could I have made?
- How complete is data collection?
- How accurate and reliable is my information?
- How well do I understand my patient's perceptions?
- Have I considered what data I need from both nursing and medical perspectives?

Diagnosis and Outcome Identification
- Were the patient and the key stakeholders involved in the process as much as possible?
- Have I included the patient and the key stakeholders in determining realistic outcomes?
- Are my outcomes clearly stated in measurable terms?
- How sure am I of the conclusions I've drawn (inferences I've made)?
- Should I be reporting some signs and symptoms immediately—could this be a medical problem that requires more qualified management?
- How well does the patient's data support that the problems I identified are the correct ones?
- Have I missed any other problems that could be indicated by the patient's data?
- Am I clear about the underlying causes and risk factors?
- How clearly and specifically are the problems and outcomes described?
- Am I clear about the definitive diagnoses?
- Have I identified "muddy issues" that may have to be clarified?
- Have I identified both nursing problems and problems requiring a multidisciplinary approach?
- Were client strengths and resources identified?
- Have I determined the priority risks and problems that must be recorded on the plan of care?

Planning
- Were the patient and the key stakeholders involved in setting priorities and developing the plan as much as possible?
- What immediate priorities could have been missed?
- Have I missed any problems that must be addressed in the plan of care?
- How well do the outcomes reflect the benefits I expect to see?
- Are the expected outcomes realistic, clear, and client-centered?
- Have I considered the *undesired responses* and identified interventions to reduce the likelihood of getting them?
- Did I consider both the problems and the outcomes when identifying interventions?
- Did I consider client preferences when developing the plan, and did I use client strengths and resources?
- Have I predicted patient responses and individualized interventions to this specific patient and situation?
- Have I decided where we'll record the priority problems and risks and the corresponding interventions?

Continued

REFLECTING ON VARIOUS PHASES OF THE NURSING PROCESS—cont'd

Implementation
- Were the patient and the key stakeholders involved in the process as much as possible?
- Are the problems still the same?
- Am I missing any new problems?
- Am I keeping the focus on client responses?
- Should I be doing anything differently? Are the interventions still appropriate?
- Have I identified and recorded changes we need to make?

Evaluation
- Where does the patient stand in relation to achieving major desired outcomes?
- How accurately and completely have I completed each of the previous phases?
- What do the patient and the key stakeholders have to say about their progress?
- What suggestions do the patient and the key stakeholders have for improvement?

There are no practice exercises for this skill, since opportunities for evaluating and correcting thinking have been provided throughout the other skills sections.

17. DETERMINING A COMPREHENSIVE PLAN AND EVALUATING AND UPDATING THE PLAN

Definition
Ensuring that the priority problems and corresponding outcomes and interventions are recorded on the patient record; keeping the plan up to date

Why This Skill Promotes Clinical Judgment
Developing a comprehensive plan and ensuring that the major care plan components are recorded (1) forces you to think about the most important aspects of giving care, (2) promotes communication between caregivers, and (3) provides data for evaluation, research, legal, and insurance purposes.

Ongoing evaluation—continually reflecting on how the plan is working and what changes must be made—helps you make adjustments *early*, making care safer and more efficient.

Guidelines: How to Develop a Comprehensive Plan/Update the Plan
1. Being able to determine a comprehensive plan requires all of the skills listed in this section and knowing the purpose and components of the recorded plan (Box 5-5).

BOX 5-5	PURPOSE AND COMPONENTS OF THE RECORDED PLAN OF CARE

Purpose of Recorded Plan
1. Promotes communication between caregivers
2. Directs care, interventions, and documentation
3. Creates a record that can later be used for evaluation, research, legal, and insurance purposes

Components of Recorded Plan (Use the Memory-Jog EASE)
Expected outcomes
Actual and potential problems that must be addressed to reach the overall outcomes
Specific interventions designed to achieve the outcomes
Evaluation statements (progress notes)

---

2. Identify the major problems and interventions yourself. Then:
   - Check the patient record to see whether the problems and interventions are addressed by preestablished plans, policies, or doctor's orders.
   - Compare your patient's situation with the interventions on preestablished plans. Modify or add interventions if needed.
3. To evaluate and update the plan, compare what's recorded in the plan with what you *actually find* when you assess the patient.
   - Determine progress toward expected outcomes. For example, if the expected outcome states *will be free of signs of infection around incision,* assess the incision for signs of infection (e.g., redness, drainage, heat, and tenderness).
   - Monitor problems closely; watch closely for new risk factors or problems. If risk factors or problems change, update the patient record as indicated.
   - Monitor patient responses to interventions. If you aren't seeing the expected results, together with the patient, decide what needs to change to improve results.
   - Modify interventions as needed, changing the record as needed.
4. Remember the following rule.

RULE

You are responsible for looking for care variances (a care variance is when a patient hasn't achieved outcomes by the time frame noted on a plan of care). If you identify a care variance, ask, (1) *What additional assessment do I need to do to determine whether this delay is justified? (2) What can be done to improve the likelihood that the person will achieve the outcomes of the plan? and (3) What resources and multidisciplinary approaches might help?* Then take appropriate action.

Practice Exercises: Determining a Comprehensive Plan and Updating the Plan

Note: Example responses are on pages 261-262.

1. Consider each of the expected outcomes and the corresponding patient data and decide whether the outcome has been achieved, partially achieved, or not achieved.

    a. **Expected outcome:** Will be ready for discharge by day three after surgery as evidenced by ability to demonstrate how to manage wound packing. **Data:** Patient says that managing wound packing shouldn't be his concern and feels he's incapable of doing so.

    b. **Expected outcome:** Will drink at least 4 quarts of fluid as evidenced by keeping a written record of fluid intake. **Data:** Patient's record indicates 5 quarts of fluid intake daily.

    c. **Expected outcome:** The baby will be discharged home with parents able to perform CPR. **Data:** Father demonstrates CPR well. Mother has trouble establishing airway.

2. Develop a comprehensive plan, identifying two priority diagnoses for the following scenario. Include an overall expected discharge outcome, outcomes for each diagnosis, and specific interventions.

Scenario

It's Monday, June 27. You admit Mrs. Edmunds, who has just suffered anaphylactic shock after a bee sting. She is expected to be discharged by Wednesday, June 29. The doctor gives Mrs. Edmunds an emergency epinephrine injection kit and tells her, "The nurse will teach you how to use it." Mrs. Edmunds still has hives all over her body and says her itching feet are driving her crazy. You find that placing her feet in cool water every so often helps her discomfort. She is still slightly wheezy from the bee sting reaction.

When you ask her about using the injection kit, she replies, "No way!" Her husband, who is retired, says, "I'll be glad to learn." It's decided that it's satisfactory to discharge Mrs. Edmunds on June 29, with her husband able to demonstrate how to give epinephrine in an emergency.

3. Suppose you're using a critical pathway to guide your patient's care, and it states that on the first day after surgery, the patient should have the Foley catheter out and be voiding normally. It's now the second day after surgery, and when you check the intake and output record, you see that she is voiding 30 cc every hour. What should you do, and why?

4. Suppose you're reviewing someone's chart to determine if a comprehensive plan of care is present. What four care plan components will you look for?

5. The next time you go to the clinical setting, get a patient chart and determine whether the four components of the plan of care are recorded somewhere on the record.

REFERENCES

1. Matz, C. E. (December 2006). Mail communication.
2. Silver, D. (January 2007). e-Mail communication.

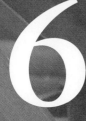

6

Mastering Common Workplace Skills

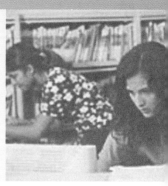

This chapter at a glance...

1. Navigating and Facilitating Change (page 199)
2. Communicating Bad News (page 203)
3. Dealing with Complaints Constructively (page 206)
4. Developing Empowered Partnerships (page 209)
5. Giving and Taking Constructive Criticism (page 212)
6. Managing Conflict Constructively (page 216)
7. Managing Your Time (page 221)
8. Preventing and Dealing with Mistakes Constructively (page 226)
9. Transforming a Group into a Team (page 233)
10. Accessing and Using Information Effectively (page 238)
11. Outcome-Focused Writing (Writing to Get Results) (page 243)

PRECHAPTER SELF-TEST

Decide where you stand in relation to the learning outcomes at the beginning of each skill in this section.

How to Use This Chapter

This chapter helps you gain key workplace skills that you need to work in any position that's highly relational (any position that demands a lot of interaction with others). When you know how to build positive relationships with patients and other professionals, you spend less time getting sidetracked by interpersonal and "human nature" problems—and more time fully engaged in progress.

Each skill is presented in the following format: (1) name of the skill, (2) definition of the skill, (3) learning outcomes, (4) thinking critically about the skill, (5) how to accomplish the skill, and (6) critical thinking exercises.

To complete many of the critical thinking exercises, you should partner with at least one other person. Content is presented in a way that can help you plan a seminar for each skill to promote in-depth discussion and learning. As part of the seminar requirements, each participant should read at least two up-to-date articles on the topic. *Note: Because the critical thinking exercises are intended to be done with a partner or in groups, there are no example responses in the* Response Key *in the back of the book.*

1. NAVIGATING AND FACILITATING CHANGE

Definition
Knowing how to chart a course to making changes and help others to do the same

Learning Outcomes
After completing this section, you should be able to:
- Explain your reaction when faced with change.
- Identify strategies to help you navigate change.
- Describe how to facilitate change in others.

Thinking Critically about Change

As someone once said, "Even if you're on the right track, you still get hit by the train if you don't keep moving." Change is a part of life. Knowing how to plot a course through the many changes we face on a daily basis is essential to thriving in this rapidly changing world. When you know how to navigate change—and how to help others do the same—you can move from feeling disrupted and frustrated to feeling a sense of progress and accomplishment.

How to Navigate and Facilitate Change

This section first addresses how to personally navigate change, and then it addresses how to facilitate change in others.

Navigating Change

- Curb the tendency to keep the status quo because it's easy and comfortable.
- When first faced with change, suspend judgment and fairly explore reasons for the required change. Navigating change doesn't mean embracing change uncritically—it means clarifying the pros and cons and making reasoned decisions about whether the change is worthwhile.
- Make sure you understand why the change is being made and how you feel about it. If you can get something out of the change, it helps you accept it. If you have strong feelings against making the change, you need to explore and work through them.
- Identify barriers to making the change and find ways to deal with them. For example, make yourself a "cheat sheet" when learning new technology.
- Ask for help. If you express the problems you have, others may be able to help. You may also identify concerns that are bothering everyone.
- Expect the following natural sequence of events often associated with adapting to change.

Stages Associated with Adapting to Change

1. **Losing focus**. Expect some confusion, disorientation, and forgetfulness at first. You may be unsure about boundaries and responsibilities. Ask for clarification, keep notes, and use to-do lists.
2. **Denial**. You may want to minimize or deny the effect the change has on you. However, *connecting with and dealing with feelings* helps you move forward. Acknowledge how you feel about what you lose and gain by making the change.
3. **Anger or Depression**. If you feel angry, discouraged, or frustrated:
   - Vent your anger in a safe place. Be careful with whom, how, and where you ventilate. Your words can come back to haunt you. Find someone who'll listen empathetically without being affected by your feelings (e.g., someone who has gone through the change you're experiencing, not someone who also is struggling and who may be pulled down by your negativity).
   - Use stress management strategies (e.g., exercise helps diffuse anger and frustration).
   - Keep away from negative people, because their thoughts might influence you.

- Stay focused on what you'll gain from making the change. Be patient with yourself, let go of the past, and take it one step at a time. Make a conscious effort to think critically and not emotionally.

4. **Moving forward**. Seek opportunities to use the new skills and procedures you've learned. Celebrate small successes, recognizing how far you've come and what you learned along the way.
   - Share your experience with those who may not have come as far as you have.
   - Remember to represent your organization positively in public, even if you don't feel that way at the moment.

Facilitating Change in Others

- Including key stakeholders, determine how the change will affect those involved. Be clear about the positives and negatives *from their perspectives.*
- Clearly describe both the required changes and the expected benefits.
- Clarify changes in roles and responsibilities.
- Get support from formal and informal group leaders (they can help or deter the process).
- Allow people to explore how the change will affect their daily lives. Encourage their involvement in finding ways to make the change easier.
- Convey an understanding of negative feelings and extra work associated with having to make a change. Provide necessary resources and support (for example, technical support) until the change has been fully implemented.
- Ask for ownership of responsibility for change (both leaders and subordinates own some of the work).
- Involving key stakeholders, identify barriers to making the change and find ways to deal with them. For example, if workers are expected to take time to practice using a new computer system, provide extra personnel to do ordinary chores.
- Be clear about time lines: Key players must know exactly what change is expected to occur and by when.
- Be patient. Going through the stages of adapting to change takes time.

OTHER PERSPECTIVES

HOW TO CHANGE THE WORLD
"We must be the change we wish to see in the world."—*Mohandas Gandhi*

CRITICAL MOMENTS

TRANSFORM RATHER THAN CONFORM
When facilitating change, aim to transform rather than conform. Inspire, show benefits, encourage, and support. When people are transformed, they change because they *want* to.

CRITICAL THINKING EXERCISES

With a partner, in a group, or in a journal entry, as appropriate:

1. Share your best and worst experiences with navigating and facilitating change. Discuss the factors that made them your best and worst experiences.
2. Describe a personal or work change that you experienced that wasn't of your choice (e.g., moving to a new home, a change in job description).
   - Think about how you felt at the time and the effect it had on your ability to make the change.
   - Identify some things you could have done to make the change easier.
3. Share a time you tried to help someone else change.
   - How successful were you?
   - What, if anything, would you do differently?
4. Study Box 6-1 *(Four Ways We Change)*. Explain why paradigm change facilitates critical thinking.
5. Explain the difference between change that transforms and change that conforms.
6. Determine whether you can achieve the learning outcomes listed at the beginning of this skill.

RECOMMENDED

Harrington, S. (2002). How RNs can meet the challenge of self-change. Retrieved September 1, 2007, from http://community.nursingspectrum.com/Magazine Articles/article.cfm?AID=5928.

Johnson, S., & Blanchard, K. (1998). *Who moved my cheese?* New York: Putnam Publishing Group.

BOX 6-1 | FOUR WAYS WE CHANGE

Four Ways We Change
1. Pendulum change: I was wrong before, but now I'm right.
2. Change by exception: I'm right, except for...
3. Incremental change: I was almost right before, but now I'm right.
4. Paradigm change: What I knew before was partially right. What I know now is more right, but still only part of what I'll know tomorrow.

Paradigm Change Is Transformational
Paradigm change combines what's useful about old ways with what's useful about new ways, and keeps us open to looking for even better ways. We realize:
- Our previous views were only part of the picture.
- What we now know is only part of what we'll know later.
- Change is no longer threatening: It enlarges and enriches.
- The unknown can then be friendly and interesting.
- Each insight smoothes the road, making the change process easier.

Adapted and summarized from Ferguson, M. (1980). *Aquarian conspiracy: Personal and social transformation in our time.* New York: GP Putnam's Sons.

Menix, K. (2000). Educating to manage the accelerated change environment effectively: Part 1. *Journal for Nurses in Staff Development, 16*(6), 282-288.

2. COMMUNICATING BAD NEWS

Definition
Knowing how to convey honesty, empathy, and responsibility when giving someone information that will have a negative impact on them

Learning Outcomes
After completing this section, you should be able to:
- Explain what can happen when you avoid giving bad news.
- Identify strategies to minimize the impact of bad news.
- Determine how you can reduce your stress when faced with giving bad news.

Thinking Critically about Giving Bad News
No one likes to give bad news. All too often, people who have bad news to give tend to avoid this unpleasant chore altogether, making things worse. When you communicate bad news at an appropriate time, in an appropriate place, and with honesty, empathy, and responsibility, you can soften the blow by minimizing the common feelings of anger, disappointment, and betrayal. How you handle giving bad news can make the difference between escalating an already difficult situation and building positive relationships in spite of adversity.

The following are guidelines for giving bad news in the context of giving bad news related to health status, and related to customer service issues.

CRITICAL THINKING EXERCISES

With a partner, in a group, or in a journal entry, as appropriate:

1. Describe the following:
   - Your best and worst experiences with how someone gave you bad news.
   - The emotions you feel when giving bad news.
   - How people you know have responded to bad news situations and why you think they responded that way.
2. Imagine that you have to tell someone that their mother has been admitted to the intensive care unit after a car accident. Using the steps for giving bad news related to health status on the next page, develop a plan for how you will do this.
3. Imagine you have to tell someone that they have to wait 2 hours to see the doctor because of other urgent problems. Using the steps for giving bad news related to customer service issues on page 206, develop a plan for how you will do this.

GIVING BAD NEWS RELATED TO HEALTH STATUS: TEN STEPS

Steps	Rationale
1. **Determine who has the authority and qualifications to give the bad news.** Usually this is the primary care provider, such as the doctor or nurse practitioner.	**Ethically, and sometimes legally, health care providers are responsible for ensuring that patients have proper support when they get bad news.** Depending on the impact of the news (e.g., if the news is about biopsy results, severe illness, or death), the patient and family is likely to have questions that must be answered by the most qualified professional. Always check your facility's policies regarding patient confidentiality and HIPAA privacy laws.
2. **Have the professional who is best qualified (or who has developed the best relationship with the person) give the news.**	**The messenger matters.** Bad news is often met with powerful emotions of disappointment and anger. Receiving bad news in a caring way from trusted professionals softens the blow. It's easy to feel that a provider who is too busy to give the bad news has betrayed you. It takes a strong, logical mind not to want to "shoot the messenger." Making sure that those who know the patient best—for example, a trusted nurse or a chaplain—are present helps reduce feelings of being abandoned or helpless.
3. **Choose the setting—ensure privacy, and don't use the phone.**	How and where the person gets bad news is key. Using the phone doesn't allow for appropriate assessment and support.
4. **Find out what the person already knows or suspects.**	**This simplifies the process and helps clarify what you need to say.**
5. **Give a warning shot.**	Saying things like, "This isn't what we wanted to hear," "I have bad news," or "I'm sorry to have to tell you this" prepares people for the emotional blow they are about to receive.
6. **Be direct, tell the news, and give time for it to sink in. (Silence is golden.)**	**Being direct helps people to get the main information first, in a logical way.** Bad news takes time to digest—patients often need to get through shock and anger, before they can move on to dealing with the impact of the news. Sometimes, all that is needed is someone to remain present, listening quietly as feelings are sorted out. You have to name the feelings before you can tame them.
7. **Respond to emotions with empathy.** Continue to use silence as a strategy. Use nonverbal gestures, as appropriate (e.g., put a hand on the person's shoulder). Help the person deal with feelings of blame.	**Each person is unique, with a range of emotional responses that depend on circumstances.** Letting people know that their emotions are *understood* helps them deal with strong feelings. Think about this analogy: An antiinflammatory drug reduces fever and associated physical discomfort. Being allowed to express emotions and feeling understood reduces anxiety and psychologic discomfort. **Bad news often brings feelings of blame. Examples of what to say:** "I'm sorry this is happening." "There's nothing that could have been done", "This is no one's fault"; "It's not worth blaming right now… it will only make things worse… we need to deal with the problem"; or "We'll help you through this." **Things *not* to say:** "I know how you feel"; "It's God's will"; or "God only gives you what you can bear."

GIVING BAD NEWS RELATED TO HEALTH STATUS: TEN STEPS—cont'd

Steps	Rationale
8. **Ask about special requests, especially related to spiritual and cultural needs.**	**Nurses are responsible for giving culturally competent care.** Asking patients and families what's most important helps them know that you care about their unique needs, and gets everyone on the same page about patient priorities. **Examples:** "Tell me what we can do to help." "Is there someone we can call?" "Do you have a specific religion; or can I get the hospital chaplain?"
9. **Be realistic, keep a positive tone, and give hope.** End with a plan, and be sure the person has a printed list of resources.	**Having hope and hearing a realistic positive attitude sets the tone for dealing with the bad news.** Hope is the "tonic" that sustains people through difficult times. **Examples of what to say:** "This is tough news… but having a positive attitude is important"; "Don't jump to conclusions or let yourself be driven by 'worst-case scenarios'."; "We're here for you, no matter what"; "Don't give up hope yet… we'll use all our resources." **Having a plan mobilizes the patient and team toward dealing with the problem.** A printed list of resources is essential for later, when the patient goes home, the information sinks in, and the patient starts thinking independently about how to handle the problem.
10. **Follow up, once there's been time for the news to sink in.**	**You don't "drop a bomb" without following up.** Some people may be mobilized in positive ways, and others may need more direction and support. Don't assume. Find out how they're doing.

HIPAA, Health Insurance Portability and Accountability Act.

4. Determine whether you can achieve the learning outcomes listed at the beginning of this skill.

RECOMMENDED

Goleman, D. (2006). *Emotional Intelligence: 10th Anniversary Edition; Why It Can Matter More Than IQ.* New York: Bantam Books.

Lachman, V. Delivering bad news. Retrieved August 27, 2007, from https://nursing.advanceweb.com/common/Editorial/Editorial.aspx?CC=20699.

Orlovsky, C. Workshops train providers to deliver bad news, difficult discussions. Retrieved August 26, 2007, from www.nursezone.com/job/Medical News-Alerts.asp?articleID=15504.

Weisinger, H. (2000). *Emotional intelligence at work.* New York: John Wiley & Sons.

See also Recommended *in the following section,* Dealing with Complaints Constructively.

GIVING BAD NEWS RELATED TO CUSTOMER SERVICE ISSUES

Steps	Example
1. **Give the bad news in a timely way.** Offer an apology, and don't try to obscure the situation.	"I'm sorry to tell you we won't be able to do your x-ray today."
2. **Showing concern, explain what happened and why.**	"Your appointment card says today, but somehow we have you scheduled in our book for next week. I'm not sure how this happened, but you can be sure that I'm going to find out."
3. **Present alternative solutions and give pros and cons of each.** Get the patient's point of view.	"I could schedule the x-ray for later today, but we get better pictures if you fast for 12 hours before the x-ray. I realize you'd have to go home and come back, and that you'd like to get it over with. I think it's worth waiting to be sure we get a good quality x-ray. Would that be OK for you?"
4. **Recommend a course of action.** Include (a) how the plan addresses the problem, and (b) how the plan addresses hardships resulting from what happened.	"I think the best solution is to schedule the x-ray as soon as possible. Since you've already had enough problems, I'll do my best to schedule you whenever it's convenient for you. I'll also find out who made this mistake and see what we can do to prevent this from happening again."
5. **Reaffirm your goals and vision for the future.** Include (a) key points that give confidence to those involved, and (b) time frame for expected results.	"We're here to serve you the best way we can. Soon we'll have a system that allows you to confirm appointments over the phone. We hope to have the system in place by May. Everyone will be encouraged to call and confirm their appointments when they get home."
6. **Follow up to see if results were satisfactory.**	"I'll send your name to our community relations department. They will call you to see if everything was resolved to your satisfaction. Please feel free to call and discuss anything you'd like with them as well. We want you to feel satisfied with your experience with us. Please let me know if you still have problems."

3. DEALING WITH COMPLAINTS CONSTRUCTIVELY

Definition
Using complaints as an opportunity to improve consumer satisfaction

Learning Outcomes
After completing this section, you should be able to:
- Explain the value of complaints.
- Express more confidence about dealing with complaints.

- Observe an improvement in how your patients respond when they come to you with a complaint.

Thinking Critically about Complaints

Dealing with complaints makes most of us uncomfortable. However, complaints are opportunities to improve. Think about the last time you complained about service. Was it just because you wanted your situation corrected, or did you think it might help them improve their service for *others?* Complaints help you:

- Correct problems before they become worse or happen to someone else.
- Identify trends in unmet needs of consumers.
- Find out about complaints before people start complaining to others.

Like all businesses, health care organizations thrive when consumers are happy. Satisfied consumers tell others about their experience and return as needed. The opposite is also true: If your consumers are unhappy, they tell others and take their business elsewhere. When someone complains, *listen* and do something about it.

How to Deal with Complaints Constructively

1. Don't take things personally. Rein in the natural tendency to be defensive, and assume there's a very good reason for the complaints (these reasons may be unclear at first).
2. Take a deep breath and remain calm in the face of anger. People requiring health care often have extenuating circumstances that cause them to have a "short fuse." Some examples:
   - Previous bad experience with health care providers or treatment plans
   - Effects of illness or disability on self, family, and work
   - Problems of being "in limbo" (the patient may not be responding as quickly or favorably as expected)
   - Family reaction to illness or disability
3. Find out what the person really values and needs.
   - Ask the person to clarify the issue; listen carefully, giving your full attention.
   - Repeat what you hear to be sure that you're clear on the issues.
   - Aim to give the person what he needs or values (this requires that you get a clear understanding from your boss about what rules you can bend or break to immediately resolve issues).
   - If you come in late to the situation, remain quiet, listen, and ask to verify your understanding of the problem.
4. Focus *on the patient's issues* and try to learn from them.
5. Swallow your pride and bite your tongue. Apologize, and avoid weak excuses (e.g., we're shorthanded, nobody's perfect). Successful apologies require you to be humble, specific on the issues, and sincere. If anger explodes:
   - Keep your own anger in check.
   - Don't defend yourself. Listen completely; focus keenly on what is being said.

- Keep in mind that some people cope in ways you consider negative (abrasive or manipulative).
- Think about whether having your manager come and talk with the person would help.

6. Involve the person in problem solving (ask for solutions). Report and record special needs.
7. Take an immediate step to resolve the problem. Explain what you're going to do and let people feel like they're winning in some way.
8. Keep the person informed (e.g., I promise to let you know the minute I know more about this). Follow up to see if solutions are working.

CRITICAL THINKING EXERCISES

With a partner, in a group, or in a journal entry, as appropriate:

1. Share your feelings about making complaints (e.g., anger, guilt, frustration).
2. Give an example of a time when you thought about complaining but decided it just wasn't worth it. How did this make you feel? Who lost the most in this situation?
3. Describe your best and worst experiences with making a complaint.
4. Explain how you usually deal with other people's complaints, and then determine some ways to improve your response.
5. Discuss the implications of the following *Other Perspectives.*

OTHER PERSPECTIVES

GIVE FIVE-STAR SERVICE
"Treat every patient or customer as though they were your favorite celebrity, hero, friend, or neighbor, or your grandma."—*Author unknown*

6. Determine whether you can achieve the learning outcomes listed at the beginning of this skill.

RECOMMENDED

Wetter, D. Why nurses need to know customer service. Retrieved September 1, 2007 from http://www.corexcel.com/html/customer.service.title.ceus.htm.
See also Recommended *in the sections* Giving Bad News, Developing Empowered Partnerships *and* Dealing with Conflict Constructively.

4. DEVELOPING EMPOWERED PARTNERSHIPS

Definition
Building mutually beneficial relationships based on the belief that people have the right and the responsibility to make their own choices and to grow in their own way

Learning Outcomes
After completing this section, you should be able to:
- Compare and contrast a parental model* and an empowered partnership model.
- Explain the benefits of empowered partnerships.
- Build empowered partnerships with patients, families, colleagues, and peers.

Thinking Critically about Empowered Partnerships
Developing empowered partnerships with peers, colleagues, and patients requires a shift in thinking from a parental model* ("I'll take care of you") to an empowered partnership model ("It's your life—you have rights and responsibilities as well as I do, and we both should grow and learn from our experience together"). Table 6-1 lists phrases that demonstrate these two models.

TABLE 6-1 PARENTAL VERSUS EMPOWERED PARTNERSHIP MODEL	
Parental Model	**Empowered Partnership**
I want to look after you.	How can I empower you to be able to be independent?
I know what's best for you.	You know yourself best. Tell me what you'd like to see happen, what's most important to you.
You should do as I say.	I want you to be able to make informed choices.
I'm responsible for you.	We share a common purpose, and we're both responsible for what happens.

Remember from the map of key elements of critical thinking on page 66 that *partnering with patients and families, clarifying outcomes,* and *getting patients involved early in the care process* is central to critical thinking and getting the results you

---

*Some people call this a paternal model. "Parental" is used to avoid sexism.

need. From getting mutual agreement on desired outcomes to identifying care approaches, apply the saying, "nothing about me without me."* Keep patients involved in all decision making.

How to Develop Empowered Partnerships

1. Be sure you can explain the concept of an empowered partnership. Although you can't completely balance power in all relationships, the aim of an empowered partnership is to balance the power *as much as possible.*

Examples of Empowered Partnerships

Nurse–patient or client	Staff nurse–nurse manager
Educator or Mentor–Learner	Nurse-pharmacist
Expert-Novice	Nurse–unlicensed worker
Nurse-Nurse	Nurse-physician

2. Partners must agree to the following statements:
   - We're both clear about our joint purpose, and we're both responsible.[†]
   - I can be trusted; I promise to be honest.
   - We should make decisions together as much as possible.
   - We'll both agree to rules for resolving conflict between us.
   - We both should expect to grow and learn from our experience together.
   - We're each responsible for our own emotional well-being (if I feel bad about something, it's my responsibility to do something about it).[†]
   - We both have the right to say no, so long as no harm is done.[†]
   - I choose to be here, so nobody's to blame.[†]
   - If one of us sees the other engage in unsafe or unethical conduct, we have the responsibility to address it appropriately.
   - We're both responsible for the outcomes (consequences) of our actions.[†]
3. An empowered partnership requires choosing to do the following:
   - Rise to the challenge of taking charge over the comfort of remaining dependent.
   - Give up some of the power; take calculated, thoughtful risks; and be willing to do the work needed to be independent.
4. It also requires the following:[2]
   - Nonjudgmental acceptance
   - Space for self-expression

---

*The South African disability movement began the slogan "Nothing about me, without me" in the 1990s. Search this slogan on Google and you will find multiple citations.
[†]**In the context of the nurse-patient relationship,** these statements aren't always so: Nurses are often held more accountable than patients. Nurses don't have the right to say *no* if it jeopardizes patient care (they must find a replacement). Patients often have few choices about where they are.

- Structure for conflict resolution
- Respect for each other's boundaries
- Support and encouragement for growth in the areas where one is limited
- Coaching skills that transform (coaching that truly affects the learner's attitudes and skills)
- Growth of partners

5. Many people are uncomfortable in an empowered partnership for the following reasons:
   - They are used to being taken care of and aren't accustomed to taking responsibility.
   - They are unwilling to accept the responsibility that comes with power.
   - They are unwilling to give up some of the power they're accustomed to having.
   - They haven't made the required shift in thinking (they don't truly believe in the benefits of partnership).

6. Change takes time. Coach those who aren't accustomed to the roles and responsibilities of being in a partnership.

7. Remember that continual focus on *mutually agreed upon outcomes* is path to success. Without it, the partnership is doomed.

OTHER PERSPECTIVES

PATIENTS MUST BE PARTNERS
"Patients have to be partners, equally responsible for treatment."
—*Tommy Lasorda, former Los Angeles Dodgers' manager*

CRITICAL THINKING EXERCISES

With a partner, in a group, or in a journal entry, as appropriate:

1. Discuss how establishing partnerships with peers is different from establishing partnerships with patients.
2. Address how establishing an empowered partnership is affected by the following:
   - The duration of contact you have with a patient
   - The patient's health state
   - Growth and development (e.g., How do you partner with a child or an elderly person?)
3. Explain what is meant by the following statement: Partnership is an attitude as much as a model for relationships.

4. The next time you have to do a presentation with someone else, follow the strategies listed in this section. Pay attention to the dynamics of empowered partnerships.

5. Determine whether you can achieve the learning outcomes listed at the beginning of this skill.

RECOMMENDED

Block, P. (1996). *Stewardship: Choosing service over self-interest.* San Francisco: Berrett-Koehler.

Yoder, L., & Restifo, V. Partnership: Making the most of mentoring. Retrieved August 28, 2007, from www.nurse.com/ce/syllabus.html?CCID=3111.

See also Recommended *in the sections* Giving and Taking Feedback, Managing Conflict Constructively *and* Transforming a Group into a Team.

5. GIVING AND TAKING CONSTRUCTIVE CRITICISM

Definition
Being able to give (and respond to) constructive criticism appropriately

Learning Outcomes
After completing this section, you should be able to:
- Discuss the effect of emotional responses to criticism.
- Determine how you can turn criticisms you receive into opportunities to grow.
- Identify strategies for giving constructive criticism.

Thinking Critically about Giving and Taking Constructive Criticism
How we think and behave is a complex issue that's closely linked to self-esteem. Being told we could be better thinkers, improve in some way, or approach things differently often brings up intensely uncomfortable feelings of being wrong or not good enough. These gut reactions cloud key issues and paralyze our ability to be objective. Knowing how to provide constructive criticism in a supportive way can make the difference between alienating others and motivating them to improve. Knowing how to respond to criticism—to be objective and work through the negative aspects of criticism—reduces our stress and helps us grow.

OTHER PERSPECTIVES

MAKE THE BEST OF PIERCING CRITICISMS
"Poor speaker... Too nervous... Your writing is too vague... There was a time when barbs like these went straight to my heart, piercing it through and through. For days and sometimes weeks, I walked around mortally wounded, sure I would never dare to write or speak in public again. It was only after the sting subsided that I began to think about the criticism. And once I did, if I thought it hit the mark, I acted on it, and as a result often ended up a better editor or writer. [When you get criticism,] distance yourself and give yourself time. Thank the person if it's valid.... Someone cared enough to take time... Let's face it. Compliments feel good, but they're often fleeting and may be about as sincere as, "Love your dress." It's criticism that has the potential to make you grow. I doubt that any of the world's great ideas came as a result of the statements, "You're doing a great job" or "I wouldn't change a thing."[6]

—*Phyllis Class, RN*

Giving Constructive Criticism*

- Be sensitive to personality differences (personalities of both the giver and the receiver greatly affect feedback).
- Keep in mind that *without mutual trust,* criticism is unlikely to be viewed constructively.
- Give feedback frequently and in a timely way (this way it's viewed as being more sincere).
- Start with what's being done right (e.g., "Here are the things I see you do right"). Next, focus on what could be improved (rather than on what's wrong).
- Stay fully engaged in the communication; listen actively to avoid misunderstandings and making false assumptions.
- Give positive feedback often to reward growth ("catch" people being effective, and surprise them with positive feedback).
- Be aware that constant negative feedback can hinder progress by making the person afraid of failure.
- Learn how to be assertive without being aggressive (Box 6-2 on the next page).

---

*Developed with the help of Barbara A. Musinski, RNC, BS.

BOX 6-2	BEING ASSERTIVE WITHOUT BEING AGGRESSIVE*

What Assertive Behavior Means
- Expressing your feelings, ideas, and needs calmly and openly
- Standing up for your own rights while showing respect for the rights of others
- Confronting fairly, being sensitive to when others feel threatened
- Valuing yourself and acting with confidence
- Owning responsibility and speaking with authority
- Building equal relationships and finding common goals

Using Assertive Behavior
1. Accept the anger or discomfort you have as your own. Don't blame others.
   - You own the problem!
   - Identify the key components of the situation and how you feel about them.
   - How do you think others who are involved feel about the issue?.
   - Decide which of your needs were not met.
2. Be cognizant of your own behavior. Keep a lid on anger (no easy task!).
3. Meet privately with the person(s). Listen first—actively commit to the other person; concentrate your attention so you accurately hear feelings, opinions, and wishes.
4. Try to understand completely before responding. Paraphrase to be sure you understand.
5. State your own feelings, thoughts, and needs clearly, in a nonthreatening way.
   - Use eye contact, a direct body posture, and a controlled voice volume and tone.
   - Using "I" messages, be clear about behavior that disturbs you and how you feel (for example, I was very embarrassed and hurt when I saw you walk away from our conversation. Rather than, You made me feel like such a jerk when ...).

*Developed with the help of Barbara A. Musinski, RNC, BS.

Taking Constructive Criticism

- Remember that negative feedback is likely to bring forth intense negative feelings. For example, say to yourself, *I'm getting upset. I'd better take a deep breath, calm down, and listen. If I work to be objective and not take things personally, I might learn something when I think about this later when I'm less stressed.*
- Befriend criticism, evaluating it objectively. Someone wants you to succeed, or she would not have bothered to share her thoughts.
- Ask yourself, *Have I heard this same criticism from other people?* If so, it's most likely true.
- Keep in mind that not all criticism is given constructively, but try to focus on what you can learn.
- If you agree with the criticism, acknowledge that the critic is right and begin to think about what you can do about it.
- Don't make excuses for yourself, don't be defensive, and sincerely try to see the benefits of the criticism.
- Practice personal feedback by monitoring your own behavior and paying attention to how others respond to you.

- Don't let false pride, rationalization, or other negative factors get in the way of your growth.
- Remember that no one's perfect, but we can all improve. Be prepared to expend some physical and emotional energy to change.
- Don't dwell on negative criticism when you're tired—wait until the next day when you're refreshed and more likely to be objective.

OTHER PERSPECTIVES

CRITICISM: DEAL WITH IT
Constructive criticism helps us improve. We all need to know how to give it, take it, deal with it, and accept it.[7]

—*Barbara A. Musinski, RNC, BS*

CRITICAL THINKING EXERCISES

With a partner, in a group, or in a journal entry, as appropriate:

1. Share what happened when you tried to give feedback to someone to help him improve. What happened and how did you feel? Would you do it differently if you had to do it again?
2. Think about a time when someone gave you criticism. What happened and how did you feel? What made things easier or harder? What did you learn in the long run?
3. Think about the following statement and decide what you would do if you had to give feedback to someone you don't get along with.
   Without mutual trust, feedback is unlikely to be viewed constructively.
4. Study the following *Other Perspectives*. Practice using some other phrases for "I want to give you some constructive criticism."

OTHER PERSPECTIVES

IS IT CRITICISM OR ADVICE? WORDS MATTER!
"Replace the term *constructive criticism* with *words that express the intent to help.* For example, say something like, 'May I give you some practical advice?' instead of 'May I give you some constructive criticism?' Try to replace *constructive* with *practical, helpful,* or *useful.* Try to replace *criticism* with *advice, recommendation, suggestion, observation,* or *opinion.*"

—*Suggestions from author's workshop participants*

5. Determine whether you can achieve the learning outcomes listed at the beginning of this skill.

RECOMMENDED

Walters, J. The 4-1-1 on constructive criticism. Retrieved August 28, 2007, from www.inc.com/articles/2001/08/23257.html.

Zurlinden, J. (2002). Preparing for a performance review. Retrieved August 28, 2007, from http://community.nursingspectrum.com/MagazineArticles/article.cfm?AID=5672.

See also Recommended *in the sections* Developing Empowered Partnerships *and* Managing Conflict Constructively.

6. MANAGING CONFLICT CONSTRUCTIVELY

Definition
Being able to make conflict work in positive ways (e.g., learning, growth, improvement)

Learning Outcomes
After completing this section, you should be able to:
- Identify your usual approach to dealing with conflict.
- Determine ways to improve your ability to make conflict work in positive ways.

Thinking Critically about Conflict
Conflict arises from human instinct. From the beginning of mankind, when survival of the fittest reigned, humans instinctively protected their territory and reacted with suspicion to people different from themselves. Today, many of us subconsciously protect our territory and react negatively toward others when things aren't going the way we expect.

Conflict can be mild, taking the form of subtle opposition to an idea or action, or it can be severe, taking the form of sharp disagreement and fighting. For many, the word *conflict* has negative connotations, bringing feelings of discomfort and dread. Most of us want to live in a world where everyone gets along and everything goes smoothly. Critical thinking requires being able to understand and exchange different viewpoints, wants, and needs and to come to a sincere agreement about what's most important. Knowing how to make conflict work in positive ways helps you grow. When you know how to manage conflict constructively, you are more likely to have positive outcomes and spend less time dealing with the negative outcomes of conflict (Table 6-2).

How to Manage Conflict Constructively
You can manage conflict constructively by following six key steps:
1. Gain insight into your natural style of dealing with conflict (Box 6-3). Make a commitment to use your strengths and work on weaknesses in an objective, purposeful way.

TABLE 6-2   OUTCOMES OF CONFLICT

Negative Outcomes of Conflict	Positive Outcomes of Managing Conflict Constructively
Increased stress	Reduced stress
Decreased productivity	Increased harmony and productivity
Poor relationships and feelings of isolation	Better relationships and more interaction
Wasted time and energy	Better understanding of others involved
Frustration, anger, and hopelessness	Improved ability to clarify main issues and find creative solutions
Lack of growth	Improved self-esteem
Poor self-esteem	Opportunity to improve bothersome things

BOX 6-3   MANAGING CONFLICT: WHAT'S YOUR STYLE?

AVOIDERS pull away. They ignore issues or withdraw from people they feel are causing conflict. Avoiders often get along well with others because they focus on promoting peace and harmony. However, they tend to allow problems to persist and place little importance on their own needs. As a result, they miss opportunities to make improvements and tend to "explode" when things finally get to be too much, even though the trigger issue may be minor.

ACCOMMODATORS or SMOOTHERS give up their own needs and try to make others feel better. Members of this group often struggle with inner conflicts because they secretly wish to speak their minds. They, too, can explode, damaging relationships because of failure to honestly confront issues that are important to them.

FORCERS try to get THEIR way even if it means others have to give up what they want or need. They're minimally interested in or aware of what others need and don't really care if they are liked.

COMPROMISERS give up part of their wants and needs and persuade others to give up part of their wants and needs. They think they get win-win solutions but may be settling for minimally acceptable solutions that continue the conflict (because they assume everyone has to lose something in negotiations rather than persisting to find answers that fully satisfy everyone involved).

COLLABORATIVE PROBLEM SOLVERS make it a rule to fairly face issues together. This group has equal concern for both the issues and the relationship. They see conflict as a means of improving relationships by gaining understanding and reducing tension. They look for solutions that allow everyone to win by identifying areas of agreement and differences. They evaluate alternatives, and choose solutions that have the full support of the key parties involved.

2. Learn to recognize patterns and appearances of conflict early. Become cognizant of verbal and nonverbal behaviors that signal that conflict may be developing (for example, withdrawal, verbalization of problems with current state of affairs).
3. Practice using conflict management strategies (Box 6-4 on the next page).
4. Develop skills you need to function more comfortably when faced with conflict (e.g., being assertive without being aggressive; see Box 6-2 on page 214).

BOX 6-4	MAD ABOUT YOU: MANAGING CONFLICT CONSTRUCTIVELY

☐ Listen with the intent to understand the other person's points of view before presenting your own.

☐ Take a deep breath, and keep a lid on your emotions. It's hard to think clearly when your adrenaline is flowing.

☐ Using "I" messages and a nonthreatening tone of voice, clearly explain how the problem is affecting you and what you'd like to happen.
  - "I feel [name the feeling]."
  - "When I see or hear [state the problem]."
  - "I would like [state the change you want to happen]."

☐ Ask yourself, What can I find in this situation that *I'm* doing to contribute to the problem? You have more control over things that *you're doing* to contribute to the problem than over things that *others are doing* to contribute to the problem.

☐ Get rid of old baggage (feelings and preconceptions you have because of things that have happened in the past); for example, thinking, *I'm just not the type of person who can handle conflict, so she knows she can get her way.*

☐ Look for deep issues. For example, say, "Tell me what's really bothering you" (keep repeating this if the answer is "I don't know").

☐ Be willing to hear things you don't like to hear. You need honest feedback to work through the issues.

☐ Ask for help from those involved. For example, "Can we agree to not be so hard on one another?"

☐ Change your approach to managing conflict depending on the situation rather than using the style you're most comfortable with. For example, many nurses use avoidance as their main approach to resolving conflicts.
  - **Use collaborative problem solving** as the overall, optimum way to manage conflict. Because this approach takes more time than you may have at the moment, initially you may need to use one of the following approaches. You also may need to use all the methods below as stepping stones to collaborative problem solving.
  - **Use avoidance** only when trying to delay confrontation until a more appropriate time, when a time-out is required, or when issues are of minor importance in relation to overall goal.
  - **Use accommodation or smoothing** when the goal is to preserve relationships or encourage the others to express themselves.
  - **Use compromise** when time is too limited for a full collaborative approach and there are two equally empowered sides that must reach agreement yet maintain a positive relationship. Find a common ground to achieve temporary settlement that at least satisfies each side's main objectives.
  - **Use forcing** only when there isn't time for discussion (for example, in an emergency), when you must implement unpopular changes, or when all other strategies have failed and the change is required.

5. Use a comprehensive approach to assessing and managing conflict:
    ■ Don't jump to conclusions: Hold opinions until you're sure of all the facts.
    ■ Choose an appropriate time and place to open discussion (ensure privacy, and find a convenient time for those involved).
    ■ Be willing to persevere until you clearly understand the issues, the values, and the goals of the key players involved.
    ■ Foster an atmosphere of trust and sincere desire to face issues fairly together; encourage free exchange of ideas, feelings, and attitudes.
    ■ Stay focused on common values and goals; look for win-win solutions (some compromising may be needed).
    ■ Look for several solutions to the problems, evaluating each solution with the key players involved.
    ■ Make a conscious effort to stay calm, help others stay calm, and keep the focus on the positive outcomes of resolving the conflict.
    ■ Take a break, or get help from outside sources as needed. Allow for time out, but keep interacting until all parties agree to the solution.
    ■ Set up a time to revisit issues to see if the solutions are actually being carried out and helping reduce the problem.
6. Apply principles of negotiation (Box 6-5).

OTHER PERSPECTIVES

IT TAKES COURAGE TO CONFRONT
"Confrontation takes considerable courage, and many people would rather take the course of least resistance (belittling and criticizing, betraying confidences, or participating in gossip about others behind their backs). But in the long run, people will trust and respect you if you are honest and open and kind with them. You care enough to confront."[8]

—Stephen Covey

BOX 6-5	**HOW TO NEGOTIATE**

- Clarify the results you want to achieve.
- Build and maintain a communication climate that supports problem solving under stress.
- Let other parties know your interests, and actively work to discover theirs.
- Be willing to explore the needs of all parties and find mutually agreeable solutions.
- Determine common interests as well as conflicting needs and desires.
- Think about various proposals, and decide whether to reject, reframe, or accept them.
- Decide the worst-case scenario (what you're willing to accept even if it's not exactly what you want). Don't accept anything that's below your worst-case scenario. Consider and discuss any offer that's less than you'd like but better than your worst-case scenario.

CRITICAL THINKING EXERCISES

With a partner, in a group, or in a journal entry, as appropriate:

1. Gain insight into how you tend to respond to conflict and how you feel about others' styles for resolving conflict:
   a. Describe two or three conflicts that you can remember in some detail.
   b. Review the styles in Box 6-3 (on page 217) and honestly consider what styles you used while in conflict. Once you've considered your own style, think about what styles the other person(s) used and how they affected you.
   c. How could you have handled the situation differently? What style(s) may have achieved a better outcome?
2. Share your stories about conflict with others, asking for a different viewpoint on what was going on in the conflict and what styles and strategies might have been helpful.
3. Find out about your tendencies related to assertiveness by taking the assertiveness test at www.humanmetrics.com/#Jtype.
4. Practice using "I" messages. Change the following statements to ones that send "I" messages.
   a. You never listen to me.
   b. I wish you wouldn't be so sloppy all the time.
   c. You make me feel like I'm the one who causes all the problems.
   d. You make me feel insignificant when you ignore me like that.
   e. Why are you always attacking me?
5. Imagine this: Someone tells you one of your patients has numerous complaints. You go straight to the room, introduce yourself, and inquire about the problem. The patient's wife immediately becomes hostile and tells you to "just get out." What do you do and why?
6. Use role playing to practice assertive communication and conflict resolution. Get a partner. Have one of you be the manager in the following situation and the other, the staff nurse. Here's the situation:
   A staff nurse is angry because he didn't get a specific day off, even though he had put in a written request well ahead of time. He needs the weekend off for his daughter's birthday. The manager spent hours trying to find proper coverage but couldn't honor his request because two other nurses also needed to be off and were turned down for their requests the previous month.
7. Determine whether you can achieve the learning outcomes listed at the beginning of this skill.

RECOMMENDED

Caputi, L. (In press). Conflict resolution: A multimedia program for health professionals. Glen Ellyn, IL: College of DuPage Press (www.dupagepress.com/).

Clark, W. (2006). Managing conflict constructively (PowerPoint presentation). Retrieved August 28, 2007 from www.uua.org/ga/ga06/2076.ppt.

Restifo, V., & Jackson, M. Surviving and thriving with conflict on the job. Retrieved August 28, 2007, from www.nurse.com/ce/syllabus.html?CCID=3961.

See also Recommended *in the sections* Communicating Bad News *and* Giving and Taking Feedback.

7. MANAGING YOUR TIME

Definition
Knowing how to use time effectively through prioritization and organization

Learning Outcomes
After completing this section, you should be able to:
- Explain how an activity diary (or log) helps you manage your time.
- Describe how to set priorities based on your personal and professional goals.
- Identify ways to organize your work to make the most of your time.

Thinking Critically about Managing Your Time
You might sometimes feel that your days seem like an endless race to catch a fast-moving train. But you need to be on that train at the controls! Taking control to manage your time helps you avoid stress and frustration. It also improves self-confidence, results, and job satisfaction because you work smarter, not harder.

How to Manage Your Time
This section is organized by the following headings: *Determining What Must Be Done, Ranking Priorities, Organizing Your Schedule and Work,* and *Streamlining Work in the Clinical Setting.*

Determining What Must Be Done
1. Develop and record your personal, professional, and work goals. Keep them in a readily accessible place. These goals serve as a guide to help you prioritize and organize.
2. Start an activity diary (or log). For several consecutives days, write down everything you do. Include what you do, the amount of time you spend doing it, and the time of day you do it. It should look something like this:

Activity Log

Time	Activities and Tasks
8-8:30 AM	Drive to health club
8:30-9 AM	Work out
9-9:45 AM	Drive to class
10-11:15 AM	Go to class
11:15 AM-1 PM	Have lunch, hang out with friends
1-2:15 PM	Go to class

3. After a few days, analyze your log, and arrange each of the activities and tasks according to the following categories:
   - Must do (essential) activities and tasks
   - Should or could do (or could be delegated to someone else) activities and tasks
   - Nice to do (if you had more time) activities
   - Not necessary (time waster) activities and tasks
4. Be sure that things under your "must do" category reflect your personal and professional or work goals. If they don't, decide whether you truly *must* do them.
5. Decide whether there are things missing on your "must do" list. Add these to the list.
6. Find ways to spend most of your time each day on the "must do" list. Figure out how to get rid of time wasters. For example, in the activity log under point 2 of this section, you could get rid of an hour's driving by working out at home instead of at the health club.
7. Review the list of "nice to do" activities. Ask, *Are there things on this list that I could or should be delegating to someone else?* If so, *Who would be the best person(s) to do the tasks?* and *What would be the results in the long run?* (Box 5-4, page 182, addresses key points on delegating in the clinical setting.)
8. Consider whether you could combine some activities. For example, if you have specific educational goals, you might listen to educational tapes while driving.

Ranking Priorities. This section addresses ranking priorities in relation to everyday life. For ranking priorities in the clinical setting, see Boxes 5-2 and 5-3, pages 181 and 182.

1. Determine the following priority needs, being clear about the rationale for your choices:
   - First-order priority: Must do—important and urgent
   - Second-order priority: Must do—important but not urgent
   - Third-order priority: Nice to do—not as important and not urgent

2. For each priority, consider the following:
    - How much time you have
    - Whether you (and only you) can do what needs to be done, or whether you can delegate the task(s) or parts of the task(s) to others
    - Whether technology can help you be more efficient (e.g., mastering computer skills)
    - Whether paying someone to get things done better or more quickly will improve your results or give you more time to spend on tasks related to major goals
    - Whether there is a cheaper way of accomplishing the task (e.g., using a library computer is cheaper than hiring a typist)

Organizing Your Schedule and Work

- Review your personal, professional, and work goals. Organize your time to get the tasks related to your most important goals done first.
- Work on major priorities at a time when you know you perform best (e.g., some people work better in the morning; others do better at night)
- Plan break time, eat healthily, drink lots of water, and sleep regular hours. Include time for exercise and stress reduction (this helps you be more productive by avoiding low energy levels).[3]
- Organize your environment for optimum productivity.
- Make a "to do" list for each day, and estimate the time each activity on your list will require. Be sure that your list includes only those activities that you must or should do.
- Reserve time in your daily schedule for unexpected events. Life is unpredictable.
- For long-term (or large) projects, keep a master list to refer to periodically. For each project, map out interim target dates that ensure you will complete the project in a timely way or by the designated deadline.
- Avoid the human tendency to put off large projects or find excuses to evade things you don't enjoy. Procrastination is a major time waster.
- Don't expect or demand perfection. Letting go of a task once it's done is crucial for managing time. Perfectionism can also be a time waster!
- Eliminate unnecessary work or steps in the work. Look for ways to streamline work, as in the following section.

Streamlining Work in the Clinical Setting

- Reduce your stress and improve your performance: Get to work early enough to get organized and plan your day before you're "under the gun" to perform.
- Use a daily worksheet that is legible and organized.
- Custer activities before entering a room—think ahead and anticipate needs (e.g., a need for pain medication).

- Avoid charting the same thing in two places. Focus most on charting what's different—for example, use charting by exception (CBE) if allowed by charting policies.
- Organize supply and medication carts so that the commonly used items are easily found.
- Label all supply shelves and cabinets clearly for easy access.

1. Use tools and technology to organize your personal and professional work. For example:
   - Use a personal digital assistant (PDA) or another electronic organizer to keep your schedule and other important information handy.
   - A paper system, such as the Franklin-Covey planner, also works well. The advantage of a paper system is that it is usually less expensive and doesn't require interaction with a personal computer (PC).
   - Whatever organizing system you use, keep all scheduled activities within the *same* organizing system, rather than keeping multiple or duplicate systems. For example, don't keep your work schedule on a PDA and your social calendar elsewhere.
2. Set limits on what you agree to do.

CRITICAL MOMENTS

MANAGING ENERGY IS AS IMPORTANT AS MANAGING TIME

Many nurses feel guilty about making time to care for themselves. When making your list of priorities, don't forget to include health promotion activities. As stressed in *The power of full engagement: Managing energy, not time is the key to high performance and personal renewal,*[15] keep your "engine" in top form by making time for things like eating well, meditating, getting enough rest, and exercising regularly.

OTHER PERSPECTIVES

LEARN TO SAY NO!

"Learning to say "no" if the request for your time is not a "must do" or "should/could do" activity is good time management. Saying something like "I would love to help you, but I'm overloaded right now" works very well. In some cases, you may also have to say something like, "I need a bit more time if you want me to do a good job." Does this mean shirking responsibilities or procrastinating? Not at all. It means that when you have a track record of showing responsibility, and want to do a good job, asking for more time or simply saying "No" may be good time management."[9]

—*Donna D. Ignatavicius, MS, RN*

CRITICAL THINKING EXERCISES

With a partner, in a group, or in a journal entry, as appropriate:

1. Develop and record at least three personal or professional goals that you want to accomplish within the next year.
2. Keep an activity diary for 3 consecutive days during the week. Be sure to include all activities for work, school, and home, if applicable. Refer to goals you identified in number 1:
   - Determine the "must do" activities that will help you achieve your goals for the next year.
   - Identify time wasters and decide how you might eliminate them.
   - Rank the "must do" activities by assigning priorities (first-order, second-order, or third-order priorities).
   - Ask yourself whether there are some things you should be doing to achieve your personal and professional goals. Add these to the list.
3. In a group discussion or with a partner, "compare notes" on the above exercises.
4. Together with a partner, in a group, or in a personal journal, explain specific strategies you will use to organize your work. Keep organization of time and environment in mind.
5. Read the following article and decide how you can apply it to the next time you go to the clinical setting: Garcia, T. A. (2006). Life of a nurse: An oh-so-simple-tool for nurse educators, preceptors, and mentors. Retrieved August 29, 2007, from http://community.nursingspectrum.com/MagazineArticles/article.cfm?AID=20107.
6. Determine where you stand in relation to the learning outcomes listed at the beginning of this skill.

RECOMMENDED

Fuimano, J. The power of concentrated effort. Retrieved August 29, 2007, from http://nursing.advanceweb.com/common/Editorial/Editorial.aspx?CC=74616.

Loehr, J., & Schwartz, T. (2003). *The power of full engagement: Managing energy, not time is the key to high performance and personal renewal.* New York: Free Press. (Also available in audiobook format.)

Silber, L. (1998). *Time management for the creative person: Right-brain strategies for stopping procrastination, getting control of the clock and calendar, and freeing up your time and your life.* New York: Three Rivers Press.

Silber, L. (2004). *Organizing from the right side of the brain: A creative approach to getting organized.* New York: St. Martin's Griffin.

8. PREVENTING AND DEALING WITH MISTAKES CONSTRUCTIVELY

Definition
Knowing how to prevent, detect, correct, and learn from errors

Learning Outcomes
After completing this section, you should be able to:
- Define the terms *error, sentinel event, near miss, hazardous condition,* and *safety culture* using your own words.
- Explain how to determine the seriousness of a mistake.
- Identify circumstances that lead you to make mistakes.
- Develop a personal plan for preventing, detecting, correcting, and learning from mistakes.

Thinking Critically about Preventing and Dealing with Mistakes
Mistakes can be our worst nightmare, or they can be stepping-stones to learning and improvement. And sometimes, they can be both. Dealing with mistakes is a complex issue that includes considering legal consequences (in some states, it's the law that patients be informed of errors; mistakes sometimes end up in malpractice litigation). This section addresses how to know what constitutes a serious error, why errors happen, and how to prevent, detect, correct, and learn from errors.

There are two major types of errors:
1. **Commission**—doing the wrong thing
2. **Omission**—failing to do the right thing

Susan Hohenhaus and the Duke University Health Systems add the following definitions to the above.[4]
1. **Execution**—doing the right thing incorrectly
2. **Rule violation**—an action that goes against the current rules or policies, which may have been done in an effort to avoid another perceived risk
3. **Mistake**—an action that proceeds as planned, but fails to achieve the intended outcome because the planned action or original intention was wrong

Too many people have a one-size-fits-all mindset when it comes to dealing with mistakes. Deep down, they believe that all errors are bad, that all errors happen because of lack of knowledge or laziness, and that the best way to deal with people who make errors is to punish them. However, this approach shames those involved, doesn't examine the real causes of errors, and does little to reduce the *incidence* of mistakes—it only reduces the *reporting* of mistakes. When errors aren't reported, opportunities to fix related problems are missed and mistakes are likely to be repeated.

Most mistakes happen for multiple reasons and in spite of good intentions. We must change the mindset from "mistakes shouldn't happen" to "when dealing with humans, mistakes *will* happen for various reasons." We must share our mistakes freely so that we can work together to find ways to prevent future mistakes. Box 6-6 shows four common reasons that medication errors happen.

A major part of preventing errors is surveillance—monitoring closely for human and system factors that may contribute to mistakes. Examples of human factors contributing to errors are nurse fatigue and lack of knowledge. Examples of system factors are poor staffing and drugs that look alike or have similar names being stored close together on a shelf.

The following terms are important to understand in the context of maintaining in-depth approaches to error prevention.*

- **Sentinel event:** An unexpected occurrence involving death or serious physical or psychologic injury (or the risk thereof). Serious injury specifically includes loss of limb or function. The phrase "or risk thereof" means any variation from the usual process of care such that if it happens again, there is a significant chance of causing a serious adverse outcome. **Example:** a break in procedures that causes nurses to omit checking that the correct leg is marked for amputation. Whether the wrong leg is amputated or not, a sentinel event has occurred. The term *sentinel* is used because of its relationship to a sentinel guard—a soldier who stands guard to keep his people safe. Sentinel events are so serious that they signal the need for immediate investigation to ensure they don't happen again.
- **Near miss:** Anything that happens during the process of care that didn't affect the outcome, but poses a significant chance of a serious adverse outcome if it happens again. **Example:** If a physician almost operates on the wrong site, but this is caught just in time, it's a near miss. Near misses are considered sentinel events, but they may not be reviewed by the Joint Commission under its sentinel event policy.
- **Hazardous condition:** Any set of circumstances (exclusive of the disease or condition for which the patient is being treated) that significantly increases the likelihood of a serious adverse outcome. **Example:** nurses who have too many acutely ill patients to give appropriate care.
- **Root cause analysis (RCA):** The process for identifying deep underlying cause(s) of a mistake—the "root(s)" of errors. Requires examining in detail what happened, why it happened, who was involved, all factors that contribute to the mistake, and what can be done to prevent it. **Example:** not assuming a drug error was due to one nurse's lack of knowledge. Rather, the error is examined deeply to identify all possible contributing factors and deciding the deepest causes (e.g., the *root cause* of the nurse's lack of knowledge could be that

---

*Unless otherwise cited, definitions are adapted from various documents available at www. jointcommission.org/PatientSafety.

there's no policy in place to ensure that new drugs aren't introduced unless all nurses have the required knowledge; this is considered a *system* problem).

- **Failure mode effect analysis (FMEA):** An approach to error prevention that aims to build systems that promote safety and prevent accidents. FMEA assumes that errors are not only possible, but also even likely, despite knowledgeable and careful health care professionals. FMEA assumes that it's too much to ask individuals alone to be responsible for errors. Instead the responsibility is placed on an interdisciplinary group that engages in a never-ending process of quality improvement to assess and correct areas where errors are likely. FMEA also aims to design a system in which critical or catastrophic errors can't happen.[5] **Example:** wrong-site surgeries that are prevented by a strict policy that includes several "check points" to ensure that the correct surgery in the correct person in the correct body part is done.
- Be sure that you also understand the definition of a healthy workplace and culture of safety in Box 1-2 on page 4.

CRITICAL MOMENTS

FAILURE TO MONITOR AND FAILURE TO DIAGNOSE: DON'T MAKE THESE MISTAKES
Failure to monitor and failure to diagnose are common errors noted on malpractice claims. Don't skip assessments, even if they seem routine. When you perform assessments, ask questions like, *Could I be missing something here? Could I be seeing these problems incorrectly? Should I be getting a second opinion?*

BOX 6-6	FOUR COMMON REASONS FOR MEDICATION ERRORS

1. **Inadequate knowledge and skill:** Lack of knowledge of patient's diagnosis, and the names, purposes, and correct administration of medications
2. **Failure to comply with policies and procedures:** Lack of attention to safeguards in medication administration procedures intended to prevent errors
3. **Communication failure:** These include transcription errors, use of abbreviations, illegible handwriting, incorrect interpretation of physician's orders, use of verbal orders, failure to record medications given or omitted, and unclear medication administration records
4. **Individual and system problems:** These include things like the number of the nurse's years of experience, number of consecutive hours worked, rotating shifts, workload, distractions and interruptions, the practice of floating nurses to unfamiliar units, hospital and pharmacy design features, and drug manufacturing problems (e.g., look-alike and sound-alike drug names, look-alike packaging, confusing and unclear labeling, failure to specify drug concentrations on dose-calculation charts)

How to Prevent and Deal with Mistakes Constructively

1. **All mistakes aren't created equal**—in addition to knowing the difference between a sentinel event, near miss, or hazardous condition, you should know the following different types of mistakes, what things cause them, and how you can prevent them.

   - **Mental slips**: These mistakes happen when there's a lapse in your attention to what you're doing or when there's a lapse in short-term memory. **Example:** You're on the way to check an IV, but you're interrupted to help lift someone up in bed. You then forget that you were on the way to check the IV and go on to another task. **Prevention:** Keep a personal worksheet that prompts you to do important tasks (for example, check IV every hour). Get your charting done as soon as possible to help you notice when you've forgotten to do something. Checklists, protocols, and computerized decision aids all help reduce mental slips because they relieve you from relying on short-term memory, the aspect of memory that becomes most imperfect under stress or fatigue.

   - **Interaction (communication) errors**: These mistakes happen when people misunderstand each other. **Example:** You're working in the emergency department and just spoke to Dr. French about one of your patients, Mrs. Moran. A few minutes later, Dr. French comes to you and says, "Would you send her to x-ray?" nodding in the direction of another patient. You don't see him nod in the other direction and assume Dr. French is referring to Mrs. Moran. **Prevention:** Repeat what you hear to clarify verbal interactions (You want me to send Mrs. Moran to x-ray?). Check written orders to clarify verbal orders.

   - **Knowledge errors**: These mistakes are due to insufficient knowledge. **Example:** You cause unnecessary side effects by giving an IV drug too quickly because you didn't know it should be given slowly. **Prevention:** Be sure you find out the answers to who, what, why, when, and how in context of each individual patient situation before you give any drug or perform any intervention.

   - **Learning errors**: Although these mistakes often include knowledge errors, learning errors usually are related to several different factors associated with being in a learning situation (for example, doing something for the first time or being stressed). **Example:** You change sterile dressings for the first time. You contaminate your glove by slightly touching an unsterile field. You don't notice it because you're focused on assessing the wound. **Prevention:** A sure-fire way to avoid learning errors is not to try anything new, which makes no sense. Many students hide from new experiences because they're afraid of making mistakes. This just postpones the inevitable. The best way to avoid learning errors is to be prepared and to practice, practice, practice in as safe an environment as possible (for example, in a skills lab). In risky situations it's best to have a more experienced nurse guide performance, give advice, or actually handle the task at hand.

- **Relying too much on technology:** These mistakes happen when you allow technology to think for you, without wondering if there's a flaw in the system. **Example:** Someone complains that a heating pad is too hot. You check the setting and see that it's in the "low" position. Instead of carefully feeling the pad yourself, you explain that it's probably okay because it's set on low. **Prevention:** Read all instruction manuals carefully. Don't trust machines more than your own knowledge and perceptions. Don't allow technology to think *for* you: think *with* it.
- **System errors:** These mistakes are related to something wrong with the way things are accomplished within the facility as a whole. **Examples:** drugs that aren't given because the pharmacist is overloaded and unable to dispense the drug in a timely manner; errors that happen because a policy or procedure is unclear; or errors that happen because a facility uses a lot of per diem personnel who are more at risk for making mistakes. Report possible system problems to the risk management or quality assurance department. Create a multidisciplinary panel to examine possible and actual system problems.

2. **Determine how serious the error is.** Serious errors need to be examined more closely, prevented more meticulously, and detected and corrected more quickly than less serious errors.

RULE

To determine the seriousness of a mistake, answer two questions:
1. **What harm could result if the error happens?** (Primarily consider harm in terms of human morbidity, mortality, and suffering. Secondarily, consider harm in terms of inconvenience, cost, and lost time. If you're unable to decide what harm could result, get help).
2. **Should this mistake be classified as a sentinel event, near miss, or hazardous condition?**

---

3. Follow policies and procedures, and be sure you understand the rationale behind them. These are designed by experts to prevent, detect, and correct errors early.
4. When using checklists, think about each item carefully. Checklists are supposed to jog your brain, not replace it.
5. Involve patients and families in their own health care as much as possible. Educate them, and encourage them to become participants in preventing errors by verifying that they're getting the right treatments and medications and by speaking up when they have questions (see Box 3-3, page 74).

6. Never perform an intervention without knowing why it's indicated in each particular situation. Be careful about multitasking.
7. Involve experts. For example, if confused about a medication regimen, ask a pharmacist.
8. Look after yourself. If you're rested, you're less likely to make mistakes.
9. Know what to do when mistakes happen:

What to Do When Mistakes Happen

1. Determine the seriousness of the error as soon as it's recognized, and take immediate steps to prevent or reduce harm. Get help if needed.
2. Follow policy and procedures for dealing with mistakes, including how to report and record the mistake. Standards and some state laws mandate that patients be informed when mistakes happen.
3. Chart actions taken to address the error (for example, increasing the frequency of monitoring or a transfer to another unit).
4. Curb the tendency to focus too much on guilt and not enough on what can be learned from the mistake.
5. Explore the specifics of the incident objectively, examining the procedures and circumstances leading to the errors. Consider the value of sharing the mistake with others to alert them of the possibility of its happening again. If procedures were followed and a mistake still happened, maybe the procedures should be revised to make them more errorproof.

OTHER PERSPECTIVES

MISTAKES: SO EASY TO DO

"Competitive cyclists have the saying, 'If you're a cyclist, you've already crashed or you're going to.' Perhaps you could substitute any other title for cyclist. If you're a nurse, you've either made a mistake or you're going to... Crashes occur for many reasons. You can crash if you don't have the necessary knowledge, skill, or equipment. Or conditions unexpectedly become too complex, and in haste you do something you otherwise would not do. Or you or a competitor breaks the rules in an effort to gain advantage. The former would be called errors; the latter are ethical or legal violations. Sometimes that distinction is important, though not always clear... I propose that errors and ethical misconduct are not a dichotomy of unrelated entities; they are two ends of continuum. Some errors can be excused; misconduct is not."[10]—*Sue Thomas Hegyvary, PhD, FAAN; Editor,* Journal of Nursing Scholarship

"I am a nurse scientist who studies medical error... I am a critical care nurse who lives in fear of making a mistake that could harm a patient... The majority of errors are the result of system failures, not the blatant carelessness of individuals. Yet people tend to point fingers at individuals and place blame. Even when well-designed systems are in place, human errors occur. Your statement, 'I am humbled that making such an error is easy to do' will bring comfort to many clinicians and scholars who strive to do the best they can in this busy, complicated world. Acknowledging that both system failures and human fallibility contribute to errors and adverse outcomes is necessary for achieving the ultimate goal of 'improving the health of the world's people.'"[11]

—*Elizabeth Henneman, RN, PhD, CCNS*

CRITICAL THINKING EXERCISES

With a partner, in a group, or in a journal entry, as appropriate:

1. Address the implications of the following statements.
   a. Being ignorant doesn't merely mean not knowing; it means not knowing what you don't know. Being educated means knowing precisely what you don't know.
   b. As a nurse it's your responsibility to be alert not only to situations that might cause you to make a mistake but also to situations that may cause others to make a mistake.
2. Respond to the following:
   a. How do you feel when you make a mistake?
   b. What can you do to help someone else who has made a mistake?
   c. How can you help correct systems that are error-prone and increase checks to prevent medication errors?
3. Share examples of a sentinel event, near miss, hazardous condition, mental slip, knowledge error, learning error, and system error.
4. Share your personal (or a family or friend's) experiences with medical errors.
5. Discuss the challenges of creating a safety culture (see Box 1-2 on page 4).
6. Discuss the roles of the following organizations in error prevention. Also address how you might use the information given on their websites.
   - National Patient Safety Foundation: www.npsf.org
   - Agency for Healthcare Research and Quality: www.ahrq.gov/qual/errorsix.htm
   - The Joint Commission: www.jointcommission.org
   - The Institute of Medicine: www.iom.edu
7. Go to a baseball game and watch how the players cover for one another to provide "safety nets" in case someone makes an error. Discuss how this applies to what you see in the health care setting.
8. Discuss the implications of the following Critical Moments.

CRITICAL MOMENTS

THREE STEPS TO PREVENTING MISTAKES
We all share accountability for ensuring patient safety: (1) Pay attention to things you're doing that may create risks for errors. (2) Report systems that fail to adequately protect patients (for example, notify the risk management department if you think of a change in a policy or procedure that could be made to reduce chances for human error). (3) Empower your patients by teaching them what to expect and telling them that the main thing they can do to prevent mistakes is to become actively involved in managing their own care.

9. Determine whether you can achieve the learning outcomes listed at the beginning of this skill.

RECOMMENDED

Gaskill, M. (2006). Preventing errors systematically. Retrieved August 31, 2007, from http://community.nursingspectrum.com/MagazineArticles/article.cfm?AID=20376.

Kosnik, L., Brown, J., & Maund, T. (2007). Patient safety: Learning from the aviation industry. Retrieved August 31, 2007, from www.nursingcenter.com/prodev/ce_article.asp?tid=688333.

Steefel, L. (2006). Routine omissions at point-of-care delivery. Retrieved September 2, 2007, from http://community.nursingspectrum.com/MagazineArticles/article.cfm?AID=23991.

Wolf, Z. Preventing medical errors: Florida requirement. Retrieved August 29, 2007, from www.nurse.com/ce/syllabus.html?CCID=2843.

See also Recommended *in the sections* Building Empowered Partnerships *and* Communicating Bad News.

9. TRANSFORMING A GROUP INTO A TEAM

Definition
Knowing how to work together to combine efforts to achieve shared outcomes, within a specific time frame

Learning Outcomes

After completing this section, you should be able to:

- Explain the common stages of team building.
- Describe strategies that transform groups into teams.
- Participate more effectively as part of a team.

Thinking Critically about Teamwork

How well a team works together determines whether you have frustrated, unhappy patients and staff; whether the atmosphere makes you dread going to work; or whether you have great patient outcomes, job satisfaction, and a sense of good will. Yet building a team isn't easy. Team members need to be nurtured as the team evolves from being a group of diverse, relatively insecure strangers to a group that values common goals and brings together diverse talents and strengths.

True teamwork occurs when all team members are:

1. Committed to common goals and a high level of productivity.
2. Energized by their ability to work together.
3. Concerned about how team members feel during the work process.

Consider the difference between what's going on in the following groups:

Group 1 consists of several nurses who have worked together for the past 6 months. They don't feel like they're working as a team and want this to change. Their manager, Jane, is a busy person who has a demanding boss. Under pressure, Jane barks orders and personally takes over some tasks. The staff responds by doing what they are told or lying low until things calm down. There is minimal group participation in problem solving and decision making. The nurses want to execute their responsibilities in a satisfactory way. But no one has given thought to the need for group goals or concerted group action. Morale is low, and everyone talks about how unhappy they are.

Group 2 consists of several nurses who also have worked together for 6 months. By contrast, these nurses are energized and proud of their successes. Like Group 1, their manager, Terri, also is a busy person with a demanding boss. However, when the pressure is on, Terri stops the action and convenes a problem-solving discussion, focusing on common goals and getting input from team members. Better solutions are found because the pressure is channeled into a spirit of "let's fix this together." These nurses enjoy a sense of growing and improving together—work is more than just a job.

How to Transform a Group into a Team

Knowing how to communicate and build trust are the cornerstones of teamwork. Early on in the team-building process, all team members must agree to a code of conduct and be aware of messages sent by their behavior. For example, if you consistently show up late for work, shirk responsibility, give excuses, or are arrogant or defensive, you need to be aware of the messages these behaviors send to the rest of the team. On the other hand, if you use behaviors like always being on time, being willing to help, accepting responsibility and being open to suggestions, you send altogether different messages.

The following give strategies for team building first from a leadership perspective, then from the team members' perspective.

1. Team leaders should:
    -   Create a shared vision of the team's mission or purpose: Everyone must be committed to reaching clearly defined outcomes.
    -   Stress that everyone is responsible for preventing errors and improving outcomes by analyzing current practices and pointing out improvements that could be made.
    -   Turn diversity to the team's advantage (for example, assign tasks based on individual strengths and preferences as much as possible).
    -   Ask for consensus in decisions (everyone agrees to agree), rather than settling for a majority vote.
    -   Be careful not to criticize new ideas.
    -   Keep team members well-informed so that everyone understands the big picture.
    -   Recognize team members for their contributions.
    -   Be sure team members are familiar with the common stages of team building (Box 6-7 on the next page). Although not every group goes through every stage, and the duration of each stage varies, it helps to know that there are common struggles in every team.

2. Team members should:
    -   Agree about roles, responsibilities, and proper lines of communication.
    -   Work hard to meet responsibilities and deliver what they promise.
    -   Get involved and contribute to the good of the group.
    -   Stay focused on the big picture of what the team is trying to accomplish.
    -   Make a conscious effort to overcome the human tendency to focus narrowly on self; too often, team members have difficulty seeing other members' struggles because they themselves are working so hard.
    -   Use behaviors that promote trust and create a caring and energized environment:
        -   Follow the "Platinum Rule" (treat others as *they* want to be treated instead of assuming they want to be treated the same as *you* do)—and point out when it's not being followed (without blaming).
        -   Show enthusiasm—it's contagious and it energizes others.
        -   Address and resolve conflicts early—push for high-quality communication.
        -   Pay attention to group process and where the team is in relation to the stages of team building (see Box 6-7).

- Recognize individual and team efforts; be a good sport and help new teammates make entry.
- Support creativity and new ways of doing things.
- Broaden your skills; offer to try new tasks or to cross-train.
- Promote group learning by collecting, sharing, and analyzing information.
- Spend fun time together (here's where relationships grow).

CRITICAL THINKING EXERCISES

With a partner, in a group, or in a journal entry, as appropriate:

1. Share "your story" about a group you currently belong to, addressing what stage of team building you are in as a group in relation to the stages in Box 6-7.
2. Share your best and worst experiences with being part of a team. Consider what went right and why you think it went right, and what went wrong and why you think it went wrong.
3. Discuss the implications of the *Other Perspectives* on the next page.

BOX 6-7   COMMON STAGES OF TEAM BUILDING

Forming
Group members start to get to know one another, testing each other's values, beliefs, and attitudes. Basic goals and tasks are defined, roles assigned, and ideas shared.

Storming
Conflict begins, often because of misunderstandings or disagreement about what realistically can get done and how exactly things will get done. More testing goes on in this phase, with some people asking themselves questions like, How much am I willing to do? This is a time to maintain high standards, provide emotional support, and aim to get consensus (agreement from everyone). Beware of false consensus during this phase; some people will say they agree when they really don't (just to avoid further conflict). Because this is a stressful stage, you may need to take more breaks.

Norming
The group becomes more cohesive and really wants to work together in a positive way. Group members agree on rules—for example, when meetings will be held, who should attend, what the proper lines of communication are, and how problems and disagreements will be handled. At this point the leader needs to be sensitive to group values, asking for votes to determine common needs and desires.

Performing
Team members begin to bond to one another and function well together with a good understanding of roles, responsibilities, and relationships.

OTHER PERSPECTIVES

TEAMWORK REQUIRES EMPOWERMENT

"Teamwork requires empowerment, a willingness and commitment to 'let go' of self (one's own ideas, plans, strategies) to the benefit of the group. As I see it, there are five stages of empowerment: (1) Letting go of self-promotion; (2) Believing that others are capable and competent; (3) Trusting others; (4) Willingness to forgo one's own processes, plans, or strategies to give others a chance; (5) Sharing the outcomes and celebrating success."[12]—*Sylvia Whiting, PhD, RN, CS*

STEPS TO TEAM BUILDING

"One of the first things you need to do is realize and acknowledge that you and your co-workers are all on the same team—you are there to provide the best care to your patient and clients that you can. You don't have to become best friends with your co-workers; you don't even have to like them. What you do need to do is treat them with respect and work with them to accomplish what needs to be accomplished. Approach work with a positive attitude—negativity only adds to the stress and tension of your workday. Remember, your co-workers are in the same situation you are. If you have a problem with a co-worker, ask to speak to them privately... One of the most difficult tasks of collaboration, the 'big picture' approach, requires repeatedly asking, 'Will this help us achieve our goal?' Continual focus on the mutually agreed upon outcome is the most likely path to success, for without it the partnership is doomed."[13]—*Nancy Dickenson-Hazard, RN, MSN, FAAN*

FOSTERING CROSS-CULTURAL UNDERSTANDING

"Working successfully with a culturally diverse staff and patient population encompasses two sets of skills. First, nurses need the holistic skills to manage patients who are different from themselves... However, the skill that's frequently overlooked is learning to work with diversity among staff members. Embracing cultural diversity in the workplace, as well as in the community, has to be an institutional commitment."[14]—*Antonia Villaruel, RN, PhD, FAAN*

4. Practice brainstorming as a group. Get in a group of 6 to 10 persons. Name one person the recorder and have him use a flip chart or blackboard. Identify a problem you'd like to resolve or a situation that could be improved (for example, how you could get teenagers to come to a meeting on sex education). For 30 minutes, have group members each share ideas to be recorded by the recorder without interpretation. Once you're finished, spend 10 minutes discussing what happened (the group dynamics) as you brainstormed.
5. Determine whether you can achieve the learning outcomes listed at the beginning of this skill.

RECOMMENDED

Kalisch, B., Curley, M., & Stefanov, S. (2007). An intervention to enhance nursing staff teamwork and engagement. *Journal of Nursing Administration, 37*(2), 77-84.

Wenckus, E., & Teinert, D. Working with an interdisciplinary team. Retrieved September 1, 2007, from www.nurse.com/ce/syllabus.html?CCID=3869.

See also Recommended *in the sections* Developing Empowered Partnerships *and* Managing Conflict Constructively.

10. ACCESSING AND USING INFORMATION EFFECTIVELY

Definition
Knowing how to find reliable, up-to-date information that's relevant to your specific concern—and then knowing how to interpret and apply it in the context of your specific situations

Learning Outcomes
After completing this section, you should be able to:
- Access information reliable, up-to-date information from a variety of sources.
- Explain how to evaluate information resources for accuracy and reliability.
- Apply information in the context of specific situations or purposes.
- Keep your files or notes organized for easy access.

Thinking Critically about Accessing and Using Information
Knowing how to find, interpret, and apply information is an essential workplace skill. Knowing how to find and use reliable, relevant information can make the difference between drowning in TMI (too much information) and quickly getting to the most important information you need to know. In the clinical setting, it can make the difference between whether you give risky, unsafe care, or safe, efficient, care that's based on the best available knowledge (see *Evidence-Based Practice* on pages 123-129).

How to Access and Use Information Effectively
1.   Learn how to use Internet and library resources: indexes, catalogs, interlibrary loan services, the circulation and reference departments, audiovisual services, and computer databases (recommended search engines and websites are listed in Box 6-8).

BOX 6-8	RECOMMENDED SEARCH ENGINES AND HEALTH-RELATED WEB SITES

Search Engines

Google Scholar (http://scholar.google.com): Has an advanced section that allows you to limit the search to Medicine and Pharmacology

Google U.S. Government Search (www.google.com/unclesam): Lists data in the federal domain

CINAHL (Cumulative Index to Nursing and Allied Health Literature) (www.cinahl.com): Most articles are available by fax or mail

Pub Med (www.ncbi.nlm.nih.gov/entrez/query.fcgi): A service of the National Library of Medicine. Provides access to more than 11 million MEDLINE citations and additional life science journals. Includes links to many sites providing full text articles and other related resources

Other Related Sites

iHealthRecord (www.ihealthrecord.org): A free, secure interactive website that allows you to keep all your health care information organized, up to date, and in one place

NurseLinx.com (www.NurseLinx.com): Provides nurses with an easy way to access the latest advances in their field

Health on the Net (www.hon.ch) and **Healthfinder** (www.healthfinder.org): Bypass the all-purpose commercial search engines and go straight to health care portals. These portals eliminate irrelevant sources for you

Agency for Healthcare Research and Quality (www.ahrq.gov) and the **Cochrane Library** (cochrane.org/resources/brochure.htm): Best evidence-based practice (EBP) websites for updating practice standards

BIOETHICSLINE (wings.buffalo.edu/faculty/research/bioethics/bio-line.html): Provides a database of bibliographic references concerning ethical and public policy issues in health care and biomedical research

2. Get to know your human resources—for example, introduce yourself to the librarian and informatics nurses (nurses in charge of using information technology). Ask for help if you get stuck. Remember that Internet search engines have "help buttons" to assist you with questions.

3. Whether you're using printed reference or Web-based information, the following ABCDs of evaluating websites and other works gets you started thinking about whether the information is reliable.

   ABCDs of Evaluating Websites and Other Works*

Authority: How well is the author known?

- Is the author a well-regarded name you recognize? What are the author's qualifications?
- Does the document contain an e-mail address?
- Did you link to this site or document from a site you trust?

---

*Adapted from Schrock, K. ABC's of website evaluation. Retrieved September 2, 2007, from http://school.discovery.com/schrockguide/eval.html.

- Are you led to additional information about the author?
- Are there statements about the review process? (e.g., is there a peer review process?)

Bias: Does the site or document try to *persuade*, rather than *inform?*

- What organization is sponsoring the site or document?
- Is there is a link to the sponsoring organization's website?
- Is the page actually an ad disguised as information?

Citations:

- Are full citations given to support the work?
- If so did you compare the author's content with the content in the citation?

Dates:

- What dates are given?
- Does the information you need demand more current data than is given in the documents you have?

4. Additional information specifically for website evaluation:
   - The HON Code of Conduct (HONcode) is a seal of approval by the Health on the Net Foundation and signifies high standards. For information on requirements to display this seal, go to www.hon.ch/HONcode/.
   - HealthRatings.org (a joint project of *Consumer Reports,* WebWatch, and The Health Improvement Institute) also helps you identify reliable websites.

5. Whether you are using a website or a printed article, use the following strategies:
   - Always try to verify information with the primary (original) sources. For example, cite this book directly if there's no credit to another reference. But, if I give a citation for a specific sentence or idea, check that citation, since it is the primary (original) source.
   - If you're unsure about the information you have, compare it with at least two other reputable sources on the same topic. Remember, "more than one source, more likely of course."
   - When overwhelmed, ask for help. Nurse educators, pharmacists, librarians, and other professionals can point you in the right direction.
   - Develop information processing and management skills so that you can focus on what's important and keep data available in a way that helps you access the most important information quickly.
     - Never read without taking notes—your notes help you process the information so you understand and remember it better. Don't highlight your way through an article—it may be easier, but it doesn't help you process, unless you're picking out only a few key ideas.
     - Make the information your own by asking yourself questions like, *How well do I understand what's known and what's unknown about this topic? What are the relationships between key concepts?* and *What questions does this information raise for me?* Think about what you're reading!

- When faced with an overwhelming amount of reading, use the strategies listed under *Scanning before Reading Research Articles* on page 129.
- Draw maps to identify relationships between key data.
- Revise notes and maps at least once to force yourself to do more in-depth thinking about what's most important. Organizing and reorganizing information to find new relationships gives you more in-depth understanding and will help you *remember* the content better.
- Get rid of irrelevant or unimportant information.
- When you find a good article, summarize the information on a card or word processor, including the bibliographic citation you might need for future purposes. Save all this until you finish the project or graduate. In the long run, this saves time. A good free program for creating citations in APA format is located online at www.noodletools.com/.
- Develop a filing system either in a file cabinet, box, or on your computer. For example, when I read an article, I make a document with the bibliographic citation and key points on my computer. Then I put the actual articles in a file cabinet in case I need to look into more detail later.
- Put key data into the computer whenever possible. Project management programs can help you.
- Carry a pocket reference, PDA, little notebook, or "cheat sheet" with key data you need to keep with you (e.g., formulas, lab values). Know how to access the computer at any worksite where you are assigned for easy access to information.

CRITICAL MOMENTS

TURN INFORMATION INTO KNOWLEDGE
You can't equate information with knowledge. Information is simply a group of facts. Turn information into knowledge by analyzing the data, identifying patterns and relationships, and working to gain insight into what the information implies.

USE YOUR NOODLE AS WELL AS YOUR COMPUTER
Computerized information is only as good as the mind that interprets it. Computers aren't able to think. They have no common sense, and they "believe" anything anyone tells them. In fact, computers simply shuffle data around like books on a tabletop. It's up to you to discriminate and decide which "books" apply and whether they are the latest "copyright." Use your noodle (brain) to interpret the information in the context of each situation. Ask questions like, *How does this information apply to this particular case? How can I be sure this information is up to date? and Does this sound reasonable?*

CRITICAL THINKING EXERCISES

With a partner, in a group, or in a journal entry, as appropriate:

1. Share information management problems you have encountered and strategies you find helpful (include those you read in this section).
2. Discuss the advice you would give if someone comes to you and says "I have to read over 150 articles for my paper in 2 weeks!"
3. Pick a topic you'd like to know more about. Then, using the library and the Internet, find three good articles or websites related to your topic. Explain why these articles or sites are helpful and how they are better than others you found.
4. Draw a map showing the relationships between the most important information presented in this section.
5. Visit all of the Web resources in Box 6-8 (page 239). Discuss under what circumstances you might use each one.
6. Determine whether you can achieve the learning outcomes listed at the beginning of this skill.

RECOMMENDED

Medical Library Association MLANet. (2006). A user's guide to finding and evaluating health information on the Web. Retrieved August 16, 2007, from www.mlanet.org/resources/userguide.html#3.

Ormondroyd, J. (M. Engle & T. Cosgrave, Eds.). (2004). Critically analyzing information resources. Retrieved September 2, 2007, from www.library.cornell.edu/okuref/research/skill26.htm.

Schrock, K. ABC's of website valuation. Retrieved September 2, 2007, from http://school.discovery.com/schrockguide/eval.html.

Widener University. Evaluating Web resources. Retrieved September 1, 2007, from www3.widener.edu/Academics/Libraries/Wolfgram_Memorial_Library/Evaluate_Web_Pages/659/.

11. OUTCOME-FOCUSED WRITING (WRITING TO GET RESULTS)

Definition
Knowing how to write in a way that gets the results you want

Learning Outcomes
After completing this section, you should be able to:
- Use specific strategies to improve your ability to get your message across to the intended audience.
- Evaluate your writings to determine if they meet your intended purpose.
- Collaborate with others to improve writing projects.

Thinking Critically about Writing
Many of us feel like we're not getting anything done unless our pens or fingers are moving and we see our paper taking form. However, the time you take *before* you start to write your paper—gathering information, clarifying your topic, identifying exactly what you aim to do, and determining the best approach—is crucial to getting the final product you want.

Writing, like any other skill, takes practice. The more you do it in the context of various situations—whether it be writing on the job or writing for school or publication—the better you become. If you apply the information in this section consistently—refer to it and follow it each time you write a paper—you will develop habits that can significantly improve your ability to get your message across.

How to Write to Get Results
This section is organized according to the following headings: *Before You Write, As You Write, Strategies for Getting over Writer's Block,* and *After You Write.*

Before You Write
1. Determine the specific outcome (observable result) you aim to achieve. Be as *specific* as you can. For instance, consider the following examples and decide which one is the best guide to helping you decide what you need to do to get the results you want.

   Example Goal: I want to write a paper on prolonging life in terminal illness.

   Example Outcome: My teacher will read a paper that explains my beliefs on prolonging life in terminal illness and follows the criteria and guidelines she gave us in class.

2. Decide what you're trying to do with your paper:
   - Communicate (inform, instruct, or persuade)?

Examples: Essays, term papers, articles, memos, letters, charting
- Form values (clarify your own values or explain them to others)?
  Examples: Personal journals, essays, term papers, articles, letters
- Learn (sort out and remember thoughts about specific topics rather than communicate)?
  Examples: Personal journals, note-taking, mapping

3. Decide what type of writing will help you achieve your purpose.
   - Expressive writing: *This is what I see, think, and feel*
   - Persuasive writing: *This is what I believe, and this is why you should believe it*
   - Narrative writing: *This is what happened (what I observed and heard), and then this what happened next*
   - Informational writing: *This is what I know and how I know it. This is what others know and how I know they know it*
   - Instructional writing: *This is how you should do this and why*

4. Start by discovering your thoughts and ideas without being concerned about grammar, form, or spelling. Map your ideas. List key ideas and questions that come to mind. Then review your ideas and ask yourself: What questions or thoughts do these ideas raise? Write these questions and thoughts down, too.
   - Share your thoughts, feelings, and perceptions with peers. Ask them what questions or thoughts are raised for them.
   - Keep a running list of your own ideas and ideas from your readings (be sure to cite your references in your notes, or you might forget where the information came from and be accused of plagiarism).
   - Create your bibliography as you go along. When you encounter an interesting reference, immediately write down the full citation. Be sure to check the format for your citations. You can find a good free program for creating citations in APA format at www.noodletools.com/.

5. Decide what content you need to include to achieve your purpose. Develop one central idea, issue, or theme that you can explain to someone in two or three sentences. Narrow your topic down to something that is manageable based on the projected length of your paper.

6. Determine a logical progression for your paper. Make an outline or organize the headings you'll use for your paper, and remember the "Three Ts:"
   Tell them what you're going to tell them (introduction).
   Tell them (body).
   Tell them what you told them (summary).

7. Find out who exactly will read what you write. Your writing style should be *appropriate to the reader*. **Examples:** Your approach to writing for your boss or instructor should be different than writing a friendly communication. If you write for lay people, use simple language.

8. Paying attention to guidelines for the paper, make a checklist of what's most important to do, and keep this in a place where you readily see it (for example, at the front of your notebook or taped to your computer).

Example checklist:

- ❏ 25% of grade is on description of nursing theory.
- ❏ 50% of grade is on analysis and application of nursing theory.
- ❏ 25% of grade is on format (grammar, spelling, bibliography).
- ❏ Make sure to focus on how the theory can be applied today.
- ❏ Wants lots of examples.

9. Plan enough time to write at least two drafts (first and final draft).

As You Write

1. If you hate to write but are good at oral presentations, use a program that allows you to dictate the paper (e.g., *Dragon NaturallySpeaking* by Nuance Communications).

2. Develop headings to let the reader know what's coming up (see the headings throughout this book). Keep paragraphs short and focused on *one idea* at a time. After you complete a paragraph, evaluate how it relates to the headings you used.
   - Have you wandered from the topic?
   - Do you need to change the heading?
   - Can you make the headings more interesting?

3. Keep it simple: Use easy terms. If you find yourself struggling with long sentences or paragraphs, consider whether bullets or numbered points could express the information more easily.
   - See how easy it is to read these short points?
   - Our brains handle short phrases and sentences better than long ones.
   - Bulleted points are actually also easier to write.

4. Use the following to get your point across:
   - Examples and analogies to make your point and show why your information is relevant
   - Tables, maps, diagrams, and other illustrations to increase understanding
   - Active rather than passive tense (e.g., *people see different things* instead of *things are seen differently by various people*)
   - Action verbs to engage the reader (e.g., *turn the patient* rather than *the patient is turned*)

5. To make sure you pay attention to the most important criteria for your paper, refer to the criteria checklist you made frequently (see the top of this page) Stay in touch with your instructor as needed—remember he is there to help you and clarify any questions you have.

6. Develop your own style. Let your personality come through rather than sticking to strict, formal rules. However, be sure that there aren't style requirements—if so, follow the style requirements rather than your preferred style.

7. Remember the Three Ts (see item 6 under *Before You Write*)

8. Trim the fat: Get rid of unnecessary words. Wordy sentences muddle your message and dilute its impact. For example, compare the following sentences (*a* says the same thing as *b*, but has more words).

a. Altogether too many students feel that writing should be taught only to those people who want to go into journalism once they have finished school. What these students don't realize is that their efforts in practicing writing can greatly enhance their general ability to think critically.

b. Many students feel that writing should be taught only to those who want to go into journalism. These students don't realize that writing promotes critical thinking.

9. If you get writer's block, stare at the computer or your paper until beads of sweat form on your forehead and you sweat it out. Just kidding ☺! Use the following strategies.

Strategies for Getting over Writer's Block

1. Just get started. Let your ideas flow onto the paper (or the computer) in whatever order they come to you. Sometimes, writing is like exercising—you need a warm-up.

2. Dictate your ideas to a tape recorder or buy voice-activated software such as *Dragon NaturallySpeaking* so that you just talk your way through the paper.

3. Break the paper down into small tasks. For example, if you can't seem to get started on the introduction, go on to address some of your other headings. It's not unusual to write the best introduction after you complete your paper. Doing easier headings before the introduction reduces your anxiety, helps you see progress, and gets your brain in "writing gear."

4. Talk through your paper. Say to someone, "I'm stuck on a point for my paper. Can you listen so I can explain it to you?" Write down key points as you explain them.

After You Write

1. Critically evaluate your paper using the following criteria.

Evaluate Important Writings

Check your paper for each of the following categories. Rate the paper using a 0-10 scale (*0 = I'm not at all satisfied with my product; 10 = I'm very satisfied*).*

___ This gives a good first impression of my work.

___ The main purpose or objective is clearly stated at the beginning of the paper.

___ There's logical progression, including introduction, body, and summary.

___ Major headings are listed, and the paragraphs pertain to the headings.

---

*If the category doesn't apply to your paper, put N/A (not applicable).

___ The paper shows that I followed instructions for content and format carefully (compare paper with criteria given in assignment).
___ The paper is written specifically for whom I expect to read it.
___ I gave informed opinions and provided reasons and facts to support them.
___ If I pull out all the headings and list them on a piece of paper, they show logical progression.
___ I checked spelling and grammar.
___ I asked someone to critique my first draft.
___ I asked someone to proofread my final draft, even if I used computerized grammar and spelling checks.
___ Overall, I'm pleased with this work.

2. Edit and revise as needed. Here's your chance to make significant improvements with just a little more effort. If you need extension on the deadline, find out if you are penalized for extensions. If not, then take the time you need to make improvements.

CRITICAL THINKING EXERCISES

1. Pick a partner and together, choose a controversial issue.
   a. One of you, write three paragraphs supporting the issue, and the other do the same opposing it.
   b. Swap papers. Edit and improve each other's papers, keeping in mind the *original purpose* of the paper.
2. Practice brainstorming. Pick a topic you want to write about. Make a list of your ideas and thoughts, and then pair off with a partner. Swap your list of ideas and thoughts with your partner. Then:
   • Each of you, add to the other person's list of ideas.
   • Switch them back and have the original author circle three or four ideas that are closely related, including what the partner added.
   • Together, write one or two sentences connecting the ideas.
3. Keep all of your papers in a portfolio.
   a. Ask if you can improve or revise one of them to meet a course objective. Hand in both the old and the new papers.
   b. Evaluate them according to the criteria in the checklist beginning on page 246.
4. Offer to critique and proofread peers' papers. It's great practice for learning what makes a good paper.
5. Keep a journal. Practice letting your thoughts flow.

RECOMMENDED

Oermann, M. (2006). Short written assignments for clinical nursing courses. *Nurse Educator, 31*(5), 228-231.

Ruth-Sahd, L. (2006). A diamond in the rough, to a polished gemstone ring: Writing for publication in a nursing journal. *Dimensions of Critical Care Nursing, 25*(3), 113-120.

TermPaperEdge.com. Term Paper Help Center. Retrieved September 1, 2007 from www.medi-smart.com/termpaper.html.

REFERENCES

1. Block, P. (1996). *Stewardship: Choosing service over self-interest.* San Francisco: Berrett-Koehler.
2. Ibid.
3. Loehr, J., & Schwartz, T. (2003). *The power of full engagement: Managing energy, not time is the key to high performance and personal renewal.* New York: Free Press.
4. Gaskill, M. (2006). Preventing errors systematically. Retrieved March 31, 2007, from http://community.nursingspectrum.com/MagazineArticles/article.cfm?AID=20376.
5. Wolf, Z. Preventing medical errors: Florida requirement. Retrieved August 29, 2007, from www.nurse.com/ce/syllabus.html?CCID=2843.
6. Class, P. (2006). The walking wounded. *Nursing Spectrum (FL Ed), 9*(21), 3.
7. Musinski, B. (March, 2007). e-Mail communication.
8. Covey, S. (1989). *The seven habits of highly effective people.* New York: Simon & Schuster.
9. Ignatavicius. D. (April, 2007). e-Mail communication.
10. Hegyvary, S. (2006). Reflections on errors and ethics. *Journal of Nursing Scholarship, 38*(2), 107.
11. Henneman, E. (2006). Letter to the editor. *Journal of Nursing Scholarship, 38*(2), 109.
12. Whiting, S. (March, 2007). e-Mail communication.
13. Dickenson-Hazard, N. (2001). Block party. *Reflections on nursing LEADERSHIP, 27*(1), 5.
14. Campion, C. (1998). Embracing our differences. *Nursing Spectrum (FL Ed), 8*(14), 5.
15. Loehr & Schwartz, op cit.

Response Key for Exercises in Chapters 1 to 5

Note: Because the exercises are open-ended questions, the following are *example* responses, not the *only* responses (see *Instructions for Completing Critical Thinking Exercises* on page 18). If a number isn't listed below, it's because giving an example response is inappropriate for that particular exercise.

CHAPTER 1

Example Responses for Pages 19-20

1. You must clearly identify the problems, the issues, and the risks that must be managed to achieve the outcomes.
4. All three terms address confidence in *your own ability* to reason well. However, *confidence in reason* addresses the importance of having faith that *others* will reason best when allowed to approach things *in their own way.*
5. **(a)** Facts are clearly observable and easily validated as true. Opinions may vary depending on personal perspectives: They may or may not be valid. **(b)** The best way to determine if an opinion is valid is to ask for the *facts* (evidence) that support the opinion. Then determine the strength of the evidence.
6. If your frontal lobe is impaired, you are likely to be very impulsive and have impaired judgment about what is or isn't appropriate. If your hippocampus is damaged, you are likely to have problems with short-term memory, causing you to ask the same questions over and over again.

CHAPTER 2

Example Responses for Page 41

2. The *Golden Rule* and the *Platinum Rule* both aim at treating others well. The *Platinum Rule* stresses that we are all different and that others may not want to be treated the same way we do. For example, don't assume that just because you like to be "touchy-feely," others do too.

3. Feelings have a great impact on what and how we think. Those of us who are driven by feelings are likely to have more problems thinking critically, especially when situations are emotionally charged.

4. Thinking critically requires that you recognize feelings and their impact on thinking, and then use your head to apply logical and ethical reasoning principles. All too often we aren't even aware of deep, strong feelings involved in certain situations. Those of us who are able to connect with emotions and give them the attention they deserve—to make them explicit, to accept them, and to recognize their influence over thinking—can facilitate more logical, sensible thinking.

6. **(a)** 1. Gain insight and self-awareness. 2. Get agreement on a code of conduct and what critical thinking entails. 3. Make the choice to practice and develop the attitudes, the knowledge, and the skills that promote critical thinking. **(b)** Once you're aware of your thinking style—how your personality and learning preference affects your usual approaches to gaining understanding and making decisions, you can find ways to improve. **(c)** Following a code of conduct helps people trust you. Without trust in relationships, there is superficial dialogue and little open, honest discussion. People who like and trust one another think better because they don't waste brain power worrying about trust issues. **(d)** Habits are automatic. They are things we do without thinking. When we have deeply ingrained habits such as the ones that inhibit critical thinking on pages 38-40, we may believe we're thinking critically, but in fact we're blind to how our habits inhibit our reasoning. If we create new habits that promote critical thinking, like Covey's habits on page 40, we are more likely to automatically think critically.

Example Responses for Pages 56-57

1. Sometimes the terms *goals* and *outcomes* are used interchangeably. However, it's more correct to use *goals* when stating *general intent* (what you aim to do) and to use *outcomes* to clearly describe what you expect *others to observe* when the goal is observed. **Example goal:** I want to teach Juan about diabetes. **Example outcome:** After 3 weeks, Juan will be able to give his own insulin and state how he will manage his dosage based on his diet, activity level, and glucose monitor readings.

3. In the first situation you encourage creative, off-the-top-of-your-head ideas. In the second situation, because of the risks involved, you need sound, evidence-based ideas.

5. Jack and Jill are goldfish, and a cat knocked the fish tank on the floor, shattering it. You could have asked, "Who are Jack and Jill?"

CHAPTER 3

Example Responses for Pages 81-82

3. It's important to comply with *reasonable* patient requests. However, if following the patient's request is *against the plan of care* or *to the detriment of the patient's health*, explain this to the patient. Repeat the patient's request so that he knows he has been heard, and then give the reason why his request is denied. If the request is reasonable, but against the plan of care, encourage the person to speak with the primary care givers (or appropriate team members), or speak with them yourself. In this case, after a thorough assessment of the patient's condition, you may say: "I understand that you want more medication. But I've talked with the doctor, and giving you more at this point is risky and not likely to work, as you have built up drug tolerance. I'll pay attention to the time and give you your medication as soon as I can.

4. "I don't know" isn't an acceptable answer. A critical thinker would respond, "I'll find out." Finding out will help her broaden her knowledge and help Mr. Vina.

5. The CT map summarizes key features of critical thinking in nursing. Pages 65-67 give narrative descriptions of some key relationships of the CT map. All of the CT features in the box on the left are important to accomplishing the features on the right.

6. In the presence of known problems, you predict the most likely and most dangerous complications and take immediate action to (1) prevent them and (2) be prepared to manage them in case they can't be prevented. **Example:** If you're going to care for someone with a wired jaw and you aren't familiar with the care of someone with a wired jaw, you'd look it up so that you'd know the common and dangerous complications and how to deal with them (e.g., in this case, one dangerous complication is aspiration because the person is unable to open his mouth, so you would have wire cutters nearby). You also look for evidence of risk and causative factors (things we know cause problems or put people at risk for problems). You then aim to manage these factors to prevent the actual problems. Example: In the case of the wired jaw, you assess for nausea (a risk factor for aspiration). If nausea is present, ask for an antinausea drug, hold food, and keep suction equipment and wire cutters nearby. Finally, you promote health and function by asking the person how he's handling dietary and fluid intake needs, and make suggestions as needed.

7. **(a)** The terms *clinical judgment*, *clinical reasoning*, and *critical thinking* are often used interchangeably. You use clinical reasoning and critical

thinking to make a clinical judgment. Critical thinking is an umbrella term that includes thinking both in and outside the clinical setting. Clinical judgment often requires thinking on your feet. It also requires knowing when to take your time and contact experts before making a decision. Clinical judgment entails things like knowing what to look for, how to recognize when a patient's status is changing, and knowing what to do about it. It requires theoretical and experiential knowledge and application of standards, ethics, and principles of nursing process. **(b)** Managing your personal life (e.g., managing stress, managing time, making the best of your learning preferences) has a significant impact on your ability to think critically.). **(c)** See *Goals and Outcomes of Nursing* and *What Are the Implications?* on pages 68-69. **(d)** It means that care is directed at reaching specific, observable, beneficial results in the client, and that the decisions we make and treatments we plan are based on data or evidence from clinical studies or accepted references. **(e)** These terms are defined on pages 79-80. **(f)** Both DT and PPMP focus on treating problems. However, PPMP is more proactive and focused on prevention and health promotion through early intervention than the DT model.

Example Responses for Pages 106-107

1. **(a)** When you know the people you're visiting and are familiar with the surroundings, your brain isn't "bombarded" by having to get to know someone or become familiar with the environment. In familiar situations, you also spend less energy on confidence and knowledge concerns. Novices spend a lot of energy dealing with unfamiliarity and confidence concerns. **(b)** Each time you see the movie, you see more things and get better insights into the characters. This analogy relates to the clinical setting. Each time you go to the same clinical setting with the same co-workers and patients, making care decisions is likely to be easier and more "on target." Going to the clinical setting for a novice is like going to a movie for the first time—a lot of information may be missed. **(c)** Visit the setting as an observer before you have to actually function in the setting. Find references on the setting that help you determine what to expect. Answer the questions in Box 3-8, page 102.
2. You could irrigate a nasogastric tube if the facility permitted it, you've received permission from your instructor, you have the required knowledge and level of competence, the procedure is reasonable and prudent, and you're willing to assume accountability for how you perform the procedure and the patient response to the procedure.
3. It's unlikely that the off-going nurse has really assessed the family's needs. It's highly unlikely that the family is doing fine. It appears as though the family has had limited involvement in the child's care. You should assess the family's needs and begin to include interventions that meet these needs in the nursing plan (e.g., allow the family to spend more time with the child).

7. You should check with your supervisor, your instructor, and the facility's policies and procedures related to activating the chain of command.
8. You should have looked up aspirin in a drug manual and found out that you don't give aspirin to a child with a fever, because of the risk of developing Reye's syndrome
9. Always ask yourself whether the signs and symptoms you identify could be related to an undiagnosed medical or medication problem.
10. **(a)** You can find the purpose of each phase of the nursing process in the *Nursing Process Summary* on page 83. **(b)** Experts think intuitively more quickly than novices because of their breadth of knowledge and experience. They make leaps with intuition and check themselves with logic. Novices need to question intuitive decisions and check themselves closely with logic. Critical thinking requires the use of both intuition and logic. **(c)** See the *Rule* (the terms *diagnose* and *diagnosis* have legal implications) on page 92. **(d)** See *Accountability for Diagnosis* and *Frequently Encountered Diagnoses and Complications* on pages 93-97. **(e)** Decision making is guided by ethics codes and national and facility standards and guidelines. **(f)** To prevent omissions, find structured tools that are standardized and tailored to the clinical situation. Think about *why* the tools guide you to record specific things, so that you learn what's relevant to each situation.

CHAPTER 4

Example Responses for Pages 131-143
Moral and Ethical Reasoning Exercises (pages 131-133)
1. The unborn child is the fourth silent scream in the room.
2. Ask for a family meeting to make the decision, and include an ethicist, trusted friends, or clergy to help.
3. Justice, beneficence, accountability
5. **(b)** Definitions and examples of these terms can be found on page 119. *Moral reasoning* and *ethical reasoning* both deal with making decisions based on standards and aiming to be fair and to achieve the best outcomes. However, *moral reasoning* is based on *personal values and standards* and *ethical reasoning* is based on *professional values, standards, and ethics codes*.
Evidence-Based Practice Exercises (page 133)
3. **(a)** Ultimately you need to examine the *results* of nursing care (how are the patients doing in relation to desired outcomes?). But it's also important to determine whether the *process is efficient and economical*, and whether the *setting* (structure) is such that it's likely to support surveillance and care processes.
6. **(a)** See *Relationship of Research to EBP* on page 123. **(b)** See *Frequently Asked Questions about Staff Nurses' Role* on page 127. **(c)** Refereed journals have a strict review process. Therefore the articles are more likely to be reliable.

Teaching Others, Teaching Ourselves, Test-Taking Exercises (page 143)

2. By teaching people about their health care, we empower them to achieve the important outcomes of being independent and achieving optimum health.

3. See *Learning and Memorization Strategies* on page 136.

CHAPTER 5

Example Responses for Pages 148-197

1. Identifying Assumptions (pages 153-155)

1. There's not enough evidence to indicate that the patient needs instruction. Many people are fully knowledgeable about their diet but aren't able to stick to it.

2. You might waste your time teaching information the patient already knows. You might alienate the patient: Who likes to be taught things they already know? The patient gets the message that you don't understand the problem—that you jump to conclusions.

3. **Scenario One. (a)** She seems to have assumed that she can create a positive attitude for Jeff by talking about advances in diabetic care. **(b)** She needed to assess Jeff's human response to learning he's a diabetic. Jeff may be well aware of advances in diabetic care but is still having trouble coming to terms with having to regulate his diet and take insulin for the rest of his life. She didn't assess before acting. **(c)** Jeff probably thinks Anita is a know-it-all because she didn't take the time to find out what his point of view on the situation was. It's a real turn-off when someone starts trying to change your attitude before he or she finds out what your attitude is.

Scenario Two. **(a)** She seems to have assumed the mother can read and that the mother will let her know if she has questions. **(b)** If the mother can't read or is embarrassed to ask questions, the child may have inadequate care from his mother. If harm results from the nurse's failure to determine the mother's understanding, the nurse may be accused of negligence.

Scenario Three. **(a)** The assumption seems to be that he would have the desired response to the drug without any adverse reactions. **(b)** It's likely that she was concerned that Mr. Schmidt wouldn't respond to the diuretic as expected—that he might experience an adverse reaction. **(c)** She probably thought the physician wouldn't like it if she challenged his judgment.

2. Assessing Systematically and Comprehensively (pages 158-159)

1. The body systems approach to assessment (see Figure 3-3, page 104) is probably the best method. Or you may choose the head-to-toe approach and cluster signs and symptoms of medical problems after you perform the assessment.

2. A nursing model approach (see Box 3-9, page 103).

3. **Scenario One. (a)** Assess the extent of Pearl's voluntary movement (can she wiggle her toes?); color of toes and skin around cast edges; whether Pearl feels numbness or tingling in her foot or leg; whether there is any edema of the leg or toes; the quality of the dorsalis pedis pulse; whether Pearl perceives a needle prick as being sharp; and whether her toes are warm or cool. **(b)** Assessing each of the above helps you detect early signs of circulatory problems, nerve compression, or skin irritation: If you find one area that begins to exhibit abnormal assessment findings (e.g., edema), you should increase the frequency and intensity of assessment of other areas (e.g., skin color). Each area of assessment has specific relevance: checking movement, numbness, and sensation monitors for nerve compression; checking for color, edema, pulse quality, and warmth monitors circulation and skin condition. **(c)** Check circulation by assessing the dorsalis pedis pulse quality and capillary refill in toes; check for nerve compression by asking her to wiggle her toes, and ask whether there is any numbness or tingling. If these are satisfactory, you might choose to put a warm sock over the toes; encourage her to wiggle her toes frequently to increase the circulation, and continue to monitor her dorsalis pedis pulse, toe temperature, and toe sensation closely.

Scenario Two. (a) Look up digoxin in an up-to-date reference (or consult with a pharmacist). Then assess as follows. **To assess for therapeutic effect**, check to see if Mr. Wu's serum digoxin level is within therapeutic range (0.8-2 ng/ml). Determine status of cardiac symptoms, as compared with baseline (status of apical and/or radial pulse rate and rhythm, lung sounds, urine output, edema, activity tolerance). **To assess for allergic or adverse reactions**, check Mr. Wu for signs and symptoms of any of the allergy or adverse reactions listed in the drug reference. **To assess for contraindications,** check Mr. Wu for signs and symptoms of any of the contraindications listed in the drug reference. Most common contraindications for digoxin include serum potassium levels less than 3.5 mEq/L (increases the risk of toxicity); pulse rate less than 60 or below physician-prescribed parameters; and clinical signs of toxicity or overdose. **To assess for drug interactions,** get a complete list of medications (including herbal and holistic drugs) and check with the pharmacist to find out if there are any drug interactions. **To assess for toxicity or overdose**, check Mr. Wu for signs and symptoms of toxicity or overdose. Most common signs and symptoms of digoxin toxicity include serum digoxin level above 2 ng/ml; atrioventricular block (PR interval greater than 0.24 sec); and progressive bradycardia, nausea, vomiting, and/or visual disturbances (blurring, snowflakes, yellow-green halos around images). **(b)** If no therapeutic effect is achieved by giving a drug or if the person is experiencing adverse reactions, you need to question whether a change in dosage is necessary or whether the drug should be continued at all. If you identify contraindications to giving the drug, you need to withhold the drug. If you identify signs of toxicity or overdose, it's especially important to withhold the drug because you'd be adding to the toxicity or overdose problem.

Scenario Three. (a) *Vital signs:* Measure temperature, pulse, respirations, and blood pressure. *Eye opening:* Call Gerome's name. Tell him to open his eyes. If he makes no response, pinch him. *Best motor response:* Ask him to move each extremity. Use a pin prick, or pinch him and see if he can tell you where he feels it. If he makes no response, pinch him and note whether he flexes his extremity to withdraw from pain, flexes in spasm, or extends his extremity. *Best verbal response:* Ask him what his name is, where he is, and what day it is. *Pupillary reaction:* Determine the size of each pupil in millimeters before flashing a light into it. Then flash a light into each pupil and observe whether it constricts briskly. *Purposeful limb movement:* Check each extremity by asking Gerome to move it, observing for muscle contraction (attempts to move), ability to lift extremity, and ability to lift extremity even though you try to hold it down. *Limb sensation:* Prick each limb with a sterile needle and ask Gerome what he feels (this may be unnecessary for Gerome, since he has a head injury rather than a spinal cord injury). *Seizure activity:* Observe for muscle twitching. *Gag reflex:* Place a clean tongue blade in the back of Gerome's throat and see if it triggers gagging. (b) By monitoring all of these parameters, signs and symptoms of increased intracranial pressure can be detected early. Signs and symptoms of increased intracranial pressure are decreasing level of consciousness; increasing restlessness; irritability and confusion; stronger headache; nausea and vomiting; increasing speech problems; pupil changes (dilated and nonreactive or constricted and nonreactive pupils); cranial nerve dysfunction; increasing muscle weakness, flaccidity, or coordination problems; seizures; decerebrate posturing (muscles stiff and extended, head retracted); and decorticate posturing (muscles rigid and still, with arms flexed, fists clenched, and legs extended)—the latter two are both late signs of increased intracranial pressure. (c) Monitor other parameters of neurologic assessment closely for other signs of increased intracranial pressure. If there are no other changes and you can indeed arouse Gerome, you don't need to be immediately concerned; however, you should increase the frequency of assessment of all parameters until you're comfortable that the increased somnolence is merely a sign of the combined effects of fatigue and existing brain swelling (rather than increasing brain swelling). If you have any questions about how to proceed, report the increased somnolence to your supervisor. (d) Check other neurologic parameters closely, and report and record findings immediately; increase the frequency of assessment. (e) If the baseline pulse was rapid, this may be a normal finding. However, you should closely assess all the other assessment parameters to check for other reportable signs and symptoms. If the pulse is dropping to 60 beats/min, closely monitor all the other assessment parameters and report the findings immediately (may be a sign of life-threatening increase in intracranial pressure).

3. Checking Accuracy and Reliability of Data (Validation) (page 160)

1. Talk with Mrs. Molinas, and explore her feelings and concerns.
2. You may be able to turn on his blood glucose monitor and check it (some monitors automatically show the previous blood glucose level). If not, ask Mr. Nola to take it again now (quietly observe his technique). If he is proficient at performing a check for blood glucose, it's likely his previous result was correct. If the second reading is significantly different from the previous reading, consider whether there is a relationship between the change in blood sugar reading and recent food intake or peak insulin levels. I would consider the blood sugar reading the patient took with you observing as being most valid.
3. Take it in the right arm. Take it again in 15 minutes.
4. Explore with Mr. McGwire why he thinks he got his foot ulcers. Ask him to tell you what he does to avoid getting foot ulcers. He may be very knowledgeable about diabetic care and foot ulcers and still be getting these ulcers.

4. Distinguishing Normal from Abnormal/Identifying Signs and Symptoms (pages 161-162)

1. **(a)** If you assumed this was an oral temperature, you should have *S* here. You may have placed a question mark here, which is actually a more correct response. You need to ask, *How was this temperature taken?* (orally? rectally? tympanic?) **(b)** If you assumed the patient never has rales, you should have an *S* here. You may have placed a question mark here, which is actually a more correct response. You need to ask questions like, *What do the patient's lungs sound like when he's in his usual state of health? What is the respiratory rate? How far up the back can you hear the rales? Are there just a few rales or are there copious rales? When the patient coughs, do the rales clear?* **(c)** You may have put an *S* here, but you really need to *ask if this is a normal pattern for the person and why the person only sleeps 3 hours at a time* (e.g., it's not unusual for mothers of newborns to sleep only 3 hours at a time because of feeding schedules). **(d)** S. **(e)** O or question mark. This is usually a normal finding, but you may have placed a question mark because you wanted to know such things as *whether there's any drainage, whether the area is hot to touch,* and *whether the patient is afebrile.* **(f)** O. This is normal for a 2-year-old. **(g)** S. **(h)** You may have placed an *S* here, but a better response is a question mark. Ask, *What are the bathing practices of a person of this culture?* **(i)** S. This is likely to be a normal finding, since the dialysis takes over the work of the kidney. **(j)** S or question mark. The pulse is somewhat slow but might be normal for someone who is young and athletic or older and on cardiac medication. You may have wanted to ask, *What is this person's normal pulse?* or *Is the person taking any cardiac medications that slow the heart rate?*
2. The italicized words in the preceding response are examples of what else you might want to know.

5. Making Inferences (Drawing Valid Conclusions) (page 163)

1. I suspect this information indicates infection of some sort.
2. I suspect this information indicates financial problems.
3. I suspect this information indicates that the patient has trouble sticking to his diet.
4. I suspect this information indicates that the child wants to be sure his mother approves of his answer, or perhaps he is afraid.
5. I suspect this information indicates there is some medical reason for the grandmother's confusion.

6. Clustering Related Cues (Data) (pages 164-165)

Scenario One. (a) Stung by a bee on the ear an hour ago; ear has no stinger, is red and swollen; no rash or wheezing; normal pulse and respirations. (b) Afraid he might die; wants to have a Popsicle and watch TV. (c) Didn't make sure she had parents' phone number down (investigate whether this was lack of knowledge or oversight); doesn't know first aid for a bee sting.

Scenario Two. (a) 41 years old; acute abdominal pain; vomiting for 2 days and unable to keep any food down; abdomen distended; no bowel sounds; scheduled to go to the operating room at 2 PM; pain suddenly getting worse; vital signs unchanged, except pulse is increased by approximately 30 beats/min. (b) 41-year-old businessman; hates everything about hospitals; scheduled to go to the operating room at 2 PM; worried because his brother died in the hospital after a car accident; suddenly experiencing severe pain.

7. Distinguishing Relevant from Irrelevant (pages 166-167)

Scenario One. (a) May be relevant because buspirone hydrochloride can cause confusion in the elderly. (b) May be relevant because it may be a sign of infection, which can cause confusion in the elderly. (c) May be relevant because it's indicative of previous cardiovascular disease, which is a risk factor for cerebrovascular accident (stroke), which may be the cause of the confusion. (d) May be relevant because dehydration in the elderly can cause electrolyte imbalance and confusion. (e) Not relevant. (f) Not relevant.

Scenario Two. (a) Probably relevant. It takes time to adjust to a diabetic regimen. (b) Not relevant (not abnormal). (c) May be relevant (may feel constipation is caused by new diet). (d) May be relevant because she has to prepare meals for others, increasing temptation. (e) Very probably relevant. Someone who likes to cook usually takes joy in eating a variety of foods. (f) Relevant. She needs to eat even less than she will when her weight is within normal limits. (g) Not relevant (has nothing to do with sticking to a diabetic diet).

8. Recognizing Inconsistencies (page 168)

Scenario One. (a) It doesn't make sense that she has only just started coming to prenatal clinic but has been going to birthing classes. If she hasn't had prenatal care until now, you wonder whether she's really happy about the baby coming or realizes the importance of prenatal visits. You may also wonder why her mother, rather than her boyfriend, came to the clinic visit. (b) Check her records to see if there's any mention of receiving prenatal care somewhere else for the earlier part of her pregnancy; ask her where she's been going to birthing classes; ask how her boyfriend and mother feel about the baby coming.

Scenario Two. Her age is inconsistent with risk factors for a myocardial infarction (MI). The big picture here—her age, absence of pain, and previously normal electrocardiogram—is inconsistent with the big picture of an MI. Occasionally people don't have pain when they have an MI, but usually there are other risk factors and signs and symptoms present. Her signs and symptoms are more consistent with those of a panic attack.

9. Identifying Patterns (page 170)

(a) Impaired respiratory function. Signs and symptoms of respiratory function problems are present. **(b)** Normal coping pattern. There are no signs or symptoms of abnormal coping pattern. **(c)** Pattern of potential (risk) for impaired bowel elimination. There are risk factors for constipation but no signs and symptoms. **(d)** Normal sleep-rest pattern. Considering that the person works nights, there are no signs and symptoms of an abnormal sleep-rest pattern. **(e)** Potential (risk) for ineffective sexual-reproductive pattern. There are risk factors for ineffective sexual-reproductive pattern.

10. Identifying Missing Information (page 171)

(a) What are the person's other vital signs (pulse, blood pressure, temperature)? Is there a history of smoking? Is the person smoking now? How long has this pattern persisted? What does the person feel is contributing to this pattern? How does the person tolerate activity? **(b)** How does the husband feel about helping her? **(c)** Who is the major caregiver? What factors are contributing to the lack of roughage in his diet and his inadequate fluid intake? What's the patient's (or caregiver's) knowledge of how to prevent altered bowel elimination? Why does the patient spend most of his time in bed? How motivated is the patient to do the things necessary to prevent altered bowel elimination? **(d)** Does the person feel he's getting adequate rest? Are any sleeping aids being taken? If so, what are they? **(e)** What are the woman's feelings about having herpes? What does the woman know about herpes transmission? How does she feel about telling prospective partners about the herpes? How does the patient plan to prevent herpes transmission?

11. Promoting Health by Identifying and Managing Risk Factors (page 173)

1. Do you have any family history of health problems? What's your ethnic background? Do you smoke? What do your usual meals consist of? Do you exercise regularly and get enough rest? How do you manage stress? Do you drink alcohol or take drugs that aren't prescribed? Are you sexually active? Do you wear your seat belt? What do you do to stay healthy?

2. Her age puts her at risk for osteoporosis. The history of falls, together with the risk of osteoporosis, put her at high risk for fractures. You need to look closely at why she is falling (e.g., balance problems? coordination problems?

weakness or fatigue? vision problems? home hazards?). You should also assess calcium intake, which has to be adequate to prevent osteoporosis.

3. Even though this is a social interaction, rather than a professional nurse-patient interaction, he's likely to listen because you're a nurse. Reinforce that he has a good question—that we all live longer now and that it's good to do things to increase the likelihood of living longer and healthier. Give some examples, like the importance of staying active and eating well. Stress the importance of annual exams that include blood studies to monitor things like cholesterol, blood sugar, and prostate-specific antigen. Suggest doing this annual exam around a specific time (e.g., birthday, Christmas) so that he remembers.

12. Diagnosing Actual and Potential Problems (page 179)

1. Potential for (or risk for) violence related to agitation and previous history of striking caregivers.
2. Potential complications: hemorrhage, shock, vomiting with aspiration, pneumonia, infection, paralytic ileus.
3. Hopelessness related to new diagnosis of terminal cancer as evidenced by statements of hopelessness and withdrawn behavior (sleeps most of the time, doesn't want to talk to anyone). Powerlessness is also an acceptable response. There is a fine line between these two diagnoses.
4. History of smoking or lung disease, whether the fractures are stable (risk for punctured lung), whether he has pain that is preventing him from coughing and clearing his lungs (risk for pneumonia).

13. Setting Priorities (pages 183-184)

1. (a); Answer (b) is likely to be dealt with informally or at home; answer (c) is likely to be covered by protocols and standards for care of colostomies.
2. Reporting the chest pain should be your immediate priority. Myocardial infarction and pulmonary embolus, both serious problems, are potential complications of thrombophlebitis.
3. (a) (i) 2 or 3. (ii) 2 or 3. (iii) 1.
(c) (ii) Anticipatory grieving isn't a problem that must be addressed to achieve the major outcomes. It's unrealistic to try to resolve this problem in 2 days. Rather, be a good listener, provide support, and encourage him to seek support from family or counselors.

14. Determining Client-Centered Expected Outcomes (page 187)

1. Client will maintain intact skin, free of signs of redness or irritation, and have a documented record of measures taken to prevent skin breakdown.
2. After suctioning, the mouth, the nose, and the lungs will be clear.
3. After ongoing support from caregivers, the client will express feelings about powerlessness and relate increased sense of power over his situation, as evidenced by statements that he is allowed to make as many choices about his own care as possible.

4. After irrigation, Foley catheter will be patent and draining clear yellow urine.

5. Endotracheal tube will be out by [date], with patient breathing adequately on his own, as determined by advanced practice nurse (APN) or physician.

6. Will demonstrate increased activity tolerance as evidenced by ability to walk the length of the hall and back by [date].

15. Determining Individualized Interventions (pages 191-192)

1. **(a)** Monitor fluid intake every shift. Keep iced tea (patient's preference) at the bedside on ice. Encourage drinking at least 3 quarts during the day and 1 quart at night. Reinforce the importance of maintaining adequate hydration. Record fluid intake. **(b)** Monitor anxiety level. Encourage her to express feelings and concerns. Fully explain all procedures. **(c)** Monitor comfort level. After applying heat for 30 minutes, assist with range of motion exercises three times a day.

2. **Contributing factors:** Age, low weight, chemotherapy, spends a lot of time in bed. **Interventions:** Monitor skin for pressure points, especially coccyx, elbows, and heels. Put a foam bed pad on bed. Use a sheep skin for coccyx and heels. Teach the importance of (1) changing positions frequently, spending more time out of bed, keeping skin moisturized, maintaining hydration and a healthy diet, and having a family member monitor her back and heels for redness, and (2) reporting skin problems to APN or physician before each chemotherapy treatment.

3. **(a) (1)** It's quite likely the children won't report finding ticks, increasing the likelihood that the mother won't know when the children may have been bitten. It also increases the likelihood that the ticks won't be properly disposed of. I doubt that there will be benefits from using this approach (punishment). **(2)** It's possible that they may go looking for ticks, increasing the likelihood of being bitten. This approach might work, but the risks outweigh the benefits. **(b)** Determine children's understanding of the severity of the consequences of tick bites and the importance of finding ways to avoid them. Initiate teaching as indicated. Explain to the children that they can best help by asking for insect repellent to be applied before going outside, reporting ticks found on themselves and on each other, and avoiding tall grassy areas. Start a rule that the children can't go outside without first applying insect repellent. Have the mother praise good behavior (e.g., asking for insect repellent) verbally, rather than offering rewards. Instruct the mother not to offer rewards for finding ticks.

17. Determining a Comprehensive Plan and Updating the Plan (pages 196-197)

1. **(a)** Not achieved. **(b)** Achieved. **(c)** Partially achieved; focus teaching toward mother's needs.

2. **Discharge outcome:** Will be discharged home with husband able to demonstrate administration of epinephrine by June 29. **Nursing diagnosis no. 1:** *Knowledge deficit (husband): Epinephrine administration.* (You may have chosen

another diagnosis, such as *ineffective coping,* for Mrs. Edmunds, in the hope that you can help her cope with the possibility of learning how to give her own injections. However, in the interest of time, teaching the husband is first priority.) **Expected outcome:** Husband will relate knowledge of action and side effects of epinephrine and when to give epinephrine and demonstrate subcutaneous injection technique. **Interventions:** Assess husband's knowledge of epinephrine action, side effects, and administration. Give husband literature about epinephrine administration. Also determine preferred learning style. Reinforce what he already knows; teach gaps in knowledge using the husband's preferred learning style. Record husband's progress toward expected outcome after each teaching session. **Nursing diagnosis no. 2:** *Altered comfort (itching feet) related to hives as evidenced by hives over feet.* **Expected outcome:** Patient will experience improved comfort as evidenced by statements of relief of itching. **Interventions:** Assist patient to place feet in cool water as needed. Medicate as ordered as needed for itching.

3. You've identified a care variance. According to the predicted care, she should be voiding normally. Assess the patient carefully, checking for bladder distention and asking the patient about urinary symptoms. Check vital signs and bring the problem to the attention of the professional in charge of care management (e.g., APN, doctor).

4. See Box 5-5 on page 195.

Mind Mapping (Concept Mapping): Getting in the "Right" State of Mind

WHAT IS MIND MAPPING (CONCEPT MAPPING)?

Mind mapping (sometimes called concept mapping) uses the right brain (the creative hemisphere) to enhance ability to understand information and solve problems: You combine writing and drawing. Unlike outlining, which uses the left brain (the logical hemisphere), mind mapping is flexible, has few rules, and is easy to learn and teach. The next page shows a mind map of how the brain works and also gives steps for how to mind map.

WHEN DO YOU USE IT?

You can use mind mapping for a variety of purposes, including the following:
- Taking notes or learning new content
- Mapping the care planning process
- Writing papers or preparing presentations
- Preparing for exams
- Promoting brainstorming
- Facilitating group problem solving

WHAT ARE THE BENEFITS?

General benefits and specific group benefits follow:

General Benefits
- Quicker than regular note-taking
- Highlights key ideas and gets rid of the irrelevant
- Helps you quickly gather, review, and recall large amounts of information

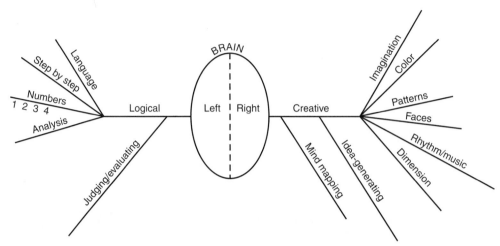

Mind map of how the brain works.

- Increases brainpower available for learning and problem solving by reducing energy used on concerns about structure and documentation
- Encourages you to identify relationships and be creative
- Helps you retain what you learn because you "play with the information" in your own way as you make your map

Group Benefits
- Promotes communication (keeps everyone focused on the main issues)
- Facilitates problem solving (generates more ideas, helps group suspend judgment)
- Makes ideas and relationships clear

HOW DOES IT PROMOTE CRITICAL THINKING?

Mind mapping facilitates the "productive and analytical phases" of critical thinking—the phase when you need to gather relevant information, identify relationships, and produce new ideas. After you complete this productive phase, you can get in touch with your left brain talents and move to the "judgment phase"—you can evaluate what your mind has produced, make judgments about its accuracy and usefulness, and make refinements.

Eight Steps for Mind Mapping to Promote Critical Thinking
1. **Put central theme or concept** in the center, at the bottom, or at the top of the page, and draw a circle around it (see the example mind map above).
2. **Place the main ideas relating to the concept** on lines (or in circles) around the central theme.

3. **Add details** by putting them on lines (or in circles) connecting them to the main ideas.
4. **Use key words or simple pictures** only; keep it legible.
5. **Make sure no idea stands alone**. If you can't connect an idea with something on the page, it's irrelevant to the central theme.
6. **Don't allow yourself to slow down** over concerns about where to place words (this is your left brain habit trying to dominate). Rather let your ideas flow and use lines to show connections.
7. **Use colors** to highlight the most important ideas.
8. **Once you've completed your mind map**, get in touch with your left-brain talents (judging and evaluating), and evaluate what you've produced. **Revise as needed**.

APPENDIX B

Patients' Rights*

Dear consumer:
State law requires that your health care provider or facility recognize *your rights* while receiving medical care, and that you respect *their right* to expect certain behavior on the part of patients. You may request a copy of the full text of this law from your health care provider or facility.

You have the following rights:
- To be treated with courtesy and respect with appreciation of dignity and protection of your need for privacy
- To receive prompt and reasonable response to questions and requests
- To be informed of the following:
  - Who is providing medical services and who is responsible for your care
  - What patient support services are available, including whether an interpreter is available if you have communication problems
  - Your diagnosis, planned course of treatment, alternatives, risks, and prognosis
  - Whether treatment is for purposes of experimental research (and to give or refuse your consent to participate in such research)
- To refuse treatment, except as otherwise provided by law
- To have impartial access to medical treatment or accommodations, regardless of race, national origin, religious, physical handicap, or source of payment
- To be given treatment for any emergency condition that will deteriorate upon failure to receive treatment
- To express any grievances about any violation of your rights as stated by state law, through the grievance procedure of your health care provider or facility and appropriate state licensing agency
- To file complaints against a health care professional, hospital, or ambulatory surgical center with the Agency for Health Care Administration (*Note:* Appropriate information for how to reach each state's agency must be listed here)
- To receive the following (upon request):
  - Full information and necessary counseling on the availability of financial recourses for your care
  - A reasonable estimate of the charges for medical care before treatment
  - Information about whether your health care provider or facility accepts the Medicare assignment rate before treatment
- To be given a copy of an itemized bill that is reasonably clear and understandable and upon request, to have charges explained

You have the following responsibilities:
- To provide your health care provider, to the best of your knowledge, with accurate and complete information about your complaints, past illnesses, hospitalizations, medications, and other matters relating to your health
- To follow the treatment plan recommended by your provider
- To report unexpected changes in your condition to the health care provider
- To keep appointments and, if you're unable to do so for any reason, to notify your provider or facility
- To ensure that the financial obligations of your health care are fulfilled as soon as possible
- To comply with health care provider and facility rules and regulations affecting patient conduct

---

*This is an example form and summary of rights. Rights may vary from state to state. Forms may vary from facility to facility.

APPENDIX C

DEAD ON!! A Game to Promote Critical Thinking

Instructions: The point of this game is to be sure that you give key parts of thinking the time and attention they require, therefore promoting thinking that's more likely to be "dead on." Get six balls; on each one, with indelible ink, put one of these letters: D, E, A, D, O, and N. Start with the "D" ball, and toss it to someone in the group. Ask the group to focus on answering the questions listed under "D" below. Once you have exhausted thoughts on the "D" ball, do the same for each of the remaining balls. Be sure to stay focused on the current ball. For example, if someone expresses feelings rather than facts (data) with the first ball, point out that the rules are that emotions are addressed only when the "E" ball is up for discussion.

D = Data
- What data (facts) do you have?
- What other data do you need?
- What assumptions have you made, and what data might validate or negate them?

E = Emotions
- What emotions (gut reactions) are there (your own, others)?
- What's your intuition telling you, and what data might validate or negate it?
- How are values affecting thinking (yours, others)?

A = Advantages
- What are the vision, the benefit(s), and the most important desired outcome(s)?
- What are the specific advantages to others (benefits and outcomes)?
- What are the specific advantages to you (benefits and outcomes)?

D = Disadvantages
- What could go wrong (what are the risks)?
- What are the specific inconveniences or risks for others?
- What are the specific inconveniences or risks for you?
- What problems or issues must be addressed to get results?
- How much work will it take, and do you have the necessary resources?

O = Out of the box
- Go out of the box—think of creative approaches!
- What can we do to reduce the disadvantages?
- What can we do to increase the likelihood of seeing the benefits?
- How can technology help?
- What research is there that might apply?
- What human resources are willing to help?

N = Now what?
- What problems, risks, or issues must be addressed?
- Who are the key stakeholders (who will be most affected)?
- What professional, community, and informal resources can help?
- What's the plan (what interventions do you need to get results and avoid risks?)
- What does all this imply?
- What did we miss when addressing the other balls? (Go through each of the balls again)

APPENDIX D
Example Critical Pathway

Clinical Pathway ■ CARE PATH NAME: TOTAL ABDOMINAL HYSTERECTOMY

☐ With Burch   ☐ Without Burch

DRG: 353-358   ELOS: 2 Days
Expected Disposition: Home

Focus	Preadmission	Day of Surgery
LABORATORY/ TESTS/ PROCEDURES	☐ Blood work ☐ <40 years Hct ☐ >40 years SMA 6, CBC ☐ EKG if >40 years ☐ CXR if >60 years ☐ Type and screen	
CONSULTS/ REFERRALS/	☐ Anesthesia Consult ☐ Nursing Consult	
PHYSICAL ASSESSMENT	☐ H & P obtained	☐ VS per post-op routine ☐ Routine post-op assessment ☐ I/O
DIAGNOSIS:		
ACTIVITY	☐ Ad lib	☐ Dangle at bedside or OOB to chair
TREATMENTS	☐ Instruction on IS ☐ Review of procedure	☐ IS/C&DB Q 1 h WA ☐ Foley ☐ SCD's ☐ Drains: **BURCH ONLY:** ☐ Suprapubic Catheter

268

Collaborative Problem List
1. Discharge Planning
2. Pain/Comfort Management
3. Coping Response to
   Surgery/Diagnosis
4. _____

Post-Op Day 1	Post-Op Day 2
☐ CBC	
☐ Primary RN	
☐ VS Q shift	☐ VS Q shift
☐ Q shift assessment	☐ Q shift assessment
☐ I/O	☐ I/O
☐ Weight	☐ Weight
☐ Fever assessment (if temp >39° C)	☐ Fever assessment (if temp >38.5° C)
☐ Exam	☐ Exam
☐ Cultures of surgical area	☐ Cultures of surgical area
☐ CBC with diff	☐ CBC with diff
☐ Blood cultures	☐ Blood cultures
☐ OOB to chair	☐ Ambulate QID
☐ IS/C&DB Q 1 h WA	☐ IS/C&DB Q 1 h
☐ D/C Foley	☐ D/C Drains:
☐ SCD's	**BURCH ONLY:**
☐ Drains:	☐ Suprapubic Catheter
BURCH ONLY:	☐ Monitor postvoid residuals
☐ Suprapubic Catheter	☐ Begin clamp routine 24 h after surgery if no hematuria

Continued

Clinical Pathway ■ **CARE PATH NAME: TOTAL ABDOMINAL HYSTERECTOMY** (*Continued*)

Focus	Preadmission	Day of Surgery
DIET	☐ NPO pre-op	☐ Ice chips ☐ Clear liquids
MEDICATIONS		☐ PCA protocol ☐ Epidural protocol ☐ IV pain meds ☐ IV antibiotics: ☐ IVF:

DISCHARGE PLANNING/ TEACHING	☐ Discharge Planning Review:
	  ☐ Pre-op checklist
	  ☐ Advanced directives
	  ☐ Client care path pamphlet
	☐ Determine services needed
	  ☐ Client lives alone
	  ☐ Client lives with others
	  Support person:
	  Phone number:
		☐ Client lives alone
		☐ Client lives with others
		Support person:
		Phone Number:

INDIVIDU ALIZED CARE FOCUS		
INTERMEDIA TE OUTCOMES	☐ Client able to explain home-going plan ☐ Client able to describe pro-cedure(s) to be performed ☐ Client states she has partici-pated in decision making and plan	☐ Afebrile ☐ Client states pain is ade-quately controlled ☐ Client shows no evidence of post-op complications

Discharge Outcomes:	Met

1. Abdominal incision approximated and healing
2. Has minimal, odorless vaginal discharge
3. Able to describe/perform pericare
4. Has functional pattern for bladder and bowel
5. Maintains adequate nutritional intake
6. Pain controlled by oral medication
7. States use of homegoing medications
8. Describes plan for follow-up care
9. Describes feeling about effects of surgery on health and sexuality
10. Identifies support systems and resources available to her after discharge
11. Afebrile or Temp <38° C with normal WBC
12. **BURCH ONLY:** Able to demonstrate clamp routine

Courtesy University Hospitals of Cleveland.
University Hospitals' carepaths have been developed to assist clinicians in patient management and clinical decision-making. The carepaths are intended to meet the needs of patients in most circumstances. They are not intended to replace a clinician's judgment or establish a protocol for all patients with that diagnosis.

Post-Op Day 1	Post-Op Day 2
☐ Advanced as tolerated	☐ House diet
☐ D/C PCA at 08:00	☐ PO meds
☐ D/C Epidural	☐ D/C HL
☐ IV pain meds to PO	
☐ IVF:	
☐ Heplock when taking PO	
Provide Homegoing Instructions:	☐ Review home-going
☐ Hysterectomy PI-128	instructions
☐ "Women and AIDS" pamphlet	
☐ Breast self exam pamphlet	
☐ Hormone replacement therapy	
☐ Instruct on pericare	
BURCH ONLY:	
☐ Clamp Routine PI Sheets	

Post-Op Day 1	Post-Op Day 2
	☐ Ambulates independently
☐ Able to void without difficulty	☐ Has had a bowel movement and/or
☐ Afebrile or temp <38°C with	passed flatus
normal WBC	☐ Tolerates house diet
☐ Tolerating PO fluids	☐ Client able to describe procedure(s)
☐ Ambulates with assistance	performed
☐ Client states pain is ade-	☐ Client able to describe pericare
quately controlled with PO	☐ Client able to explain all discharge
Pain medication	instructions
	BURCH ONLY:
	☐ Able to measure and record
	postvoid residuals

Not Met	Comments	Date/Initials

APPENDIX E

Admission Tool

☐

Main Line Hospitals

Bryn Mawr Hospital
Lankenau Hospital
Paoli Hospital

INITIAL PATIENT ASSESSMENT

Patient I.D.

Complete shaded area **OR** ☐ See 24 Hour Flow Sheet   ☐ See E.D. Triage Sheet

Date:	Height:	Weight:	Language spoken other than English:

Primary Care Physician/Specialist: _____

Reason for procedure/hospitalization: _____
_____

Procedure/Date: _____
_____

Upon entry to the Hospital: Correct ID band in place ☐ Yes

Vital Signs Temp _____   P _____   RR _____   BP _____

O2 Sat _____   O2 _____   RA _____   ☐ Not Applicable

INITIAL PAIN ASSESSMENT

Does patient have complaint of or admitting diagnosis of pain?   ☐ Patient non-verbal
    ☐ Yes (see 24 hr flowsheet)
    ☐ No
Intensity (0-10 scale) _____
Location: ☐ Head ☐ Back   ☐ Upper extremity ☐ R ☐ L   ☐ Lower extremity ☐ R ☐ L
          ☐ Chest ☐ Abdomen ☐ Other _____
Description: ☐ Sharp ☐ Stabbing   ☐ Burning   ☐ Constant   Intermittent
          ☐ Other _____
Onset/Duration of Pain _____
What makes pain better/worse? _____
Impact of ADLs: ☐ Decreased Activity/Self Care _____
☐ Decreased Appetite/Nausea/Vomiting ☐ Other _____

Allergies: Drug/Food/Latex/Tape/Dyes ☐ None Known

ALLERGIES	REACTION	ALLERGIES	REACTION

ADVANCE DIRECTIVES   ☐ NA (Patient < 18 years old)   ☐ Unable to Assess

Does the patient have an advance directive? ☐ Yes	☐ No
☐ Copy in current chart ☐ Refer to old records ☐ Patient/Family to obtain copy for record (Place reminder on Pathway until received) ☐ Patient to formulate another advance directive (sample in "It's Up To You") ☐ Substance as stated by patient: _____ _____	☐ Information Given ☐ Information Declined ☐ Patient declines stating content ☐ Patient/family declines to bring, and/or complete advance directive information ☐ Refer to Social Work

COMPLETE THIS SECTION FOR ALL PATIENTS

PAST SURGICAL HISTORY

Patient I.D

Past surgical History: _____

Previous anesthesia: □ General   □ Spinal   □ Other _____
Problems with Anesthesia? _____ □ Motion Sickness
Family history/problems with anesthesia: _____

HEALTH HISTORY   Check/Circle Applicable Boxes Only

NEUROLOGIC
- □ Stroke / TIA
  - □ Residual _____
  - □ None
- □ Blackouts/Fainting/Vertigo
- □ Seizures
- □ Migraine/Headaches
- □ Numbness/Tingling
  - ____ Arm ____ Legs
- □ Speech difficulty
- □ Swallowing/Choking
- □ Head injury
- □ Confusion/Dementia
- □ Memory changes
- □ Other _____
- □ *No identified problems*

CARDIOVASCULAR
- □ High blood pressure/Low blood pressure
- □ Aneurysm
- □ Congenital heart defect
- □ Heart attack
- □ Heart failure
- □ Murmur
- □ Chest pain/Angina
- □ Irregular pulse
- □ Circulation problem
- □ Phlebitis/Clots
- □ Pacemaker/Defib.
- □ High cholesterol
- □ Cardiovascular intervention
- □ *No identified problems*

RESPIRATORY
- □ Shortness of breath
- □ Pneumonia
- □ COPD
- □ Asthma
- □ Acute Bronchitis
- □ Cough
- □ Seasonal/Environmental allergies
- □ Snoring/Apnea
- □ CPAP/BiPAP
- □ TB
- □ Post nasal drip
- □ Other _____
- □ *No identified problems*

GASTROINTESTINAL
- □ Constipation/Incontinence
- □ Irritable Bowels/Diarrhea
- □ Last B.M.
- □ Blood in stool
- □ Recent change in bowel habits
- □ Crohn's/Colitis
- □ Diverticular disease
- □ Ostomy _____
- □ Ulcers
- □ Hiatal hernia/Reflux
- □ Hepatitis
- □ Gall bladder disease
- □ Mucositis
- □ Other _____
- □ *No identified problems*

MUSCULOSKELETAL
- □ Arthritis/DJD
- □ Joint replacement _____
- □ Osteoporosis
- □ Spinal/Back problems _____
- □ Muscle weakness/ Spasticity
- □ Fibromyalgia
- □ Quadriplegic
- □ Paraplegic
- □ Other _____
- □ *No identified problems*

GENITOURINARY
- □ Burning/Urgency/Frequency
- □ Blood in urine
- □ Recurrent UTI
- □ Kidney failure/Dialysis
- □ Kidney stones
- □ Prostate problems
- □ Incontinence
- □ Ostomy _____
- □ Other _____
- □ *No identified problems*

PSYCHOSOCIAL
- □ Alcohol use
  - Last alcohol use _____
  - Type/Amount _____
- □ Tobacco use
  - Last used _____
  - Type/Amount _____
- □ Drug use
  - Type/Amount _____
- □ Depression
- □ Panic/Anxiety attacks
- □ Bereavement
- □ Claustrophobia
- □ Physical/Psychological abuse
- □ Attention deficit disorder
- □ Other _____
- □ *No identified problems*

INTEGUMENTARY
- □ Pressure ulcers
  - location _____
  - stage _____
  - 2nd location _____
  - stage _____
- □ Multiple pressure ulcers
- □ Specialty bed
- □ Lower leg/foot wounds
  - □ Right □ Left □ Both
- □ Skin problems _____
- □ Dry skin
- □ Rash
- □ Old scars
- □ Tattoos/Body piercings
- □ Petechia/Bruising
- □ Other _____
- □ *No identified problems*

METABOLIC
- □ Diabetes type: _____
- □ Hypoglycemia
- □ Hypo/hyperthyroid
- □ Anemia
- □ Obesity
- □ Other _____
- □ *No identified problems*

GYN
- □ LMP _____
- □ Possibility of pregnancy
- □ Pregnant
- □ Breast feeding
- □ Breast Mass/Tenderness/Discharge
- □ Vaginal Discharge
- □ Pre/post menopausal
- □ Other _____
- □ *No identified problems*

CANCER/HEMATOLOGIC
Type of cancer _____

Prior Chemo/XRT _____

PICC/PORTS
  Location _____
- □ Blood/Bleeding Disorders
- □ Immunosuppression
- □ Other _____
- □ Clinical Trial Experience
- □ *No identified problems*

SENSORY DEFICITS
- □ Vision Changes
- □ Glaucoma/Cataracts
  - □ Had surgery
- □ Hearing Deficit
- □ Other _____
- □ *No identified problems*
- □ Infectious Disease/STD
  - Type _____
- □ Sexually Transmitted Disease
  - Type _____

SLEEP HABITS
Usual bed time _____
Usual wake time _____

Sleepy during day	□ Yes	□ No
Trouble falling asleep	□ Yes	□ No
Trouble staying asleep	□ Yes	□ No

- □ Other _____
- □ *No identified problems*

COMMENTS
_____
_____
_____

ASSISTIVE DEVICES/PERSONAL ITEMS: *Check appropriate boxes*

□ See personal belongings list, if applicable	PAT/POA	Brought to hospital	Left at home	NA
Glasses/Contacts				
Dentures □ Upper □ Lower □ Both □ Partial				
Jewelry: Type				
Crutches/Prosthesis/Cane/Walker				
Breathing devices: Type				
Wigs/Hairpieces				
Religious items				
Hearing Aid □ Right □ Left □ Both				

Page 2 of 4

Admission tool reprinted with permission.

○   ○   ○   ○   ○

○

COMPLETE THIS SECTION FOR ALL PATIENTS

Patient I.D.

CULTURAL/RELIGIOUS/SPIRITUAL	ACTION TAKEN

Religious Preference: _____ □ NA

Would like to see: □ Hospital Chaplain / Representative
                    □ Personal Religious Leader
                    (Name) _____ (Phone #) _____
                    □ No visits

Any cultural, spiritual or religious requests while in the hospital?
    □ No □ Yes Specify: _____

ACTION TAKEN
□ Refer to Chaplain

Enter consult and place on pathway

SOCIAL/DISCHARGE PLANNING	ACTION TAKEN

□ Lives Alone □Lives with spouse/significant other/family/caretaker
□ Stairs _____ □ Bathroom on same level as living quarters
□ Lives in nursing home/assisted living ❶ _____
□ Unable to return to previous living arrangement ❷
□ Compromised in ADLs and /or lack of support network ❶
□ Insurance concerns ❶ □ Financial concerns ❷
□ Received services prior to admission: □unknown □home care □med equip ❶
□ Evidence of physical/emotional abuse or neglect or domestic violence ❷
□ Current substance abuse ❷
□ Special discharge needs _____
□ Patient plans to be discharged to: _____
□ Discharge Transportation
    (Name) _____ (Phone#)_____
□ *No discharge planning needs identified*

ACTION TAKEN
□Assist With ADLs
□Patient Education

❶ □ Refer to Case
    Manager/Home Care

❷ □ Refer to Social Work

Enter consult and place on pathway

NUTRITIONAL STATUS	□ No Identified Problems	ACTION TAKEN

Diet prior to admission _____
If any of the following are present, send computer order to Nutrition Services
□ Unintentional weight loss/gain ≥10 lbs in the last 6 months ❶
□ Vomiting/diarrhea for the last 3 days or longer ❶
□ Poor appetite for the last 5 days or longer ❶
□ Reliance on Nutrition support/tube, feeding/TPN ❶
□ Newly diagnosed pt. with diabetes need for education ❶,❷
□ Pressure ulcer stage II or greater ❶
□ Pregnant or breastfeeding

ACTION TAKEN
❶ □ Nutrition Referral

❷ □ Community Educator/
    Diabetes Referral

SMOKING STATUS	□ No Identified Problems

□ Smoking cessation information given
□ Smoking cessation information declined
□ Community Educator/Smoking Cessation Referral

Enter consult and place on pathway

EDUCATION NEEDS ASSESSMENT	ACTION TAKEN

Learning Readiness: □ Willing to Learn □ Unable to Learn □ Resists/refuses at this time
Barriers to Learning: □ No Barriers □ Cognitive □ Cultural
                          □ Educational □Emotional □ Language
                          □ Motivational □ Financial □ Physical □ Religious
    □ Comments/Other_____
Plans to Overcome Barriers to Education: □Family involvement □Reinforcement
                                            □Written Materials □ Audiovisual Aids
                                            □ Interpreter
    □ Other_____
Specific Educational Needs: □ Disease Process □ Activity Level □ Diet
                                 □ Procedures □Hygiene
                                 □ Medications (including Drug and Food Interactions)
                                 □ Medical Equipment/Assistive Devices
                                 □ Skin/Ostomy □ Pain Management
                                 □ Other _____
Teaching to be directed primarily to: □ Patient □ Family
    □ Other_____

ACTION TAKEN
□ Education Initiated

□ Unable to initiate
   education

Information obtained from/completed by: _____ Date/Time:_____

Completed by: _____ Date/Time:_____

Reviewed by RN:_____ Date/Time:_____

COMPLETE THIS SECTION FOR INPATIENTS ONLY

Patient I.D.

Patient Folder Given?   ☐ Yes   ☐ No

| Patient Information May be Given To/Emergency Contact: |
| Name:_____ |
| Phone Number:_____ |

☐ Patient Handbook/Patient's Rights and Responsibilities reviewed.
☐ Patient/family oriented to room

RESPIRATORY STATUS ☐ No Identified Problems	ACTION TAKEN
☐ Patient is pre-op for upper abdominal or thoracic surgery <u>and</u> has a history of Emphysema, Bronchitis, Asthma, or Pulmonary Fibrosis	**Requires Physician Order** ☐ Respiratory Care Referred **Enter consult and place on pathway**

PHYSICAL THERAPY/OCCUPATIONAL THERAPY/SPEECH THERAPY ☐ No Identified Problems	ACTION TAKEN
☐ Recent loss of function affecting Activities of Daily Living (ADL) ☐ Decreased strength and/or range of motion that could be resolved with therapy ☐ Difficulty swallowing and/or signs of choking while drinking/eating	**Requires Physician Order** **Enter consult and place on pathway**

REMINDERS:

COMPLETE MEDICATION RECONCILIATION FORM FOR ALL MEDICATIONS

COMPLETE VACCINE SCREENING/STANDING ORDER FORM

<u>COMMENTS</u>

_____
_____
_____
_____
_____
_____
_____
_____
_____
_____
_____
_____
_____
_____
_____
_____
_____

Completed by RN _____ Date/Time _____

APPENDIX F

Nursing Interventions Classification (NIC) and Nursing Outcomes Classification (NOC) Examples

EXAMPLES OF NURSING INTERVENTIONS CLASSIFICATION (NIC) LABELS*

Abuse Protection Support
Acid-Base Management
Acid-Base Monitoring
Active Listening
Activity Therapy
Acupressure
Admission Care
Airway Management
Airway Suctioning
Allergy Management
Amnioinfusion
Amputation Care
Analgesic Administration
Bed Rest Care
Behavior Management
Bibliotherapy
Biofeedback
Birthing
Bladder Irrigation
Bleeding Precautions
Calming Technique
Cardiac Precautions
Caregiver Support
Case Management
Cast Care: Maintenance
Circulatory Precautions
Code Management
Cognitive Restructuring
Decision-Making Support
Delegation
Dementia Management
Discharge Planning
Documentation
Dying Care
Electrolyte Management
Emergency Cart Checking

Emotional Support
Endotracheal Extubation
Hair Care
Hallucination Management
Immunization/Vaccination
   Management
Impulse Control Training
Incident Reporting
Intravenous (IV) Therapy
Kangaroo Care
Leech Therapy
Milieu Therapy
Mood Management
Multidisciplinary Care
Mutual Goal Setting
Nail Care
Nausea Management
Oral Health Maintenance
Oxygen Therapy
Pain Management
Patient Contracting

EXAMPLES OF NURSING OUTCOMES CLASSIFICATION (NOC) LABELS†

Acceptance: Health Status
Adherence Behavior
Aggression Control
Ambulation: Walking
Ambulation: Wheelchair
Anxiety Control
Asthma Control
Blood Glucose Control
Body Image
Breastfeeding: Weaning
Cardiac Pump Effectiveness
Caregiver Stressors
Caregiver Well-Being
Circulation Status

Coagulation Status
Cognitive Ability
Comfort Level
Community Competence
Concentration
Decision Making
Depression Control
Dignified Dying
Distorted Thought Control
Endurance
Family Coping
Fear Control
Fetal Status: Intrapartum
Fluid Balance
Grief Resolution
Growth
Health Beliefs
Health Promoting Behavior
Health Seeking Behavior
Hearing Compensation Behavior
Hope
Hydration
Immunization Behavior
Joint Movement: Passive
Knowledge: Disease Process
Leisure Participation
Loneliness
Medication Response
Memory
Neglect Recovery
Newborn Adaptation
Pain Control
Quality of Life
Risk Control
Safety Behavior: Personal
Self-Direction of Care
Self-Esteem
Skeletal Function
Spiritual Well-Being
Suffering Level
Symptom Control
Thermoregulation

*For a comprehensive list, see the most up-to-date edition of McClosky, J., & Bulechek, G. (2004). *Nursing interventions* (4th ed). St. Louis: Mosby.
†For a comprehensive list, see the most up-to-date edition of Moorhead, S., Johnson, M., & Maas, M. (2004). *Nursing outcomes classification* (3rd ed.). St. Louis: Mosby.

American Nurses Association (ANA) Standards of Practice and Professional Performance Related to Registered Nurses

STANDARDS OF PRACTICE

Standard 1. Assessment: The registered nurse collects comprehensive data pertinent to the patient's health or situation.

Standard 2. Diagnosis: The registered nurse analyzes the assessment data to determine the diagnoses or issues.

Standard 3. Outcomes Identification: The registered nurse identifies expected outcomes for a plan individualized to the patient or the situation.

Standard 4. Planning: The registered nurse develops a plan that prescribes strategies and alternatives to attain expected outcomes.

Standard 5. Implementation: The registered nurse implements the identified plan.

    Standard 5a. The registered nurse coordinates care delivery. The registered nurse employs strategies to promote health and a safe environment.

    Standard 5b. Health Teaching and Health Promotion: The registered nurse employs strategies to promote health and a safe environment.

Standard 6. Evaluation: The registered nurse evaluates progress towards attainment of outcomes.

STANDARDS OF PROFESSIONAL PERFORMANCE

Standard 7. Quality of Practice: The registered nurse systematically enhances the quality and effectiveness of nursing practice.

Standard 8. Education: The registered nurse attains knowledge and competency that reflects current nursing practice.

Reprinted with permission from American Nurses Association. (2004). *Nursing: Scope and standards of practice*, Silver Spring, MD: Nursesbooks.org.

Standard 9. Professional Practice Evaluation: The registered nurse evaluates one's own nursing practice in relation to professional practice standards and guidelines, relevant statutes, rules, and regulations.

Standard 10. Collegiality: The registered nurse interacts with and contributes to the professional development of peers and colleagues.

Standard 11. Collaboration: The registered nurse collaborates with patient, family, and others in the conduct of nursing practice.

Standard 12. Ethics: The registered nurse integrates ethical provisions in all areas of practice.

Standard 13. Research: The registered nurse integrates research findings into practice.

Standard 14. Resource Utilization: The registered nurse considers factors related to safety, effectiveness, cost, and impact on practice in the professional practice setting and the profession.

Standard 15. Leadership. The registered nurse provides leadership in the professional practice setting and the profession.

NCLEX® Practice Questions[*]

Note: Correct answers and rationales can be found on pages 283-286)

1. Which of the following play activities would be appropriate for a toddler?
   1. Musical mobile above bed
   2. Rattle
   3. Jigsaw puzzle
   4. Wagon

2. If a client who was under a local anesthetic during recent surgery is slurring speech, what would be the nurse's priority action?
   1. Check intravenous (IV) placement, blood pressure, pulse, and respiratory status.
   2. Recognize this as a symptom of anxiety, and encourage the client to sleep off the effect.
   3. Determine whether the client consumed a large quantity of alcohol before surgery.
   4. Do nothing, because this frequently occurs in clients who receive large doses of local anesthetics.

3. Which of the following tasks should the charge nurse delegate to an experienced licensed practical nurse (LPN) working on the adult medical unit?
   1. Teaching a client about the preprocedure preparation for a gastric endoscopy

2. Inserting a nasogatric (NG) tube for gastric acid analysis
3. Administering IV midazolam hydrochloride (Versed) during endoscopy
4. Developing a nursing care plan for a client having a cystoscopy

4. Which of the following clients is likely to be predisposed to an adverse reaction to a medication?
   1. A 5-year-old with an eye infection
   2. A 20-year-old with a fracture
   3. A 4-year-old with an upper respiratory tract infection
   4. A 70-year-old woman with liver disease

5. A client is experiencing respiratory alkalosis as a result of hyperventilation. The nurse would expect the blood gas values to reflect what changes?
   1. Decreased pH, decreased P_{CO_2}
   2. Decreased pH, elevated P_{CO_2}
   3. Increased pH, decreased P_{CO_2}
   4. Increased pH, increased P_{CO_2}

6. A client with human immunodeficiency virus (HIV) has been receiving antiviral medication for the past 3 months. When he calls the clinic complaining of polydipsia, polyuria, and polyphagia, the nurse understands that which of

---

*Practice questions borrowed from the companion CD for Zerwekh, J., & Claborn, J. (2006). *Illustrated study guide for the NCLEX-RN Exam.* St. Louis: Mosby (questions 19 and 20 adapted here). To order this book with companion CD, go to www.elsevierhealth.com or call (800) 545-2522.

the following is most likely the reason for the symptoms?
1. Pancreatic infiltration by HIV virus leading to diabetic-like symptoms
2. Allergic reaction to the non-nucleoside reverse transcriptase inhibitor medications
3. Nonadherence with the antiviral medication regimen
4. Hyperglycemia caused by the protease inhibitor

7. When assessing a client for possible side effects of vincristine, the nurse should observe for which toxic side effect?
1. Diarrhea
2. Alopecia
3. Hemorrhagic cystitis
4. Peripheral neuropathy

8. A 9-year-old client with leukemia asks, "Will I die?" What is an initial therapeutic response based on the needs of the dying child?
1. "Think about getting well instead of dying."
2. "Tell me what you are thinking about dying."
3. "You need to ask your doctor."
4. "I really don't know."

9. The nurse is assessing a client who may be experiencing auditory hallucinations. Which client activity would assist the nurse to confirm that a hallucination is occurring?
1. Client mumbling to self; tilted head; eyes darting back and forth
2. Client performing obsessive-compulsive rituals such as turning a radio off and on; talking to self

3. Client is hyperactive and very easily distracted; avoids contact with other clients
4. Client is cool, aloof, and unapproachable; avoids enclosed areas

10. A client has extensive burns with eschar on the anterior trunk. What is the nurse's primary concern regarding eschar formation?
1. It prevents fluid remobilization in the first 48 hours after burn trauma.
2. Infection is difficult to assess before the eschar sloughs.
3. It restricts the ability of the client to move about.
4. Circulation to the extremities is diminished because of edema formation.

11. The nurse is assessing the hearing of a client with Bell's palsy. What would be the best way to determine the hearing of the client?
1. Stand out of sight of the client and ask the client to move or do something.
2. Use a tuning fork to test for lateralization of sound.
3. Stand in front of the client and whisper, "Raise your hand."
4. Snap your fingers next to the client's ear and ask if the sound was heard.

12. The nurse is caring for a client postoperative thyroidectomy. What would be an important nursing intervention?
1. Have the client speak every 5 to 10 minutes if hoarseness is present.

2. Provide a low-calcium diet to prevent hypercalcemia.
3. Check the dressing at the back of the neck for bleeding.
4. Apply a soft cervical collar to restrict neck movement.

13. A client in sickle cell crisis is admitted to the emergency room (ER). What are the priorities of care?
    1. Nutrition, hydration, electrolyte balance
    2. Hydration, pain management, electrolyte balance
    3. Hydration, oxygenation, pain management
    4. Hydration, oxygenation, electrolyte balance

14. A client with intractable asthma develops Cushing's syndrome. Development of the complication can most likely be attributed to long-term use of which of the following?
    1. Prednisone
    2. Theophylline
    3. Metaproterenol (Alupent)
    4. Cromolyn (Intal)

15. While discussing her diagnosis of hypertension, a client asks the nurse how long she is going to have to take all of the medications that have been prescribed. On what principle is the nurse's response based?
    1. The client will be scheduled for an appointment in 2 months; the doctor will decrease her medications at that time.
    2. As soon as her blood pressure (BP) returns to normal levels, the client will be able to stop taking her medications.

3. To maintain stable control of her BP, the client will have to take the medications indefinitely.
4. The nurse cannot discuss the medications with the client; the client will need to talk with the doctor.

16. An older client is admitted who is experiencing congestive heart failure. What observation by the nurse indicates the client's condition is getting worse?
    1. Arterial blood gases show a significant decrease in the pH and P_{CO_2}.
    2. Blood pressure is 160/98 mm Hg; pulse is 110 beats/min.
    3. Urinary output is 60 ml/hr, and crackles are heard at the base bilaterally.
    4. The client is showing increasing irritability and confusion.

17. A client returns to the unit after surgical creation of a continent (Kock's) ileostomy. What will the care of ileostomy include?
    1. Postoperative irrigations through a drain in the stoma
    2. Irrigating it with normal saline solution after 24 hours
    3. Attaching an ostomy bag with careful checking for watertight seal
    4. Assessing for skin excoriation and increased drainage caused by location of stoma

18. A client is scheduled for paracentesis for ascites. Which statement by the client would indicate to the nurse that the preprocedure teaching has been successful?

1. "I will need to lie flat in bed during the procedure."
2. "I believe this is a surgical procedure."
3. "I need to drink two glasses of water right before the procedure to maintain a full bladder."
4. "The doctor will slowly remove fluid from my abdomen to relieve the swelling."

19. The nurse is administering mannitol (Osmitrol) to a client who had a craniotomy for a pituitary tumor the previous day. What nursing observation would indicate that the medication is having the desire effect?
    1. The serum blood sugar level is within normal range.
    2. There is a significant increase in urinary output.
    3. There has been a weight loss of 3 lb since the previous day.
    4. The neurologic signs indicate reduction in intracranial pressure.

20. The nurse is preparing health teaching for adult women regarding the prevention of osteoporosis. What would be important to include in the teaching plan? Select all that apply.
    1. Daily walking for 15-30 minutes
    2. Supplemental calcium intake
    3. Reduction of caffeine intake
    4. Increased intake of water
    5. Avoiding sunlight because of photosensitivity
    6. Increased intake of fresh fruit and vegetables

21. After a transurethral resection of the prostate (TURP), a client has a three-way urinary catheter with continuous bladder irrigation. The nurse is preparing to hang another container of solution to the bladder irrigation. The nurse would obtain what type of solution?
    1. Isotonic sterile irrigating solution
    2. Distilled, sterile water
    3. Normal saline solution with 2000 units of heparin
    4. Nonsterile saline irrigating fluid

22. What specific directions are given to the client who is taking phenazopyridine (Pyridium)?
    1. The medication may discolor contact lens; if the sclera begin to turn yellow, return to clinic.
    2. Always take the medication on an empty stomach to increase absorption.
    3. Do not take any medication containing aspirin or salicylates.
    4. The medication may interfere with the effectiveness of the mini pill for birth control.

23. The nurse understands that combination oral contraceptive pills prevent pregnancy primarily by which of the following mechanisms?
    1. Decreasing fallopian tube motility
    2. Thinning of cervical mucus
    3. Suppressing ovulation
    4. Causing inflammation of the endometrium

24. The nurse admits a client in active labor. Her assessment reveals 9 cm dilation with complete effacement, +2 station. The woman asks the nurse to give her something for pain. Which of the following would be the best nursing action?

1. Administer a placebo of normal saline solution and tell her it's for pain control.
2. Tell the woman to wait just a little bit longer.
3. Call the anesthesiologist to insert an epidural.
4. Stay with the woman and assist her to breathe with the contractions.

ANSWERS TO NCLEX PRACTICE QUESTIONS

1. **Correct answer**: 4
Rationale: Toddlers enjoy motion toys, such as pull toys, riding toys, and wagons. Because they promote fine motor movement, play activities such as finger paints, interlocking blocks, and large piece puzzles would help these skills. Musical mobiles and rattles are better suited as toys for infants.

2. **Correct answer**: 1
Rationale: It is important for the nurse to recognize that this is an abnormal symptom. A nurse should check the IV for patency in case rapid treatment is needed and should obtain a complete set of vital signs to assess for cardiovascular effects. The nurse should complete the appropriate assessments, given the change in the client's condition. Client alcohol consumption should be determined before the procedure; it might lead the surgery to be cancelled. The client's change in condition should be assessed appropriately, and the nurse should contact the health care provider and provide a condition report after the assessment.

3. **Correct answer**: 2
Rationale: NG tube insertion is included in LPN education and is an appropriate task for an experienced LPN. Client teaching, administration of IV hypnotic medications, and developing the plan of care are more appropriate for registered nurse (RN) practice.

4. **Correct answer**: 4
Rationale: A 70-year-old woman has multiple factors that can predispose her to an adverse reaction, including age and liver disease, and the liver is where most drugs are metabolized. A 20-year-old has no predisposing factors, such as genetics, pathophysiologic dysfunction, or drug allergies, that could identify him as high risk. A 40-year-old with a respiratory tract infection has no predisposing factors that would identify him as high risk. A 5-year-old, although a child, may have an adverse reaction to topical eye medication but is not as likely as an older adult to have such a reaction.

5. **Correct answer**: 3
Rationale: The blood gas indications for respiratory alkalosis are increased pH and decreased P_{CO_2} (Remember the mnemonic "respiratory opposite, metabolic equal" when referring to direction of pH and P_{CO_2}.)

6. **Correct answer**: 4
Rationale: Protease inhibitors have been associated with hyperglycemia, new-onset diabetes, abrupt exacerbation of existing diabetes, and diabetic ketoacidosis. This usually occurs after 2 months of use. Polydipsia, polyuria,

and polyphagia are symptoms attributed to diabetes, rather than to an allergic reaction. These symptoms are not an indication of nonadherence to the antiviral regimen, although nonadherence can be attributed to many factors, including the complexity of the treatment regimen.

7. **Correct answer**: 4
Rationale: Peripheral neuropathy is toxic, has long-term consequences, and is specific to use of vincristine. This is a good example of how a test question asks for a distinction between a toxic effect and a side effect. The other options all occur but are adverse side effects with the majority of chemotherapy drugs.

8. **Correct answer**: 2
Rationale: The child usually has a fairly accurate evaluation of a situation, and the nurse needs to respond to his questions about dying in a way that allows him a chance to express his concerns, which would be by making an open-ended statement.

9. **Correct answer**: 1
Rationale: The client experiencing the auditory hallucination will often look out into space and act as if he is listening to someone talking. This is associated with behaviors such as tilting the head, mumbling, and moving the eyes. There may be times the client actually responds verbally to the auditory hallucination.

10. **Correct answer**: 2
Rationale: The burns are on the anterior trunk and do not involve extremities; hence the problem would be in watching for infection, because the eschar makes it difficult to visually examine the healing skin. Removal of the eschar enhances healing and prevents infection, which occurs because of the moist, enclosed area under the eschar.

11. **Correct answer**: 1
Rationale: Bell's palsy involves a sensorineural hearing loss. The client must be able to hear the direction of sound without any visual prompting. The tuning fork assists in differentiating between air and bone conduction of sound. Standing in front of the client would allow him to read lips, and snapping fingers beside the ear is not a valid assessment tool for hearing.

12. **Correct answer**: 3
Rationale: If bleeding occurs, the blood will drain posteriorly, or behind the client's neck. Serum levels of calcium are important to monitor, because of possible damage to the parathyroids during surgery. Oral intake of calcium is not immediately significant. The client is often hoarse; it is important to monitor for increasing hoarseness that would be indicative of edema. A cervical collar is not indicated.

13. **Correct answer**: 3
Rationale: The priorities for care of a client in sickle cell crises are focused on providing fluid, oxygen, and pain control during the crisis. Electrolyte management is not a priority, nor is nutrition.

14. **Correct answer**: 1
Rationale: Cushing's syndrome results from excessive use of glucocorticoids. This can occur from frequent or long-term use of corticosteroids such as prednisone. Theophylline, metaproterenol, and cromolyn do not cause Cushing's syndrome.

15. **Correct answer**: 3
Rationale: Noncompliance with the blood pressure medication regimen is a common problem in the treatment of hypertension. The client must understand that the only way to keep her blood pressure under control is to continue to take her medications. She is not going to be able to discontinue the medications unless there is a significant change in her condition as a result of weight loss, an exercise program, and/or decreased stress.

16. **Correct answer**: 4
Rationale: Increasing irritation and confusion are early indications of hypoxia. The P_{CO_2} usually goes up, and the blood pressure and pulse are within expected levels. Crackles at the base of the lungs are a common finding in clients with congestive heart failure.

17. **Correct answer**: 1
Rationale: A catheter is placed in the stoma during surgery and is irrigated every 2 to 4 hours postoperatively. The catheter may be left in place for about 4 to 6 days. The client is taught how to catheterize his stoma every 2 to 4 hours to remove any drainage or urine. The potential for fluid and electrolyte imbalance is decreased. The stoma should not leak.

18. **Correct answer**: 4
Rationale: After signing an informed consent form for the procedure, the client will need to sit upright at the side of the bed, with feet propped on a stool, while fluid is removed to relieve acute symptoms of ascites. The fluid is drawn out slowly and checked for amount, color, and characteristics of drainage. Rapid removal can lead to decreased abdominal pressure, which can contribute to shock and vasodilation. A compression bandage will be needed for the puncture site, and the site must be monitored.

19. **Correct answer**: 4
Rationale: Mannitol is an osmotic diuretic and is given to clients who have undergone a craniotomy to decrease or to prevent an increase in cerebral pressure. The improvement in neurologic signs and the reduced intracranial pressure indicate the medication is achieving the desired effects. An increase in urine output and weight loss may occur but is not specific to neurologic implications.

20. **Correct answers**: 1, 2, and 3
Rationale: These are the most common preventive measures in women at increased risk for osteoporosis. Some sunlight is encouraged to facilitate production of vitamin D and absorption of calcium intake. Increased intake of water, fruits, and vegetables is important to prevent the constipation frequently associated with increase in calcium intake, but this relates to *constipation*, not what the question is asking about: preventive measures for *osteoporosis*.

21. **Correct answer**: 1
Rationale: The isotonic sterile irrigating solution is critical to prevent absorption of the irrigation fluid, which could result in fluid overload. Distilled water should never be used for irrigations, and the solution for a continuous bladder irrigation should always be sterile. Heparin would not be used.

22. **Correct answer**: 1
Rationale: The nurse should advise the client that if she notices yellow discoloration of the sclera while taking

phenazopyridine (Pyridium), she should return to the office immediately. This may indicate poor renal excretion and requires follow-up with the physicians. Phenazopyridine should be administered with food, and there is no drug interaction with aspirin or with birth control pills.

23. **Correct answer**: 3

Rationale: The primary mechanism of action of oral contraceptives is suppression of ovulation. Ovulation is suppressed in 95% to 98% of clients. Should ovulation occur, other mechanisms of action are likely to prevent conception; cervical mucus thickens and the endometrium becomes atrophic, making the uterine environment unfavorable for implantation.

24. **Correct answer**: 4

Rationale: The woman is too far along in the labor process to be given any pain medication; it would significantly depress the neonate. The best approach is to stay with her and coach her through breathing and relaxation techniques during the contractions. The delivery of this infant will most likely occur within the next hour.

Glossary

accountable Being responsible and answerable for something.

advanced practice nurse (APN) or advanced practice registered nurse (APRN) A nurse who, by virtue of credentials (usually completion of a master's program and certification), has a wide scope of authority to act (may include treating medical problems and prescribing medications).

air embolism An air bubble that gets into the bloodstream. Can be fatal.

amenities Hospitality services (includes delivering food, meal setup, making beds, cleaning the care environment).

analysis A mental process that aims to get a better understanding of the nature of something by carefully separating the whole into smaller parts. For example, if you want to know more about someone's physical health, you examine each organ and system separately.

anaphylactic shock Extreme hypotension caused by an allergic reaction; requires immediate treatment or can be fatal.

assessment tool A printed or computerized form used to ensure that key information is gathered and recorded during assessment.

assumption Something that's taken for granted without proof. (Compare with *hypothesis* and *inference.*)

attitude A way of acting, feeling, or thinking that shows one's disposition or opinion (e.g., a threatening attitude).

baseline data Information that describes the status of a problem before treatment begins.

benchmark A standard or point used to measure quality.

best practices A term referring to ways certain problems are best prevented and managed from an outcome and cost perspective.

care variance When a patient hasn't achieved activities or outcomes by the time frame noted on a critical path.

caring behavior Behavior that shows understanding and respect for another's perceptions, feelings, needs, and desires.

circumstances The conditions or facts accompanying an event or having some bearing on it.

classify To arrange or group together data according to categories, thereby increasing understanding because relationships become more obvious.

client-centered outcome (1) A statement that describes the benefits the client is expected to experience from nursing care. (2) A statement or phrase that describes what the client or patient is expected to be able to do when the plan of care is terminated. For example, "Will be discharged home able to walk independently using a walker by 8/24."

clinical judgment (1) Nursing opinion(s) made about a person's, family's, or group's health at a certain point in time. (2) Nursing decisions made about things like what to assess, what to do first, and who should do it.

clinical reasoning The process used to make a clinical judgment.

collaborative actions Nursing actions prescribed by a physician or facility protocol (e.g., administering IVs). (Compare with *independent nursing actions.*)

competence Having the necessary knowledge, skill, and attitude to perform an action.

context See *circumstances.*

critical Characterized by careful and exact evaluation; crucial.

critical pathway (clinical pathway) A method of care management of a well-defined group of patients during a well-defined period of time. A clinical pathway explicitly states the goals and key elements of care based on evidence-based practice (EBP) guidelines, best practice, and patient expectations.

critical thinking indicator (CTI) Short description of behavior that demonstrates the knowledge, the characteristics, and the skills that promote critical thinking.

cues Patient data that prompt to you suspect a health problem (e.g., signs and symptoms are cues)

data Pieces of information about health status (e.g., vital signs).

data base form See *assessment tool.*

database assessment Comprehensive data collected upon initial contact with a patient.

deductive reasoning Drawing *specific* conclusions from *general* facts. For example, "If *all* Greeks have beards, and George is a Greek, George must have a beard." (Compare with *inductive reasoning.*)

defining characteristics The signs and symptoms usually associated with a specific problem.

definitive diagnosis The most specific, most correct diagnosis.

definitive interventions The most specific actions required to prevent, resolve, or manage a health problem.

diagnose To identify and name health problems after careful analysis of evidence from an assessment.

diagnostic error When you miss a health problem or identify it incorrectly.

diagnostic reasoning Specific, deliberate use of critical thinking to reach conclusions about health status.

diagnostic statement A phrase that clearly describes a diagnosis; includes the problem name, related (risk) factors, and any evidence confirming the diagnosis.

diaphoretic The condition of being sweaty, usually suspected to be a sign of a health problem (e.g., shock).

disposition A person's usual attitude or tendency toward behaving.

diuretic A drug given to enhance kidney function to improve urine elimination.

efficiency The quality of being able to produce a desired effect safely, with minimal time, risks, expense, and effort.

emboli More than one embolus. (See *embolus.*)

embolus A clot that has moved through one vessel and lodged in another. (Compare with *thrombus.*)

empathy Understanding another's feelings or perceptions but not sharing the same feelings or point of view. (Compare with *sympathy.*)

empiric Relying solely on practical experience, ignoring science.

epidemiology The body of knowledge reflecting what is known about a specific health state.

esthetics An idea of what is pleasing to the senses.

ethics The study of the general nature of morals and of the specific moral choices to be made by individuals in relationships with others.

etiology The cause of or contributing factors to a health problem.

expected outcome See *client-centered outcome.*

expedite To make something happen in a quick way.

explicit Clearly and specifically expressed or described.

evidence-based practice (EBP) See page 123.

focus assessment Data collection that aims to gain specific information about only one aspect of health status.

guidelines Documents that delineate how care is to be provided in specific situations (e.g., procedure manuals, care standards, protocols).

habits of inquiry Habits that enhance the ability to search for the truth (e.g., following rules of logic).

hospitalist A doctor who specializes in the care of hospitalized patients.

human responses Reactions of individuals or groups to health problems or changes in life.

humanistic A way of thought or action concerned with the interests or ideals of people.

hypothesis (1) A hunch. (2) An assertion subject to verification or proof. (Compare with *assumption* and *inference.*)

imply To suggest.

independent nursing actions Nursing actions performed independently, without need for physician's orders or facility protocols (e.g., ensuring adequate oral intake to prevent dehydration). (Compare with *collaborative actions.*)

independent nursing interventions See *independent nursing actions.*

indicator A criterion for evaluating progress toward a goal.

inductive reasoning Drawing general conclusions by observing a few *specific* members of a class. For example, "If every Greek you ever see has a beard, you may conclude that all Greeks have beards." (Compare with *deductive reasoning.*)

infer To suspect something or to attach meaning to information. For example, if someone is frowning, we may infer that he or she is worried.

inference Something we suspect to be true, based on a logical conclusion after examination of the evidence. (Compare with *assumption* and *hypothesis.*)

informatics The study of the application of computer and statistical techniques to the management of information.

intervention Something done to prevent, cure, or control a health problem (e.g., turning someone every 2 hours is an intervention to prevent skin breakdown).

intubation The process of inserting a tube into an individual's bronchus to facilitate breathing.

intuition Knowing something without evidence.

irrigate To flush something with normal saline solution or water.

life processes Events or changes that occur during one's lifetime (e.g., growing up, getting married, losing someone).

logic A system of reasoning that leads to valid conclusions.

malpractice When a patient is harmed by professional conduct (e.g., by something a professional did or omitted doing).

measurable Capable of being clearly observed so that the quality or quantity of something can be determined.

medical domain Actions a physician is legally qualified to perform.

mentor A knowledgeable, insightful, and trusted person who helps someone grow personally and professionally.

myocardial infarction Partial or complete occlusion of one or more of the coronary arteries, causing death of coronary tissue.

nasogastric tube A tube inserted through the nose, down the esophagus, and into the stomach.

negligence Failure to provide the degree of care that someone of ordinary prudence would provide under the same circumstances. To claim negligence, it is necessary that there be a duty owed by one person to another, that the duty be breached, and that the breach cause harm.

nursing action Something done by a nurse to achieve an outcome.

nursing intervention See *nursing action.*

nursing domain Actions a nurse is legally qualified to perform.

nursing process The professional, systematic approach to ensuring complete care. The process includes assessment diagnosis, outcome identification, planning, implementation, and evaluation.

objective data Information that you can clearly observe or measure (e.g., a pulse of 140 beats per minute).

outcome The expected result of interventions.

paradigm (pa'-ra-dim) A model or way of doing things.

patent Open, so as to allow the flow of fluid or air.

phenomena Issues, concerns, or experiences (e.g., pain is a phenomena that nurses are responsible for managing).

policies See *guidelines.*

potential diagnosis A health problem that may occur because of certain risk factors present (e.g., someone who's on prolonged bed rest has a potential [or risk] for impaired skin integrity).

potential problem See *potential diagnosis.*

preceptor An experienced, more qualified nurse assigned by a facility to facilitate learning for a less experienced nurse.

proactive (comes from *act before***)** A way of thinking and behaving that accepts responsibility for one's actions and takes initiative to plan ahead to anticipate and prevent problems before they happen.

procedures See *guidelines.*

protocols See *guidelines.*

pulmonary embolus A clot that has blocked off circulation and oxygenation to lung tissue. Considered to be life-threatening.

QA *See quality assessment.*

QI *See quality improvement.*

qualified Having the competence and authority to perform an action.

quality The degree to which patient care services increase the probability of achieving *desired* outcomes with the decreased probability of *undesired* outcomes.

quality assessment (QA) Ongoing studies designed to evaluate quality of patient care and services. Just as assessment is the first step of the nursing process, QA is the first step of QI (quality improvement).

quality improvement (QI) Ongoing studies designed to identify ways to promote achievement of desired outcomes in a timely, cost-effective fashion while decreasing the risks for undesired outcomes.

rales Abnormal breath sounds (crackles) caused by the passage of air through bronchi containing fluid.

related factor See *risk factor.*

response A reaction.

risk factor Something known to contribute to (or be associated with) a specific problem. (See also *etiology.*)

signs Objective data that cause you to suspect a health problem.

somnolent Overly sleepy; difficult to arouse.

standards of care See *guidelines.*

standard of nursing care The degree of skill, care, and diligence exercised by members of the nursing profession practicing in similar situations and settings.

subjective data Information the patient states or communicates; the patient's perceptions (e.g., "My heart feels like it's racing")

supervision The active process of directing, guiding, and influencing the outcome of someone's performance of a task.

sympathy Sharing the same feelings as another. (Compare with *empathy.*)

symptoms Subjective data that cause you to suspect a health problem.

synthesis The process of putting pieces of information together to make a whole. For example, nurses put signs and symptoms together to make a diagnosis.

thrombi More than one thrombus. (See *thrombus.*)

thrombus A clot that threatens blood supply to tissues. If the clot moves, it becomes an embolus.

tubal ligation Surgery performed to sterilize a woman by cutting and suturing her fallopian tubes.

UAP (unlicensed assistive personnel) Workers who are trained to function in an assistive role to registered nurses. The term includes, but is not limited to, nurses' aides, medication aides, orderlies, and attendants or technicians.

validation The process of gathering more data to determine whether the information or data you've already collected are factual or true.

validity The extent to which something can be believed to be factual and true.

variance in care See *care variance.*

wellness diagnosis A clinical judgment about an individual, family, or community in transition from a specific level of wellness to a higher level of wellness.

Index

A

AACN. *See* American Association of Critical Care Nurses
Abnormal function, CTIs for, 48
Accommodators, conflict and, 217b
Accountability, 120
　nursing diagnosis, 93
Accuracy, checking, 159-160
ACE Star Model of Knowledge Transformation, 124-125, 124f, 144
Acrostic, 136-137
Activity diary, time management, 221-222
Admission tool, 272-275
Advance directives, 121, 122b
Advanced practice nurses (APNs), 89
Advise, criticism *v.*, 215
Age/maturity, critical thinking, 36
Agency for Healthcare Research and Quality (AHRQ), website, 131
Aggressive behavior, assertive behavior *v.*, 214b
AHRQ. *See* Agency for Healthcare Research and Quality
Allergies, problem diagnoses, 177
Ambiguity, 179
American Association of Critical Care Nurses (AACN), 98
American Nurses Association (ANA), 66
　Code of Ethics, 120-121
　nursing diagnosis, 92
　standards, 22
　standards for practice, 100, 144, 277-278
ANA. *See* American Nurses Association
Analysis. *See* Failure mode effect analysis; Root cause analysis; Systemic problem analysis worksheet
Analyzing data, 12-13
　data collecting *v.*, 88
Anger, 200
　change and, 200
　complaints and, 207
Anger management, potential, 174
Anxiety, 37-38
APNs. *See* Advanced practice nurses
Assertive behavior, aggressive behavior *v.*, 214b
Assess, 52
Assessment, 83
　charting and, 105
　systematical/comprehensive, 155-156
　　practice exercises, 158-159
Association of Rehabilitation Nurses (ARN), 98

B

Assumptions
　avoiding, 153
　critically ill, 110
　identifying, 57, 152-155
Attitudes, critical thinking and, 10b
Authority, information and, 239-240
Autonomy, 120
Avoiders, conflict and, 217b

Baseline data, 152
Bedside, dynamic thinking, scenario, 84
Behavior(s). *See also specific i.e. assertive behavior*
　health and, 75
　over time, 52
　PPMP and, 75
Beneficence, 120
Benner, P., novices *v.* experts, 71b
Biases, 39
　critical thinking, 36
Bibliography, writing skills, 244
Birth order, thinking style and, 29-31
Body systems assessment, 104f, 156
　data and, 112
Brain, 108
　"boot camps" for, 20
　clinical judgement and, 86
　exercises, 20
　injuries, 20
　parts, thinking and, 17
"Brain drain," technology and, 104
Brain-based learning, 3-5
Brainstorming, writing skills, 247

C

Canadian Nurse Registered Examination (CNRE), 2
Care management, standards for practice, 100
Care plan, 89
　components, 89b
Care practices, questioning, 129-130
Caring, 105
　compassion and, 64
Causative factor, 151
CBE. *See* Charting by exception
Certification tests, 82. *See also* Canadian Nurse Registered Examination; National State Board Examinations; NCLEX
　critical thinking and, 2

Page numbers followed by *f, t,* and *b* indicate figures, tables, and boxes, respectively.

Chain of command
   activating, 99-105
   malpractice suits and, 183
Change
   associated stages, 200-201
   critical thinking exercises, 202-203
   navigating, 200-201
   in others, facilitating, 201
   resistance to, 39
   thinking critically, 200
   ways to, 202b
   workplace skills and, 199
Character, developing, 51
Charting, 112
   critical thinking and, 105-107
Charting by exception (CBE), 224
Charts, errors and, 231
Checklists
   errors and, 230
   writing skills, 245
Choices, 39
Chronic diseases, 76
Circumstances. *See* Context
Citations, document information, 240
Client-centered outcomes (Patient-centered outcomes)
   clinical judgment, 185
   determining, 184-187
      guidelines, 185-187
   expected, 187
   guidelines, 185-187
   practice exercises, 187
   rule, 186
Clinical decision-making, 90f
   algorithm, 97
Clinical function, 111
Clinical judgment (Clinical reasoning), 64, 110, 112
   brain and, 86
   critical thinking, 15, 15f, 64-65
      research, 67b
   developing, 101
   "getting most" from, 151
   separate skills, 150
   skills, 99
      practicing, 148-197
Clinical outcome, quality of care and, 79-80
Clinical practice, indicators in, 10
Clinical practice guidelines (CPGs), EBP and, 126b
Clinical reasoning. *See* Clinical judgment
Clinical setting
   delegation principles, 182b
   questions in, 102b
   streamlining work in, 223-224
Clinical summaries, to EBP, 124
Clinical thinking exercises, empowered partnerships, 211-212

Clustering related cues skills, 163-165
   clinical judgment and, 164
   information and, relevant *v.* irrelevant, 165
CNRE. *See* Canadian Nurse Registered Examination
Code of conduct, 27
Code of Ethics, ANA, 120-121
Collaborative problem solvers, conflict and, 217b
Collaborative thinking, 14
Commission, mistakes and, 226
Common sense, 7-8
Communicating bad news, 203-206
   customer service issues, 206b
   health status, 204-205b
Communication
   bad news, 203-206
   Chain of Command, 99-105
   effective, 66
   strategies, critical thinking, 34-35b
   teamwork skills, 234
   writing and, 243-244
Competence, caring *v.*, 64
Complaints, dealing with, 206-208
   constructive thinking, 207-208
Complications
   medical diagnoses, 96b
   technology, 75
   treatments/invasive procedures, 97b
Comprehensive assessment tools, 102
Comprehensive plan. *See* Plans of care
Compromisers, conflict and, 217b
Computerized decision-support tools, 88
Computers, 111. *See also* Internet resources
   decision making and, rule, 88
   document information, 241
   NCLEX, 141
Concept mapping. *See* Mind mapping
Conclusions
   charting and, 105
   drawing, 13
Confidence, 2
Confidentiality, 120
Conflict management, 216-221
   constructive, 216-217, 218b, 219
   style, 217b
Conflict outcomes, 217
Conformity, 39
Consideration, nurses and, 2
Constructive criticism, 212-216
   giving, 213, 214b
   taking, 214-215
Context (Circumstances), 110
   attention to, 70-71
   critical thinking strategies, 44
Control, 5
"Courses of Action," 122
Covey, S, 40

CPGs. *See* Clinical practice guidelines
Creativity, 86
Critical moments
  mistakes, 228
  time management, 224
Critical pathways, 109, 268-271
Critical thinkers, characteristics, 8-9, 11b
Critical thinking, 9-14, 12b, 15, 15f, 112
  age/maturity, 36
  applied definition, 6, 7b
  attitudes and, 10b
  bad news, 203
  barriers, 38-40
  care and, 1-23
  charting, 105-107
  clinical judgement and, 15, 64-65
    research, 67b
  common sense v., 8
  communication strategies, 34-35b
  complaints, 207
  conflict management, 216
  constructive criticism, 212
  descriptions, 6, 7b
  empowered partnerships, 209-210
  EQ, 36, 36b
  factors influencing, 34, 36-38
  familiar, 9-14
  focusing on, 2-3
  habits and, 38-40
  how to, 24-60
  improving, advances in, 14b
  information, accessing and using, 238
  learning outcome, 1, 25
  learning questions, 117
  mistakes, preventing/dealing with, 226-228
  nurses, 64-65, 66f
  nursing research, 125-129
  outcome-focused writing, 243
  strategies, 43-48
  summary/key points, 22
  teamwork skills, 234
  thinking v., 5
Critical thinking exercises, 18-19, 41, 55-57, 81,
    106-107, 131-133
  change and, 202-203
  complaints, 208
  conflict and, 220
  errors and, 231-232
  instructions, 18-20
  teaching, 143
  time management, 225
  writing skills, 247
Critical thinking indicators (CTIs), 9, 22, 25, 40, 53, 110
  4-circle CT model, 68
  behaviors, 10b

Critical thinking indicators (CTIs) *(Continued)*
  intellectual skills, 48-51, 50b
  knowledge, 48-51, 49b
  perspectives, 55-56
Critical thinking potential, questions evaluating, 18
Critical thinking skills, studies of, 51b
Critical thinking strategies, context (Circumstances), 44
Critically ill, assumptions and, 110
Criticism, critical thinking exercises, 215
Cross-cultural understanding, teamwork skills, 237
CTIs. *See* Critical thinking indicators
Cues, 151. *See also* Data
Culture
  assumptions and, 153
  thinking style and, 29-31
Customer service issues, communicating
    bad news, 206b

D

Data, 151
  body systems assessment, 112
  classifying, 13
  key, document information, 241
Data collecting, analyzing data v., 88
Database assessment, 152
Dates, document information, 240
DEAD ON!! game, 267
Decision making, 13, 37, 119-120, 122
  computers and, rule, 88
  interventions, 188
  nursing standards/guidelines, 100
Decision trees, 46
Defining characteristics, 152
Definitive diagnosis, 151
Delegation principles, 101, 112
  in clinical setting, 182b
Denial, change and, 200
Depression, 200
Diabetes, 76
Diagnose and treat approach (DT approach),
    PPMP v., 74-76
Diagnoses, 109. *See also* Medical diagnoses; Nursing
    diagnosis; specific i.e. definitive diagnosis
  failure to, 228
  health problems, 95
  invasive procedures, 174
  legal implications, 92, 112
  nursing process, 89-99
Diagnosis/outcome identification, 83b
Diagnostic statement, problem diagnoses, 177
Diagrams, 46
  problem diagnoses, actual/potential, 174f
Direct patient assessment, 102
Direct-care interventions, 190
Discovery, 125

Disease management, 111
 PPMP and, 76-77
Distractions, critical thinking and, 38
Document body, writing skills, 244
Document information
 inform *v.* persuade, 240
 key data, 241
Documentation
 nursing instructor and, 102
 tools, 112
DT approach. *See* Diagnose and treat approach
Dynamic thinking
 at bedside, scenario, 84
 nursing process, rule, 85

E

EBP. *See* Evidence-based practice
Editing, writing skills, 247
Educated guesses, test-taking and, 140b
"80/20 rule," priorities and, 183
Einstein, A., 21
Elderly, 110
Emotional intelligence (EQ), critical thinking,
 36, 36b
Emotions, naming, 54
Empowered partnership model, parental partnership
 model *v.*, 209t
Empowered partnerships, 73-74, 74b
 clinical thinking exercises, 211-212
 developing, 209-212
 "how to," 210-211
 examples, 210
Empowerment, teamwork skills, 237
End-of-life issues, 132
Energy management, time management, 224
EQ. *See* Emotional intelligence
Error(s)
 critical thinking exercises, 231-232
 prevention, new thinking, 13
 seriousness of, rule, 230
Ethical codes, 120-121, 144
Ethical principles, 120
Ethical reasoning, 118-123
 exercises, 131-133
 moral reasoning *v.*, 119-120
 principles, 144
 steps for, 122-123
Ethics, 123
 perspectives, 119
Evaluate, 52
Evaluation, 84b, 125
 early, 37
 plan of action, 194-197
 writing skills, 246-247
Evaluative styles, 38

Evidence
 identifying assumptions, 152
 individualized interventions, 190
Evidence summary, 125
Evidence-based care, 77-82, 79
 creativity and, 86
 evolving, 82
Evidence-based communication, 66
Evidence-based practice (EBP), 123-129
 clinical practice guidelines in, 126b, 128
 exercises, 133
 nursing research, critical thinking and, 125-129
 websites, 126b
Evidence-based thinking, 14
Execution, mistakes and, 226
Exercise, PPMP and, 77b
Expected outcome, plan of care and, 196-197
Experience, 17
 clinical reasoning, 150
 past, 37
 thinking-in-action, 16
Expert thinking
 novice thinking *v.*, 69-70, 72t
Experts, 71b, 111
 errors and, 231
 novices *v.*, 107
 organization for, 5

F

Face-saving, 39
Facione and Facione's Critical Thinking
 Dispositions, 11b
Facts, relationships in, 136
Failure mode effect analysis (FMEA), 228
Familiar, new *v.*, critical thinking and, 9-14
Families
 decisions and, 2
 empowering, nurses and, 73-74, 74b
Fatigue, 37-38
Female thinking, male thinking *v.*, 31-32
Fidelity, 120
Flaws, critical thinking, 47
FMEA. *See* Failure mode effect analysis
Focusing
 on details, big picture *v.*, 46
 outcomes and, 55
Forcers, conflict and, 217b
4-circle CT model, 15-16, 22, 51, 59, 110
 CTIs and, 68
Frontal lobe, 17
Function
 behaviors and, 75
 individualized interventions, 190
Functional outcome, quality of care and, 79-80

G

Goals
  nursing outcomes and, 68-69
  outcome-focused thinking and, 42
  writing skills, 243-245
Golden rule, Platinum rule *v.*, 41
Gordon's Functional Health Patterns,
    103, 103b, 112
Group leaders, change and, 201
Guidelines. *See also* Clinical practice guidelines;
    Decision making
  client-centered outcomes, 185-187
  EBP, 126b, 128
  inconsistencies, 167-168
  individualized interventions, 188-190
  information and, 165-166
  missing information identification skills,
    170-171
  patient data, 161
  plans of care, 194-195
  problem diagnoses, 175
  risk factors, 171-172
  setting priorities, 180
  writing skills, 244-245

H

Habits, critical thinking, 38-40
Habits of inquiry, 48
Hazardous condition, 227
Health, behaviors and, 75
Health care
  changes in, thinking and, 71-82
  environment, 121
Health care decisions, patients and families, nurses
    and, 73-74, 74b
Health Insurance Portability and Accountability
    privacy laws (HIPAA privacy laws), 104
Health problems, diagnoses rule, 95
Health status
  assessment, 156
  communicating bad news, 204-205b
Healthy People 2000, 75
HIPAA privacy laws. *See* Health Insurance Portability
    and Accountability privacy laws
HON Code of Conduct (HONcode),
    240
HONcode. *See* HON Code of Conduct
Human potential, maximizing strategies, 13
Human resources
  information, 239
  learning from, 103
Humor, 3
Hypothalamus, 17
Hypotheses, testing, 13

I

Identification patterns. *See* Pattern identification skills
Impaired skin integrity, accountability and, 93
Implementation, 83-84b
Inconsistencies, recognizing, 167-168
  guidelines, 167-168
  practice exercises, 168
Independence
  accountability and, 93
  behaviors and, 75
  teaching, 134-135
Independent learning skills, 144
Indirect-care interventions, 190
Individualized interventions, 188-192, 189b
  clinical judgment, 188
  guidelines, 188-190
  practice exercises, 191
  rule, 189, 190
Infection, 94
Inference, 152
  clinical judgment and, 162-163
Inform, persuade *v.*, 240
Information
  accessing and using, 238-242
    how to, 238-241
  critical thinking, 48
  to knowledge, 241
  organizing/reorganizing, 137
  relevant *v.* irrelevant, 165-167
    guidelines in, 165-166
    practice exercises, 166-167
  revisiting, 48
Information management skills, 240
Information processing skills, 240
Insight, gaining, 26-32
Institute of medicine (IOM), 111
  competencies, 71-73
  Quality of care, 72-73
Instruments, CTIs and, 53
Integration, 125
Intensive care unit, blog, 91
Interaction errors, 229
Internet resources
  information, 238
  NCLEX, 141
Interpersonal skills, 14
Interventions, 103
  charting and, 105
  client-centered outcomes, expected, 186
  errors and, 231
  specific, 188-190
Introduction, writing skills, 244
Intuition, 45
  logic *v.*, 85-86, 107-108

Intuitive thinking, 111
  rule, 86
Invasive procedures
  complications, 97b
  diagnosis and, 174
IOM. *See* Institute of medicine

J

Job satisfaction, 2
Judgemental styles, 38
Justice, 120

K

Key data, document information, 241
Kidney disease, 76
Knowledge
  critical thinking strategies, 44
  CTIs for, 48-51, 49b
  to EBP, 124
  inconsistencies and, 168
Knowledge errors, 229
Knowledge, previous, thinking-in-action, 16
Knowledge-based communication, 66

L

Leaders. *See* Group leaders; Leadership
Leadership, 108
Learners, 108
Learning, strategies for, 136-137
Learning environments, 4b
Learning errors, 229-230
Learning outcome(s)
  change, workplace skills and, 199
  clinical judgment skills, 149
  communicating bad news, 203
  complaints, dealing with, 206-207
  conflict management, 216
  constructive criticism, 212
  critical thinking, 1, 25
  information, accessing and using, 238
  nursing, critical thinking judgment, 62-115
  outcome-focused writing, 243
  teamwork skills, 234
  time management, 221
Learning preferences, strategies for, 58b
Learning questions, critical thinking, beyond
  judgment, 117
Learning rule, 28
Learning skills, 37
Learning style inventories, 28
Learning style questionnaire, 28
Learning styles, 13
  connecting with, 26, 28
  preferred, 137
Library, information, 238

Limbic system, 17
Logic, 45
  intuition *v.*, 85-86, 107-108
Logic-sound reasoning, 59

M

M & M (Medical or Medication problems), signs and
  symptoms, 163
Male thinking, female thinking *v.*, 31-32
Malpractice suits, chain of command and, 183
Mapping critical thinking, 65-67
Maps, 46
  document information, 241
  problem diagnoses, 177
    actual/potential, 174f
Maslow's human needs, setting priorities
  and, 182b
Medical diagnoses, potential complications, 96b
Medical or Medication problems. *See* M & M
Medical-surgical nursing, nursing diagnosis
  and, 95b
Medication errors, 227
  reasons, 228b
Medication regimens, accountability and, 93
  rule, 94
Medications, problem diagnoses, 177
Memorizing, 144
  strategies, 136-137
Memory hook, 136
Mental images, memory and, 134
Mental slips, 229
"Mentee," 33
Mentoring, partnerships and, 33
Mentors, 108
"Mind games," 20
Mind mapping (Concept mapping), 13, 18, 46,
  263-265, 264f
Missing information identification skills, 170-171
  guidelines, 170-171
  practice exercises, 171
Mistake(s), 226-227
  critical thinking exercises, 231-232
  opportunities *v.*, 48
  preventing/dealing with, 226-233
    constructive, 229-231
Mnemonics, 136
Monitoring. *See also* Patient monitoring
  failure to, 228
  individualized interventions, 189
Moral dilemma, 120
Moral distress, 120
Moral reasoning, 118-123
  ethical reasoning *v.*, 119-120
  exercises, 131-133
Moral uncertainty, 120

Motivating factors, 38
Motivation, 54
Mouth care, research, 125
Myers-Briggs indicator, thinking style, 29b

N

National Council Licensure Examination.
    See NCLEX
National Practice Safety Goals (NPGS), 97
National State Board Examinations, 54
NCLEX (National Council Licensure Examination),
    54, 82, 112
  critical thinking and, 2
  preparation strategies, 142
  test-taking strategies, 141-142
Near miss, 227
Negative feedback, 214
Negative "talk," 38
Negotiation, "how to," 219b
Neurologic focus assessment guide, 157b
New, familiar *v.*
  critical thinking and, 9-14
Normal function, CTIs for, 48
Note taking, document information, 240
Novice, 71b
  experts *v.*, 107
  organization for, 5
Novice thinking, expert thinking *v.*, 69-70, 72t
NPGS. *See* National Practice Safety Goals
Nurses
  consideration and, 2
  critical thinking in, 64-65, 66f
  families, 73-74, 74b
  patients and, learning needs, 94
Nursing diagnosis, 92
  accountability for, 93
  definitions, 112
  medical-surgical nursing, 95b
Nursing classification labels, 276
Nursing interventions, writing, individualized
    interventions, 190
Nursing outcomes. *See* Outcomes
Nursing practice
  critical thinking
    beyond judgment, 116-147
    judgment and, 62-115
  decisions, scope of, 100
  exercises
    assumptions and, 153-155
    clustering related cues skills, 164-165
    individualized interventions, 191
    missing information identification skills, 171
    patient data, normal *v.* abnormal, 161-162
    pattern identification skills, 170
    plan of care, 196

Nursing practice *(Continued)*
    risk factor identification and management
        skills, 173
    risk problems, 179
    setting priorities, 183-184
    systematical/comprehensive assessment,
        158-159
  improvement, nurses and, 67-68
  major outcomes, 69
    implications of, 69
  performance, nurses and, 67-68
  responsibilities, 89-92
  roles, health problem management, 94
  standards, 144
    principles, 144
Nursing process, 13, 37, 111, 193-194b
  changing, 82-89
  clinical judgment, 15, 15f
  dynamic thinking, 84, 85
    rule, 85
  outcome-focused, 84
  proactive, 84
  roles in, diagnosis and management, 89-99
  summary, 83-84b
Nursing research, EBP and, critical thinking and,
    125-129
Nursing term standardization, organizations for, 98b

O

Objective data, 151
Observing, 13
Occipital lobe, 17
Omfer, 152
Omission, mistakes and, 226
Opportunities, mistakes *v.*, 48
Organizations
  nursing term standardization and, 98b
  values, 118
Outcome evaluations, QI and, 130
Outcome measurement, 14. *See also* Clinical
    outcome
Outcome-focused care, 77-82
Outcome-focused thinking, 42-43
  problem-focused thinking *v.*, 7
  rule, 80
Outcome-focused writing, 243-248
Outcomes, 52, 110. *See also* Client-centered outcomes
  clarifying, rules for, 42
  classification labels, 276
  critical thinking strategies, 43
  focusing, 55
  learner and, 134
  outcome-focused thinking and, 42
  problems and, dynamic relationship of, 80-81
  writing skills, 243-245

P

Parental partnership model, empowered partnership model *v.*, 209t
Parietal lobe, 17
Partnerships. *See also* Empowered partnerships
  mentoring, 33
Patient(s)
  decisions and, 2
  empowering, nurses and, 73-74, 74b
  nurses, learning needs, 94
  restraining, 126-127
Patient bill of rights, 144
Patient care decisions, charting, 105
Patient chart, plan of care and, 196-197
Patient data
  guidelines, 161
  normal *v.* abnormal
    guidelines, 161
    practice exercises, 161-162
Patient harm, Chain of Command, 99
Patient monitoring
  problems, 174
  technology, 75
Patient outcomes, 2
Patient-centered outcomes. *See* Client-centered outcomes
Patients rights, 120-121, 266
Pattern identification skills, 169-170
  practice exercises, 170
Paul and Elder's Intellectual Traits, 11b
PDA. *See* Personal digital assistant
Peer review, 53
Personal digital assistant (PDA)
  document information, 241
  time management, 224
Personal feedback, monitoring, 214
Personal role, decision making and, 122
Personal thinking style, 59
Personal values, 118
  decision making and, 122
Personality
  thinking and, 28
  types
    colors for, 30
    sensitivity to, 29b
Perspectives
  change and, 201
  complaints and, 208
  conflict and, 219
  constructive criticism, 213
  critical thinking, 106-108
    strategies, 44-45
  criticism, 215
  CTIs, 55-56
  empowered partnerships, 211

Perspectives *(Continued)*
  errors and, 231-232
  ethics, 119, 123
  moral/ethical reasoning, 131
  nursing, critical thinking judgment, 62-115
  teaching, 143
  teamwork skills, 237
  time management, 224
PET scans. *See* Positron Emission Tomography scans
Physicians treatment plan, accountability and, 93
Plan of action
  determining and evaluating, 194-197
    clinical judgment, 194
  monitoring, 123
Planning, 83b
Plans of care
  guidelines for, updating, 194-195
  individualized, 111-112
  practice exercises, 196
  recorded, purpose and components, 195b
  rule, 195
"Platinum rule"
  Golden rule *v.*, 41
  teamwork skills, 234
Pneumonia, accountability and, 93
Pocket reference, document information, 241
Policies and procedures, errors and, 230
Positive reinforcement, 37-38
Positron Emission Tomography (PET) scans, 20
Potential problem. *See* Risk problems
PPMP. *See* Predict, prevent, manage, and promote
Practice. *See* Nursing practice
Predict, prevent, manage, and promote (PPMP), 76-77
  DT approach *v.*, 74-76
  elephant and, 76
  individualized interventions, 190
  requirements of, 75
Predictive model, PPMP as, 74
Prejudices, critical thinking, 36
Prevention, treatment and, 74
Principle-centered creativity, 111
Privacy laws, 108
Problem diagnoses. *See also* Risk problems; Systemic problem analysis worksheet
  actual/potential, 173-179
    clinical judgment, 173-174
    diagrams and maps, 174f
    guidelines, 175
    identification checklist, 176b
Problem-focused thinking, outcome-focused thinking *v.*, 7
Problems
  client-centered outcomes, expected, 186
  expected outcome, 191-192
  identifying, 175, 176b, 177

Problems (*Continued*)
  outcomes and, dynamic relationship of, 80-81
  predicting, 174
  setting priorities, 180-184, 181b
  solving, 7
Problem-solving skills, 12, 37, 45, 110
  complaints and, 208
  critical thinking and, 12
  reasoning in, 150
Process
  evaluation, QI and, 130
  outcomes and, 52
Professional organizations, 121
Proofreading, writing skills, 247
Protective factor outcomes, 80

Q

QI. *See* Quality improvement
Quality improvement (QI), 144
  surveillance, 130-133
Quality of care
  clinical outcome and, 79-80
  IOM and, 72-73
Quality of life outcomes, 94
  symptom severity, 79
Questions, 20
  in clinical setting, 102b
  critical thinking, beyond judgment, 117
  critical thinking potential, 18
  critical thinking strategies, 43-45
  document information, 241
  identifying assumptions, 152
  staff nurses, 127-129
  teaching, 135
  test, components of, 139b

R

RCA. *See* Root cause analysis
Reading skills, 37
Reasoning, 6, 15, 15f
  nursing and, 118
  related factors and, 37-38
Recognized terminology, standard terminology
    v., 97-98
References, writing skills, 244-245, 246
Reflective thinking. *See* Thinking back
Registered nurse (RN) staffing, inadequate, 125
Related factor, 151
Relationships, 59
  trust in, 32-33
Reliability (Validating data), checking, 159-160
Research. *See also* Nursing research
  critical thinking, clinical judgment and, 67b
  EBP *v.*, 123-124
Research articles, scanning, 129

Resource(s)
  awareness, 37-38
  critical thinking strategies, 44
Restraining patients, 126-127
Revising, writing skills, 247
Risk awareness, 37-38
Risk factor(s)
  identification and management skills
    clinical judgment and, 171
    guidelines, 171-172
    practice exercises, 173
    promoting health by, 171-173
  individualized interventions, 189
  problem diagnoses, 176
  systemic problem analysis worksheet, 178b
Risk management, 76-77, 110
  strategies, 172
Risk problems
  practice exercises, 179
  predicting, 177
Risk reduction outcomes, 79-80
RN. *See* Registered nurse
Root cause analysis (RCA), 227-228
Rule violation, mistakes and, 226

S

Safety, 4b, 94
  empowered partnerships, 73-74, 74b
Satisfaction outcomes, 80
Scanning, research articles, 129
Scenario, critical thinking, 81
Schedule organization skill, 223
Scheffer and Rubenfeld's Habits of Mind, 11b
Scientific method, 13
Search engines, 238, 239b
Self awareness, 59
  gaining, 26-32
Self-assessment, 53
Self-confidence, critical thinking, 36
Self-deception, 40
Self-discipline, 137
Self-focusing, 39
Self-quizzing, 137
Self-regulating skills, 192-194
Sentinel event, 227
Setting priorities, 180-184
  guidelines, 180
  Maslow's human needs, 182b
  practice exercises, 183-184
  principles, 181b
  rule, 180
Signs and symptoms, 151
  identifying, 161
  problems and, 175, 176b
Simulated learning experiences, 47, 59

"Sixth sense," 107
Skills, 51. *See also teamwork skills;* specific i.e. writing skills
  critical thinking strategies, 44
Special needs, reporting, complaints and, 208
Staff nurses, role of, questions, 127-129
Stakeholders, 122, 123
  change and, 201
Standard terminology, recognized terminology *v.*, 97-98
Standard tools, 111
  thinking and, 87-89
Standards, 120-121
Standards-based communication, 66
Stereotyping, 40
Stewardship, 111
Strategies
  communication, critical thinking, 34-35b
  critical thinking, 43-48
    context, 44
    knowledge, 44
    questions, 43-45
    resources, 44
    skills, 44
  human potential, 13
  learning, 136-137
  learning preferences, 58b
  memorizing, 136-137
  Perspectives, critical thinking, 44-45
  risk management, 172
  stress management, 200
  team building, 235-236, 236b
  test-taking
    NCLEX, 141-142
    preparing for, 137
  "What-if," 13-14
Stress, 37-38
Stress management strategies, 200
Structure evaluation, QI and, 130-131
Structured tools
  rule for, 88
  thinking and, 87
Sttrategies, critical thinking, outcomes, 43
Studies. *See* Research
Subjective data, 151
  assessment and, 156
Summary
  teaching and, 134
  writing skills, 244
Support, anxiety and, 134
Surveillance
  error prevention and, 227
  QI and, 130-133
Symptom severity, quality of life outcomes and, 79
System errors, 230
Systemic problem analysis worksheet, 178b

T
Task-oriented thinking, 109
Teaching
  others, steps for, 134-135
  yourself, 135-137
Team
  group to, 233-238
  group transformation, 234-236
Team building
  stages of, 236b, 237
  strategies, 235-236, 236b
Team members, 235-236
Teamwork skills, 233-238
Technology
  "Brain drain," 104
  errors and accuracy, 75
  relying on, errors and, 230
Temporal lobe, 17
Terminology. *See* Recognized terminology; Standard
  terminology
Test(s)
  CTIs and, 53
  questions, components of, 139b
  standard, 54
Test-taking
  actual, 138, 139
  after, 140
  preparing for, 138
  skills, 54
  strategies, 137-143
    preparing for, 137
Thalamus, 17
Therapeutic alliance outcomes, 80
Therapeutic effect, accountability and, 94
Thinking, 28. *See also* Critical thinking
  assessing and evaluating, 52-58
  brain parts involved, 17
  charting and, 105
  critical thinking *v.*, 5
  evaluating, principles of, 52
  health care, changes in, 71-82
  improving, 3-5
    steps, 59
  influencing factors, 45
  other persons, evaluating, 53
  situational factors, 37-38
  standard tools for, 87-89
  trends influencing, 78-79b
Thinking ahead, 16
Thinking back (Reflective thinking), 16
Thinking style, 41
  Myers-Briggs indicator, 29b
  personality, 28
  upbringing, 29-31

Thinking-in-action, 16
Time limitations, motivation and, 38
Time lines, change and, 201
Time management, 221-225
    activities in, 221-222
    critical thinking, 221
    nursing care and, 105
    priorities, 222-223
Transforming, conforming *v.*, change and, 201
Translation, 125
Treatments, 174
    accountability and, 93
    complications, 97b
Trends, thinking and, 78-79b
Trial and error, 45, 46, 59
Trust, 59
    relationships and, 32-33
    rule, 33
    teamwork skills, 234
Truth telling. *See* Veracity
Tunnel vision, 39

U
"Umbrella term," critical thinking as, 22
    map of, 65
Upbringing, thinking style and, 29-31
"Use it or loose it" rule, 136
Use of Services outcomes, 80

V
Valid conclusions. *See* Inference
Values, clarifying, 118-119
Veracity (Truth telling), 120

Violence, potential, 174
Vital signs, assessment, 156
Vocabulary, nursing, required, 151-152b
Voice-activated software, writing skills, 246

W
Websites
    AHRQ, 131
    document information, 240
    EBP, 126b
    information, 238, 239, 239b
Well-being, 94
    behaviors and, 75
    individualized interventions, 190
"What-if" strategies, 13-14
Work organization skill, 223
Workplace skills, 2, 3b
    mastering, 198-248
    prechapter self-test, 199
Workplaces, healthy, 4b
Writers block, writing skills, 246
Writing. *See also* Outcome-focused writing
    before, 243-245
        goals and outcomes, 243-245
        type, purpose and, 244
Writing skills, 37
    "after you write," 246
    "as you write," 245-246
    for results, 243-247
Written outcomes, client-centered outcomes,
    185-186

ABOUT THE AUTHOR

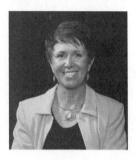 Known for making difficult content easy to understand, Rosalinda Alfaro-LeFevre, RN, MSN is an energetic presenter and an *AJN Book of the Year* and a *Sigma Theta Tau Best Pick* award recipient. Her work has been translated into 7 languages. She has over 20 years clinical experience (mostly in ICU, CCU, and ED), has taught in associate degree and baccalaureate nursing programs, and is the recipient of the *Hospital of the University of Pennsylvania Distinguished Alumnus Award* and the *Villanova University Distinguished Contribution to Nursing Education Medallion*. Rosalinda ("Roz") is the president of Teaching Smart/Learning Easy in Stuart, Florida, a company dedicated to helping people acquire the intellectual and interpersonal skills needed to deal with today's personal and workplace challenges. Born in Buenos Aires, Argentina, to a British mother and Argentine father, Roz immigrated to the United States from Argentina via Canada as a child. Although Roz is an American at heart, she points out that she is blessed with multicultural experiences, presenting nationally and internationally and enjoying close relationships with her family in Spain, Argentina, and the United Kingdom. You can learn more about Rosalinda at *www.AlfaroTeachSmart.com*.